second edition

Bedside
Nursing
Techniques

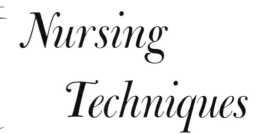

in medicine and surgery

AUDREY LATSHAW SUTTON, R.N.

Case Reviewer, Hospital Division of Blue Cross of Philadelphia; Nursing Consultant, James Associates Medical Advisors, Swarthmore, Pa. Formerly, Instructor, Wilmington General Hospital, Wilmington, Delaware and H. Fletcher Brown Vocational School, Wilmington, Delaware; and Director of Nursing Service, Edgewood General Hospital, Berlin, New Jersey.

W. B. Saunders Company
Philadelphia · London · Toronto

W. B. Saunders Company: West Washington Square
Philadelphia, Pa. 19105

12 Dyott Street
London, WC1A 1DB

833 Oxford Street
Toronto 18, Ontario

Listed here is the latest translated edition of this book together with the language of the translation and the publisher.

Japanese *(1st Edition)* — Igaku Shoin,
Tokyo, Japan

Spanish *(1st Edition)* — Nueva Editorial Interamericana, S.A., de C.V.,
Mexico

Bedside Nursing Techniques   ISBN 0-7216-8666-4

Print No.:   9   8   7

Dedicated to

the nurse whose career is
interrupted by those sometimes
joyful and sometimes distressing
events which accompany being
a wife and mother

Preface to the Second Edition

Preeminent among the rewards of authorship is the satisfaction of learning that one's book has served the purpose for which it was intended. As the Preface to the First Edition points out, *Bedside Nursing Techniques* "is designed to serve as a handbook of practical information for the bedside nurse," and comments from nurses who have used the book indicate that it has satisfactorily performed that function. An additional source of gratification has been the extent to which instructors and students in schools of nursing have found it useful as a compilation of practical techniques for which the theoretical basis of principle has been laid down in textbook and lecture.

This second edition contains descriptions and illustrations of techniques that were not previously included; some were requested by users of the first edition, others were added because the introduction of new equipment has required the development of new techniques and procedures. Among the chapters that received most extensive revision are those on hypothermia, on administration of oxygen (now incorporating a new section on hyperbaric oxygen therapy), and on diseases of the digestive system. The information concerning use of respirators has been rewritten to describe recent innovations in design and functioning of this type of equipment.

Once again I express the hope that the reader will find this volume truly useful in helping to solve the everyday problems that arise in trying to provide high quality individualized care for the patient.

AUDREY LATSHAW SUTTON, R.N.

Preface to the First Edition

This book is designed to serve as a handbook of practical information for the bedside nurse. It is a reference for all those occasions when the nurse knows what to do but can't quite remember how to go about doing it. Every nurse encounters such occasions.

This book gives the answer to that frequent question, "What's new?" The newest concepts of hospital care, the recent designs in equipment, the current techniques and procedures, and the latest diagnostic and therapeutic methods in medicine and surgery are included and explained in terms of the nurse's role in patient care.

This is not just another one of those "cut and dried" procedure books. It is written somewhat informally, using simple everyday nurses' language. Its simplicity is further enhanced by the numerous illustrations. The illustrations are placed actually within the text so that the nurse can immediately see what is being described.

You will see advice and suggestions on the best and easiest way to do a number of things. These are the methods which in my experience I have found to be the best and easiest either from the standpoint of nursing performance or patient satisfaction.

Not every nursing procedure is included. Basic procedures are omitted because it was felt that these are performed so frequently that they seldom need reviewing.

The book is divided into two parts: General Nursing Techniques and Specific Nursing Techniques. The first chapter in Part One gives the reader a glimpse of how the changing trends in hospital architecture and equipment and the newer trends in hospital care affect the routines of bedside nursing care. The remaining chapters in Part One are related to nursing techniques that apply to all areas of medical and surgical nursing.

In Part Two the techniques are grouped according to their relationship to specific anatomic systems. Each chapter in Part Two is organized in such a manner as to give a composite picture of all the techniques used in the care of patients in any particular specialty.

The chapters in Part Two are subdivided under the headings "Diagnostic Procedures," "Therapeutic and Rehabilitative Procedures," "Procedures to Review," "Diets to Review" and "Medications to Review." There is a complete list of diagnostic procedures. Every pertinent diagnostic method used with each group of disease conditions is listed. The normals of all laboratory tests are given along with how the results of these tests vary with given disease conditions. The preparation of the patient is given for every diagnostic test. The procedures for many tests are given either because the nurse conducts the test or because the information is pertinent to nursing care. Those procedures recommended in the laboratory manuals and textbooks listed in the bibliography were used. It should be understood that various institutions may have slight variations of these procedures.

In the section on "Therapeutic and Rehabilitative Procedures," you will find volumes of practical information on how to perform all special procedures related to disease conditions. Additional procedures that are also pertinent to the subject but are basic procedures or procedures discussed elsewhere in the book are listed under "Additional Procedures to Review." Cross references are given for procedures found elsewhere in the book. Diets and medications are listed for review so that the nurse has a total picture of what is involved in specific patient care. Newer medications that have brought about revolutionary changes in therapy are elaborated in the text.

You will notice that gynecological nursing has been omitted. This was done because it was felt that most of the gynecological nursing procedures are basic and that most nurses are familiar with these. Laboratory tests related to diseases of the female reproductive system are listed among those for endocrine disorders in Chapter 20. Other related techniques such as radiotherapy and pre- and postoperative techniques are covered in Part One.

I wish to express my appreciation for the cooperative efforts of the many individuals who have contributed to the making of this book.

I especially want to pay tribute to Ruth A. Davis, who did an excellent job of deciphering my handwriting and postscripts, and to Robert Kern, who interpreted my sketches for the illustrations.

I hope that you will find much use for this volume.

AUDREY LATSHAW SUTTON, R.N.

Contents

PART TWO ▧ SPECIFIC NURSING TECHNIQUES

PART ONE

General
Nursing
Techniques

Planning Bedside Nursing Care

Since this text is primarily concerned with the details of how to perform procedures, it seems appropriate to mention that there is more involved in bedside nursing than simply performing procedures. As you use the material throughout this text, keep in mind that although the book is procedure centered, nursing certainly is not procedure centered.

In this chapter we wish to briefly bring into focus the many aspects which must be considered in the planning and execution of competent nursing care. It is hoped that you will refer to this chapter periodically in order to keep nursing techniques in their proper perspective as related to total patient care.

The factors that must be taken into consideration in planning nursing care include: (1) the physical setup of the hospital, (2) the delegation of care, and (3) the patient's needs.

THE PHYSICAL SETUP OF THE HOSPITAL

An organized nursing plan is of necessity dependent upon the structural layout of the hospital and the equipment available. Before formulating any type of plan, the nurse must acquaint herself with the surroundings so that she knows just what she has to work with.

The recent trend in hospital design is that of simplicity. The reason for this compact structural trend is that hospital services can be more efficiently centralized, thus providing improved and more convenient patient care.

The interior decoration of hospitals has also changed. A typical modern patient room is colorfully decorated. Furniture is less bulky and can be moved easily and with less noise. A number of hospitals now have the electrically controlled hi-lo beds which can be lowered and raised by pressing a button. These beds eliminate the use of footstools for climbing in and out of bed and, in addition, save nursing time and labor because the patient can adjust the bed himself. The newer beds also are equipped with bed sides which can be raised when needed or lowered out of view when not used, and with i.v. poles that can be fastened either at the head or the foot of the bed.

Units are usually arranged so that no more than one or two patients are assigned to one room. There may be a few rooms on a floor with four or six patients to a room, but as a whole, hospitals are no longer using the big ward-type rooms.

Intercommunication systems are becoming

standard hospital equipment. With the intercom system the nurse and the patient have direct communication with each other. Both the patient and the nurse can call each other when necessary. The control unit for the patient is either built into the wall or attached to a cord on the wall. The newer type, attached to a wall cord, can be placed anywhere on the bed within convenient reach of the patient.

Many newer hospitals are completely air-conditioned, and older hospitals have installed this equipment in special departments. Heating units are automatically controlled with the unit concealed in the walls or floor.

Floor plans are such that they save steps and provide better work space for the nurse. Each clinical department usually contains a chart room, conference room, and nurses' lounge room located near the nurses' station.

Hospital equipment also has its improvements and additions. There are ice machines that make an abundant supply of chipped or cubed ice, automatic tube systems that carry written communications to any department in the hospital, piped-in oxygen and suction wall outlets in each patient unit, electronic monitoring devices that measure vital signs, and portable patient lifters that lift the patient in and out of bed and in and out of a bathtub. All of these devices of course save nursing time and labor as well as improve patient care.

One other item that has also contributed a great deal to this progress is the prepackaged disposable article. It seems as though almost every hospital supply article is now available prepackaged and disposable. Almost every kind of surgical dressing, ranging from witch hazel compresses to colostomy dressing kits, is now available in individual prepackaged sterilized envelopes. Disposable articles include needles and syringes, oxygen masks and catheters, plastic drainage tubes (urinary, rectal, and gastric), surgical gloves, plastic stopcocks, and face masks. Completely disposable sets include catheterization sets, enema sets, a preoperative shaving kit, irrigating sets, and intravenous and blood transfusion sets. All of this equipment is available individually packaged and sterilized for use.

PATIENT CARE UNITS

The modern concept in patient care is to group in one unit patients who need the same amount of care. For instance, all those patients who are critically ill and require constant supervision and intensive care are grouped in one unit, while those who are ambulatory and require little care are grouped in another unit. This approach to patient care is called "progressive patient care."

The progressive care program was recognized some years ago as being advantageous for several reasons; among these, better care can be given to patients when hospital facilities and equipment are organized to the patient's needs. A few hospitals have adopted a complete progressive care program. Such hospitals have patients grouped in three to five units designated as follows:

1. Intensive care unit (for the critically ill)
2. Intermediate care unit (for those requiring basic care)
3. Long-term care unit (for chronic disease)
4. Self-care unit (for ambulatory patients who can care for themselves)
5. Home care unit (follow-up work done after discharge)

Some total progressive care hospitals use only three units: the intensive care unit, intermediate care unit, and self-care unit. The procedure in hospitals which have adopted this program is to admit the patient to a suitable unit, and as his condition progresses, he is transferred to another unit. The typical surgical patient, for example, would go from the operating room to the recovery room to the intensive care unit to the intermediate care unit to the self-care unit and then home.

Although most hospitals have not adopted the entire progressive care program, many have recognized the importance of at least a portion of this program. This was evident when the recovery room came into existence. Some years ago the recovery room was instituted as an area to take the patient from the operating room until his recovery from anesthesia. The reason is that the patient who is recovering from anesthesia needs concentrated care and attention. This is actually a form of progressive care. Almost all hospitals now have recovery rooms. More recently a number of hospitals have also recognized the need for an intensive care unit.

THE INTENSIVE CARE UNIT

According to Public Health Service reports, more than 20 per cent of all short-term hospitals with a capacity of 100 beds or more now have intensive care units. These units are frequently called "IC units" or, more simply, ICU. Hospitals that have these units still have the ordinary medical, surgical, orthopedic, etc., services and use the intensive care unit for those selected medical and surgical patients who are critically ill. It should be stressed here that the IC unit is not used only for those patients who are expected to die. In fact, a number of institutions insist that known terminal cases be kept out of the unit.

In a survey of intensive care units published in *Modern Hospital,** some examples of conditions suitable for admission to the intensive care unit were as follows:

Surgical: emergency tracheostomy, postoperative patients who had a complicated course during surgery; patients requiring intensive preoperative therapy; selected postoperative chest and cardiac patients; severely burned patients in the acute phase of illness; acute surgical coma.
Medical: complicated myocardial infarction; acute massive gastrointestinal hemorrhage; acute renal shutdown; severe electrolyte and metabolic derangements; acute poisoning; acute medical coma; severe cardiac arrhythmias, acute pulmonary edema; status asthmaticus; and status epilepticus.

The attending physician makes the choice as to whether or not his patient is to be transferred to the intensive care unit. Emergency patients are admitted directly to the intensive care unit; other patients are transferred to the unit from the recovery room and from the medical and/or surgical department. When the patient is transferred to the unit, all his

belongings are transferred with him, and his old room is not reserved for his return.

A number of hospitals have the recovery room and intensive care unit in the same area. Some hospitals also have several types of special care units or rooms in the intensive care unit. One may be used only for coronary cases. These units are sometimes called coronary care units. Another may be the renal unit, in which the patient is placed for use of the artificial kidney. The original belief in planning the intensive care unit was to have all the patients placed in one large room, similar to a recovery room, so that the nursing staff could constantly observe every patient. The trend in thought now is to have the unit separated into windowed observation rooms of one to four patients per room so that the patient can have privacy and a quiet atmosphere.

The intensive care unit is equipped with everything needed in emergency situations and for continual care of the patient. Usual equipment includes oxygen and suction wall outlets, blood pressure apparatus attached to the wall, oxygen therapy equipment, respirators, hypothermia equipment, bronchoscope, laryngoscope, cardiac pacemakers, cardiac monitor, external-internal defibrillator, electrocardiograph machine, thoracotomy pack, intravenous cut-down set, tracheotomy set, intravenous solutions, cardiac emergency drugs, endotracheal tubes and adaptors, incision and suture materials, stethoscopes, suction catheters, waterseal bottles and tubing, and surgical dressing supplies.

A number of medical authorities predict that the recently developed monitoring devices will be brought into wider use in the near future, and with their use more coronary care units will be adopted. As mentioned previously, a few hospitals already have coronary care units set up in the intensive care area. In these units each bedridden coronary patient wears chest electrodes attached to an electrocardiograph which is connected to a monitoring system located within the nurse's view. Each heartbeat beeps on a loudspeaker, and if cardiac arrest occurs, a light flashes, and an alarm sounds on the monitor. In some units a cardiac monitor pacemaker combination is attached to each critically ill patient,

*Modern Hospital, 100:68, 1963.

and when the heart stops, the pacemaker automatically starts the heart. In other areas when the alarm in the monitoring system signals, indicating heart arrest, the nurse rushes a pacemaker to the patient's bedside. Heart fibrillation as well is signaled on an alarm, in which case an electronic defibrillator is used to slow the random-beating heart to a stop so that the pacemaker may be used.

The nursing staff in the intensive care unit may consist of registered nurses, licensed practical nurses, and nurses' aides. Some hospital staffs feel that there is no need for practical nurses and aides in this area. Registered nurses are given orientation and training prior to their assignment to the unit. The instruction program varies, but in many instances the program includes a review of current medical, surgical, and nursing practices, and techniques of using the emergency equipment. In one institution we know of, nurses are taught how to use the artificial heart machine so that they will be proficient in assisting in the event of acute coronary shock. In intensive care units which have an artificial kidney, nurses are also instructed in its use.

Most hospitals allow visiting privileges in the intensive care unit but restrict the number of visitors and length of visiting time. Only the mother and father and husband or wife are permitted to visit. The number is restricted to one or two at a time, and the length of time is usually five minutes during every hour. Flowers sent to the patient are usually placed in the visitors' waiting room.

The patient charge during the time spent in the ICU is higher than if he were elsewhere in the hospital. The intensive care unit, however, offers considerable financial savings to the patient because he does not need private duty nurses.

THE INTERMEDIATE CARE UNIT

In hospitals which have adopted a complete progressive care program, the intermediate care unit is used for patients who are ill but not dangerously so. This of course comprises the largest area of the hospital. Nurses who work in this area express the opinion that there is a definite advantage to planning and carrying out nursing duties without the usual disruptions encountered in the care of the critically ill.

THE LONG-TERM CARE UNIT

This unit is designed to care for patients who are chronically ill. It would encompass those conditions with which there is a long convalescent and rehabilitation period as in arthritis, hepatitis, and muscular dystrophy.

THE SELF-CARE UNIT

In this unit of the progressive care program, the patient is ambulatory and can care for himself. These units are operated as is a hotel. For example, the patient can mingle freely with other patients in a lounge or recreation area, and he can walk to a dining room for meals. Many patients also make their own beds.

THE HOME CARE UNIT

Some hospitals have a staff in this unit which works in collaboration with the patient, his family, and community health agencies in providing home care for those who need this service. The advantage of this service is that many patients without this help would be hospitalized for longer periods of time.

DELEGATION OF CARE

Other factors that influence the nurse's planning of patient care are (1) the type and amount of care delegated to hospital service departments other than nursing and (2) the method of assignment of care among the nursing staff.

Hospital Service Departments

Some years ago, the hospital nurse did everything connected with patient care from scrubbing the walls to making his bed. However, as medicine progressed and the hospital population increased, the shortage of nurses simultaneously grew more acute, and ways and means were concurrently designed to relieve the nurse of some of her duties.

As a result, hospital administration now attempts to eliminate from nursing all those duties not directly related to nursing; some of those duties are performed by related departments. Examples of other departmental duties that may no longer be performed by the nurse or require the supervision of the nurse are as follows:

Dietary Department
1. Passes out and collects menus
2. Delivers trays to each patient and collects them
3. Visits the patient periodically to discuss problems concerning diet
4. Gives dietary instruction before discharge
5. Prepares between meal nourishments and delivers them to bedside
6. Checks and restocks unit refrigerator and kitchen supplies

Laboratory Department
1. Takes routine admission studies before patient arrives in nursing care unit
2. Collects specimens for all blood studies early in morning so as not to require a "hold breakfast"
3. Notifies dietary department directly when studies that require "hold breakfast" have been completed
4. Instructs patient as to preparation for some studies
5. Transports patient to and from laboratory

Inhalation Therapy Department
1. Brings all inhalation therapy equipment to bedside
2. Sets up equipment for use
3. Explains equipment to patient and instructs patient regarding use
4. Visits patient on continuous therapy daily or oftener to check equipment and to make certain therapy is effective
5. Takes care of all charges to patient
6. Instructs nursing personnel regarding use of equipment
7. Removes equipment from bedside when therapy is discontinued and cleans, sterilizes, and repairs equipment

Housekeeping Department
1. Cleans room daily, including mopping floors, damp dusting all furniture, and flower care
2. Does terminal cleaning of patient unit at discharge, including making of bed and removal and sterilization of bedside utensils
3. Periodically cleans station refrigerator

X-ray Department
1. Transports patient to and from x-ray
2. Gives pre x-ray series instruction to patient when required
3. Takes care of all x-ray charges to patient
4. Notifies dietary department when x-ray studies requiring "hold meals" have been completed

Admission Department
1. Makes up patient charts and sends them with patient to unit
2. Supervises and instructs patient regarding routine admission lab work
3. Notifies physician of patient's admission
4. Instructs patient and family regarding visitation and other hospital policies
5. Transports patient from admission department to laboratory, then to room

Barber and Beautician Services
1. Give shaves, haircuts, and shampoos

Social Service Department
1. Coordinates other hospital and community services
2. Advises patients and families with problems

Physical Therapy Department
1. Conducts exercise programs at bedside
2. Transports patient to and from department
3. Instructs in crutch walking and use of other rehabilitative equipment

Central Service Department
1. Sterilizes and wraps all sterile equipment including operating room supplies
2. Daily checks and restocks all unit sterile supplies
3. Delivers all other supplies to unit

Unfortunately, not every hospital has all the service departments just mentioned. The duties and functions of service departments also vary within each hospital. The foregoing list, however, has been offered as a brief sampling of possible duties which may or may not be performed by the nurse.

ASSIGNMENT OF NURSING CARE

The role of the nurse has changed not only because of newer trends in the functions of related service, but also as a result of newer trends in nursing. Two factors within the nursing service department that affect the planning of bedside care include the variety of personnel available for assignment of nursing care and a variety of methods in assignment of nursing care.

Personnel for Assignment of Nursing Care

Those individuals who are part of the nursing service department and who assist the registered nurse in bedside care are described as follows:

The Nurse's Aide and Orderly. The nurse's aide and orderly are given a training program at the hospital which employs them. The training period may last for one week to one month, depending upon the hospital.

The nurse's aide is trained to perform tasks such as making beds, giving baths, taking temperatures, passing trays, feeding patients, transporting patients to and from other areas of the hospital, answering call bells, giving water and other nourishment, and giving bedpans.

The orderly may be assigned to perform the same tasks as the nurse's aide. He may assist with the nursing care of the male patient in specific units as well as perform duties throughout the entire hospital such as lifting and moving heavy patients.

The nurse's aide and orderly should never be solely responsible for a patient.

The Practical Nurse. The most recent addition to the nursing service team is the practical nurse. The practical nurse goes to an accredited school for a training period lasting from one year to 18 months. She receives preclinical instruction in sociology, family structures and functions, child growth and development, anatomy and physiology, materia medica, nursing arts, nutrition and diet therapy, and in some cases microbiology. She receives clinical training under the supervision of a clinical instructor in medical, surgical, obstetric, and pediatric nursing. She graduates and receives a diploma, then takes state board examinations to receive a practical nursing license. She is then called a licensed practical nurse or an L.P.N.

There are also a number of postgraduate courses now available to practical nurses in such subjects as pharmacology and operating room techniques, the result being that the practical nurse is trained to perform almost all the nursing tasks.

The Ward Clerk. Each patient unit has a ward clerk who receives on-the-job training for tasks of a clerical nature. Her duties usually include answering the phone, ordering non-treatment supplies, delivering messages, acting as a receptionist to visitors and new patients, making out forms, and charting T.P.R.'s.

The Registered Nurse. After reading the numerous nursing tasks which can be performed by other departments and nursing personnel, one may wonder what is left for the registered nurse to do. Actually, a volume can be written on this subject alone. To put it simply, the registered nurse interprets the patient's physical, mental, and social needs and sees to it that these needs are fulfilled by her and by other members of the nursing team. This brings us to a discussion of the methods used in assigning bedside care so that the patient's total needs are met.

Methods of Assignment

One of three methods of assigning patient care is usually used: the functional method, the case method, or the team method.

The Functional Method. In this system each person is assigned a specific procedure to perform, for example, one person takes T.P.R's and blood pressures, another makes unoccupied beds, another gives all medications, and another gives all treatments.

This system is the best way to get work done

but is not recommended because it eliminates the opportunity for a personal approach, leaving a great deal to be desired in meeting the psychological needs of the patient.

The Case Method. With this method several patients are assigned to a nurse who gives all the care including treatments, medications, baths, bedmaking, teaching, and so forth to that particular group of patients. Although this method of assignment is the most satisfactory to the nurse and the patient, it is frequently not possible to implement because the nurse's aide and the practical nurse are not qualified to give total care to patients.

The Team Method. With this system a group of patients are cared for by several persons. Twenty patients, for example, may be assigned to a nursing team consisting of one R.N., one L.P.N., and two nurse's aides. The R.N. is the team leader. As a team leader, she makes periodic rounds to all the patients in order to ascertain their physical, emotional, and teaching needs. The R.N. then assigns certain duties as well as patients to herself and to the members of her team. To do this, she must be acquainted with the personality and educational and technical skills of her teammates as well as know the emotional and physical needs of the patients. In addition, the R.N., acting as a team leader, is responsible for the supervision of her team members. She accomplishes this supervision by instructing and supervising and by follow-up observation.

The team leader is directly responsible to the head nurse, whom she can consult in the event of questions and problems.

THE PATIENT'S NEEDS

Before the execution of any nursing plan, one must have full knowledge of the patient's needs. The nurse must know the nature of the patient's illness and the principles relating to the treatment of that illness. She must also be alert to the patient's psychological responses to his illness. Knowledge of the nature and treatment of illness is obtained from the

patient's chart and is applied to theoretical facts learned in the classroom. The patient's phychological responses to illness can be learned only from himself. Ever since nursing began, nurses have been attuned to the fact that it is a profession involving the patient's physical needs. More recently, however, a strong emphasis has been placed on the patient's emotional needs. The nurse can help to create an emotionally therapeutic atmosphere by adjusting her own attitudes toward each patient on an individual basis and by exploring her patient's attitudes.

An emotional atmosphere conducive to helping the patient get well is the end product of good nurse-patient rapport. Rapport is established by communication. What the nurse says to the patient and the way in which it is said are important.

What should communication between the nurse and patient include?

1. *An explanation of the patient's condition.* The nurse listens to the patient and attempts to learn what the patient knows about his illness. If there are misconceptions and fears regarding his condition, she tries to correct them. The patient must also have some knowledge of his illness so that he understands why certain therapeutic procedures are important to his convalescence. In some instances the patient must be told what symptoms to watch for and what to do when they occur.

2. *An explanation of procedures.* Every procedure must be explained to the patient before it is carried out. The nurse should explain to the patient what general events will take place during his hospitalization as well as new procedures prescribed on a daily basis. All events and procedures should be explained well in advance. Patients do not appreciate being surprised by a nurse walking into the room with an armful of strange-looking equipment. This makes the patient feel ill at ease and could also make him uncooperative. The nurse should tell the patient what she is going to do before she takes the equipment into the room.

The nurse must also explain how each procedure will help the patient and what is expected of him during the procedure.

The patient should also be told the importance of other factors related to treatments, such as diet and medications.

3. *Observation of the patient and the family for further explanation and calming of fears.* Prime requisites in effective communication are observation and listening. The nurse is not expected to be an expert psychologist, but she should be alert to key statements and/or behavior signs which may portray fears and emotional stress on the part of the patient as well as his family.

BIBLIOGRAPHY

Burd, S. F.: The Application of Theoretical Knowledge in Nurse Patient Relations. Nurs. Clin. N. Amer. *1*:187, 1966.

Daly, A.: Teaching Residents and Nurses Emotional Aspects of Their Specialty. Hosp. Topics, *42*:87, 1964.

Smith, C.: Assembly Line Nursing. Nurs. Mir., *120*:13, 1965.

Weaver, K.: Good Nursing Care Is Patient Centered. R N, *28*:99, 1965.

Whittaker, J.: The Human Touch Is Still Needed. Nurs. Mir., *119*:15, 1964.

Hypothermia

The idea of cooling the body, either locally or generally, is an ancient one, but general cooling of the body has become quite popular as a useful technique. The most important effect of generalized cooling of the body is a decrease in the rate of all metabolic processes. As a result of this decrease, the rate of circulation and oxygen requirement are reduced. Hypothermia is now being used to control massive gastrointestinal hemorrhage, to reduce a persistent high fever, to prevent cerebral edema, and to facilitate surgical intervention.

There are several methods currently used to produce hypothermia. The body can be packed in ice or placed on special refrigerated blankets. This is called "surface cooling." Surface cooling is done to reduce a detrimental fever, to prevent cerebral edema and to cool the body for some types of heart surgery (see p. 246). The body can also be cooled by cooling the blood stream. Blood stream cooling is done with a special apparatus attached to an artificial heart machine and is used mainly in heart surgery (see p. 246). When hypothermia is used to control gastrointestinal bleeding, tubes are passed into the digestive tract and with the use of a special machine, cold water is circulated through the tubes. This is called "intragastric cooling."

When hypothermia is used during surgery the patient is cooled in the operating room. When hypothermia is used for other purposes the treatment is done in the patient's own room.

In surface cooling, the body temperature could be reduced to as low as 25° C. (77° F.) but for most purposes it is lowered only a few degrees. In preventing cerebral edema the temperature is lowered to around 31 to 35° C. (87.8-95° F.) and in treating a high fever the temperature is reduced and maintained at 35 to 36° C. (96 to 98° F.). Surface cooling to as low as 25° C. is used only in surgery. In blood stream cooling, the temperature is lowered still further.

SURFACE COOLING

The newer methods of surface cooling are being used on patients who are seriously ill with a high fever of 103° F. and above and on patients with central nervous system damage in which there is a danger of cerebral edema.

There are two main facets to the technique of surface cooling: cooling the body and preventing shivering.

COOLING THE BODY

The technique of surface cooling of the body is based on the principle that the body loses heat through the mechanism of radiation and conduction. Radiation heat loss is the loss of heat rays from the surface of the body to the environment. This heat loss varies with the temperature of the body and the environment. Heat loss by conduction occurs when the body comes in contact with an object; heat is then dissipated directly to the object. Large quantities of heat are lost from the body as a result of the skin's continual contact with a cold surface.

When the physician prescribes surface cooling, the orders include the temperature at which the body is to be maintained and the length of time the treatment is to be continued.

Most hospitals now have a hypothermia machine which is used to cool the patient. The hypothermia machine consists of a refrigerating machine and cooling blankets shown here.

Through the long rubber tube passing back and forth in the blanket, the machine pumps a supply of solution that can be cooled and heated to any desired temperature. The patient is simply placed on the blanket or between blankets and the blanket temperature is lowered. When the patient's rectal temperature reaches the desired level the temperature of the machine is regulated to keep it there. If the patient's temperature gets too low, the machine is simply turned off briefly. If the patient's temperature rises, the machine is turned cooler.

A number of hospitals now use an electric thermometer to check the patient's temperature during the hypothermia treatment. The electric thermometer has a probe which is inserted in the patient's rectum. The probe is in turn connected to a recording device which constantly registers the temperature. The electric thermometer looks like this:

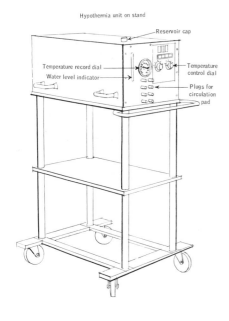

Hypothermia unit on stand

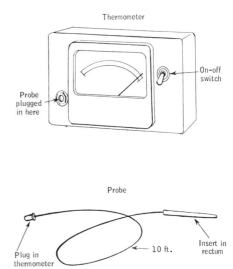

Thermometer

Probe

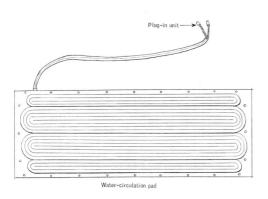

Water-circulation pad

How To Use a Hypothermia Machine

There are several hypothermia machines currently on the market. All of them operate on the same principle. The illustrations used here have been adapted from the hypothermia unit manufactured by the Gorman-Rupp Industries, Inc.

To operate the hypothermia equipment, first place the electric plug in a wall outlet, then select the number and size of the cooling blankets to be used and connect them to the unit. The cooling blankets through which the water circulates may be large or small, and may be arranged over and beneath the patient in a variety of ways depending upon the size of the patient and the physician's preference.

Protective caps should remain on any couplings not used, as shown here:

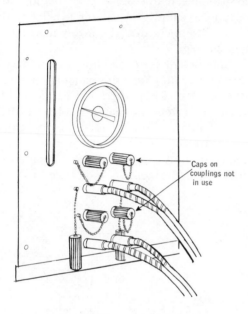

Caps on couplings not in use

Fill the unit reservoir with distilled water. (In another type of hypothermia unit, the reservoir is filled with denatured alcohol mixed with distilled water.) Watch the reservoir level indicator as a guide to how much water is still needed.

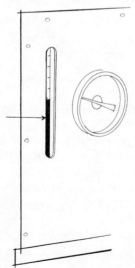

Set the cool and heat dial at 80°.

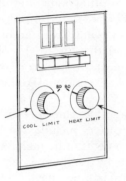

Turn on the pump by pushing the "Heat" button. This switch will start the pump, which pumps water from the reservoir into the blankets.

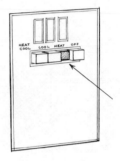

Allow a few minutes for the water to circulate into the cooling blankets, then check the water level indicator. More water may have to be added before the blankets are filled. Before adding extra water, push the "Off" button to turn the pump off.

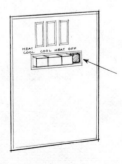

It may be necessary to start and stop the pump a few times before the cooling blankets are completely full. It is possible that the quantity of water feeding back from the blankets will exceed the capacity of the reservoir.

This will cause no ill effects while the pump is on, but when the pump is off, the water will overflow from the reservoir. To prevent spillage, the reservoir cap should be tightened when the pump is turned off. When the unit is in operation, the reservoir cap should be loosened about one quarter turn to prevent a vacuum from forming.

To cool the water, set the "Cool" dial to the desired temperature and push the "Cool" button. Here the arrows point to the "Cool" light, which is on, the "Cool" button pushed in, and the "Cool" dial turned to the desired temperature.

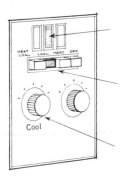

The blanket temperature should be adjusted to around 40 to 50° F. at first and then readjusted as the patient's temperature drops. Remember that the temperature dial setting and the thermometer on the hypothermia machine regulate and indicate the temperature of the water circulating through the cooling blankets, not the temperature of the patient.

The patient should now be prepared for placement on the cooling blanket. Regardless of the arrangement of blankets, it is preferable not to cover the cooling blanket with a bed sheet or blanket because the cover tends to trap warmer air between the cooling surface and the skin, thus acting as an insulating area. Before the final arrangement of the cooling blankets around the patient, the patient's temperature recording device should be put in place.

In some hospitals, a thin coat of lanolin, cold cream, or mineral oil is applied to the entire body before hypothermic induction. This protects the skin against possible frostbite, which may occur if ice forms from condensa-

tion on the cooling blanket. It also allows better contact between the skin and the cooling blanket, thus resulting in more rapid cooling.

Once the patient is on the cooling blanket, his temperature will begin to fall. The nurse should observe the patient's temperature on the electric thermometer about every 15 minutes. As the rectal temperature falls the blanket temperature should be gradually raised to 50 to 60° F. Depending on how low the patient's temperature is to be maintained, the blanket temperature can be raised even higher. Once the patient's temperature reaches about 1° F. near the body temperature desired, the blanket should be set about 15 to 20 degrees lower than body temperature. For example, if the patient's temperature is to be maintained at 96° F., wait until his temperature reaches this level and then turn the blanket temperature from the 50 to 60° F. level up to around 75° F. A blanket temperature of around 75° F. will maintain the patient's temperature at 96° F.

With one cooling blanket, it takes several hours to reduce a high temperature to around 96° F. With several blankets this time is reduced. After the temperature is lowered it can be kept down with little difficulty. As soon as the temperature begins to go up, even slightly, the blanket temperature is lowered. The physician prescribes the length of time the temperature is to be maintained.

When the treatment is to be discontinued the blankets can be warmed or the patient can be removed from the blankets and warm up on his own. The nurse also checks the patient's temperature frequently during the warming period. It is not necessary to disconnect the blankets from the hypothermia unit for storage but if additional or larger blankets are needed for the next treatment, more distilled water must be added to the reservoir.

Although the technique for keeping the patient's temperature reduced is fairly simple using the method just described, there is another device available that can be attached to a hypothermia unit. It makes the technique even simpler. That device is an automatic temperature control unit. With such a device the temperature of the hypothermia machine is automatically controlled to keep the patient's temperature at a desired level. With such a machine, the thermometer unit is attached to the hypothermia unit. It is operated like this:

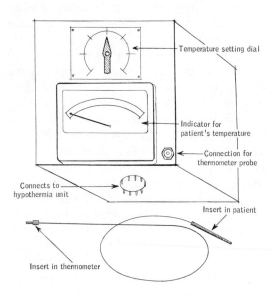

1. Connect the thermometer unit to the hypothermia unit.
2. Set the desired temperature of the patient on the dial.

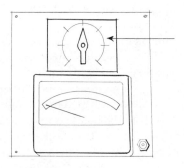

3. Push the automatic "Heat-Cool" button on the hypothermia unit.
4. The patient's temperature is indicated on

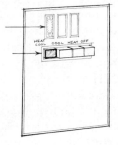

the thermometer dial. This unit automatically controls the patient's temperature.

USING ICE FOR SURFACE COOLING

In the event that a hypothermia machine is not available, the body can be cooled by placing the patient in ice. This is done by fixing a tube of ice like this:

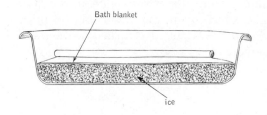

then placing the patient, wrapped in a bath blanket, on top. The bath blanket already in the tub is then folded over the patient and adjusted so that it covers the body from the neck on down. About 2 inches of crushed ice is then put on top of the patient so that he is completely covered from the neck down. Enough water is poured over the ice to make it thoroughly wet, thus improving the contact.

The patient's temperature is taken rectally and when the desired temperature is reached the patient is either removed from the tub and placed on ice bags or left in the ice water, depending on the physician's preference.

PREVENTING SHIVERING

During cooling it is important to prevent shivering because shivering elevates the metabolic rate, which in turn increases the body temperature, thereby defeating the purpose of therapy. Furthermore, it takes much longer to reduce the temperature of a shivering patient. In addition, prolonged shivering, especially in a neurologic condition, causes an increase in spinal fluid pressure, circulation rate, and intracranial pressure. Some patients, particularly the comatose, do not shiver during hypothermia therapy.

To prevent shivering, drugs such as chlorpromazine and sodium phenobarbital are given intravenously. The amount of drug given depends on how much is needed to cause the patient to stop shivering. Often these drugs are not needed after the patient's temperature has been brought down because at a body temperature of 94° F. or below, the posterior hypothalamus (the body's temperature regulating center) gradually begins losing its ability to function. Some patients, however, do require additional doses once or twice daily.

CONTINUATION OF CARE

While the patient's temperature is reduced, the temperature, pulse, blood pressure and respirations are checked frequently. In fact, vital signs should be checked prior to the treatment so that a base line can be established. During the first 20 minutes of the treatment, there will be an elevation in pulse rate and blood pressure, with no drop in temperature. This elevation is caused by peripheral vasoconstriction. When the rectal temperature drops to 95° F., the pulse rate will also decrease. In caring for neurologic conditions, it should be remembered that with increased intracranial pressure, the blood pressure increases while the pulse rate decreases; whereas hypothermia itself will cause a simultaneous decrease in blood pressure and pulse rate.

An indwelling catheter (see p. 266) is kept in place during the treatment and an accurate record of intake and output is kept. The catheter is often required because the patient's decreased level of consciousness (resulting from a neurogenic disease condition or from hypothermia itself) may lead to loss of voluntary control of voiding. Urinary specific gravity readings may be taken every 2 hours. As hypothermia progresses, urinary output becomes dilute, with no fall in urine volume. This occurs because the antidiuretic hormone is depressed.

Depending on the patient's diagnosis, condition, and depth of hypothermia, nasopharyngeal suction may be required (see p. 136), because expectoration of sputum is often difficult during a lowered level of consciousness.

Special mouth care (see p. 159) is important, since during treatment the patient is receiving nothing by mouth.

Hypothermia masks signs of infection;

therefore, the nurse should watch for symptoms such as cyanosis, pallor, irregular respirations, high white blood cell count, and rapid pulse.

Fluid and electrolyte balance are maintained by intravenous infusions (see p. 83) or gavage (see p. 161). If intravenous solutions are given, the needle should be inserted prior to the treatment because the vasoconstriction which occurs after the treatment has begun makes it difficult to insert a needle into the veins.

The stomach should be aspirated prior to gavage feeding to prevent distention and possible vomiting and aspiration of fluid into the trachea. After gavage feeding, peristalsis and emptying of the stomach may be delayed.

Careful positioning of the patient and irrigation or medication of the eyes is necessary due to the decrease in corneal reflexes and eye secretions (see Chapter 18). Eye patches may be used to keep the cornea moist.

After shivering has stopped, a muscular rigidity may occur and persist. This is important to remember when observing the neurologic patient for degree of motion and presence or absence of rigidity or flaccidity of the extremities. At temperatures of 93 to 94° F., amnesia is produced; however, the patient continues to feel pain stimuli. At 80 to 82° F. the patient cannot respond to verbal stimuli and voluntary motion is lost. At this temperature range, spontaneous respirations usually cease because of a depression in stimuli to the medulla. Respiration may then be continued by use of the intermittent positive pressure apparatus (see p. 56). At 76 to 77° F., the gag reflex, superficial skin responses, reaction of pupils to light, and deep tendon reflexes are lost. Although nervous system activity is decreased during hypothermia, it is believed by some authorities that the convulsive threshold is elevated.

How hypothermia affects the precise action of drugs is not yet fully known. It is believed that hypothermia may decrease the action time and excretion time of drugs; therefore, the nurse must be alert to symptoms of cumulative effect.

The patient's skin should be checked every 2 hours for discoloration (white, red, or blue), hardness, numbness, and prickling which may be symptoms of frostbite. The complication of frostbite occurs rarely and only when the temperature of the cooling blanket is maintained below the freezing point.

The rewarming after hypothermia may be slow or rapid. Regardless of the rewarming method used (hot water bottle, woolen blankets, or hypothermy blankets), no substance with a temperature greater than 95 to 105° F. should be placed next to the patient's skin. The nurse should definitely check the temperature of the warming agent with the physician. Active rewarming of the patient is stopped when the patient's temperature is within 1° F. of the desired level.

During rewarming it is important to continue observation of vital signs, nervous system activity, and skin changes (caused by possible frostbite).

BLOOD STREAM COOLING

Hypothermia produced by cooling the blood is used during surgery. This method is fairly new and at present is used in heart surgery via extracorporeal circulation (see p. 245). The effects of and observations made during the hypothermia that is caused by cooling of the blood are the same as those occurring during the hypothermia that is caused by surface cooling. The special nursing techniques used when the patient is recovering from heart surgery are discussed in Chapter 14.

INTRAGASTRIC COOLING

In 1958, intragastric hypothermia was introduced as a method for controlling massive upper gastrointestinal hemorrhage. It is now clearly established that by cooling the stomach wall a reduction in gastric blood flow, acid secretion and digestive activity can be achieved. There are now several machines available for use in producing intragastric hypothermia.

The current technique for intragastric cooling is as follows:

A large-bore nasogastric tube (see p. 151) is inserted into the stomach and all blood clots are removed. This nasogastric tube is left in place and attached to suction. A special latex gastric balloon attached to a plastic gastric tube is then passed into the stomach and chilled water-alcohol solution is slowly introduced into the balloon until the desired volume is attained. The special gastric balloons usually hold up to 1000 cc. of solution. The intragastric hypothermia machine keeps the solution at the desired temperature by pumping the solution back and forth between the stomach balloon and the refrigeration unit.

The nasogastric tube left in place and attached to suction serves as a monitor to further bleeding, and if the gastric balloon were to burst, it would immediately remove the circulating solution from the stomach.

During the treatment the stomach is maintained at a temperature of 10 to 14° C. (50 to 57° F.). To prevent the entire body from becoming cool, the patient is placed on a hypothermia machine blanket and the blanket is heated, supplying external heat. The patient's temperature is monitored with an electric thermometer and the blanket is heated to a level which maintains normal body temperature.

When the gastric bleeding has stopped, the balloon is generally kept in place for 12 to 24 hours following the cessation of cooling so that if bleeding recurs the treatment can be started immediately.

With this method, gastric bleeding can be stopped in about 30 minutes; however, the treatment is usually continued for longer periods of time. Some physicians cool the stomach for at least 2 days.

In instances of small hemorrhages and when the hospital does not have a special intragastric hypothermia machine, constant manual ice-water irrigations through a large-bore nasogastric tube with a syringe may be carried out.

Intragastic cooling is currently used on those patients who have proved refractory to all conservative methods of treatment and who are considered a poor surgical risk.

BIBLIOGRAPHY

Allen, E. V., Barker, N. W., and Hines, E. A., Jr.: Peripheral Vascular Disease. 3rd ed. Philadelphia, W. B. Saunders Co., 1962.

Boba, A.: Hypothermia for the Neurosurgical Patient. Springfield, Ill., Charles C Thomas, Publisher, 1960.

Cooper, K. E., and Ross, D. N.: Hypothermia in Surgical Practice. London, Cassell & Co. Ltd., 1960.

Hickey, M. C.: Hypothermia. Am. J. Nurs., 65:116, 1965.

Lewis, F. J.: The Treatment of Fever with Surface Cooling. Surg. Clin. N. Amer., 39:177, 1959.

Wangensteen, S. L.: Intragastric Cooling for Upper Gastrointestinal Hemorrhage. Surg. Clin. N. Amer., 42:1171, 1962.

Radiotherapy

Radiotherapy refers to the therapeutic use of roentgen rays (x-rays), radium and radioactive substances. The term "radiotherapy" should not be confused with the term "radiation therapy," which includes the use of radiotherapeutic substances (x-rays, radium and radioactive isotopes) in addition to radiations produced by ultraviolet rays, infrared rays and shortwave diathermy (electrotherapy).

Radiotherapy is useful because of its destructive effect on living cells. Malignant growths respond to radiation because malignant cells are more sensitive than the cells of normal tissues. The radiotherapeutic agents are administered in a manner designed to cause maximal destruction of abnormal cells and minimal destruction of normal cells. In the remaining discussion an attempt will be made to give the nurse an understanding of the nature, uses and hazards of the radiotherapeutic agents: x-rays, radium, and radioactive isotopes.

X-RAYS

X-rays are waves of energy generated by the passage of high-voltage electric current through a glass vacuum tube. The roentgen is the internationally accepted unit of measurement of the quantity of radiation. X-rays are useful diagnostically and therapeutically because of their ability to penetrate anatomical structures.

Low-voltage, high-voltage or supervoltage x-ray equipment is available for generating energies appropriate for lesions of all sizes and depths. The advantages of the newer high- and supervoltage machines are deeper penetration of the x-ray beams and a sharper focusing of the beam, which makes it possible to administer large doses to deep-seated neoplasms and avoid more vital structures.

X-ray therapy is especially successful in treating malignant lesions originating from the reticuloendothelial tissue—i.e., leukemias and lymphomas—and from embryo-type tissue such as the teratomas. X-ray therapy is notably successful in carcinoma of the larynx, nasopharynx, tongue, lips and skin. The therapy may be used instead of surgery or in conjunction with surgery.

Certain aspects of x-ray therapy may be puzzling to the patient. The nurse should be aware of these so that she can answer questions of concern to the patient. Facts which should be known are:

1. X-rays are used in treating illnesses other than malignant tumors. (Examples: hyperchlorhydria and some types of dermatitis.)
2. Although the patient is left alone in a room during the time of therapy, there is an intercommunication system over which he may talk with the technician or a window

through which he may be seen by the technician.

3. Many patients fear that the giant machine suspended above them may fall. Reassurance from the nurse should be offered.

4. Markings of indelible ink are placed on the patient's skin by the physician to designate the areas of entry for x-rays in treating an internal organ. These areas of entry are called skin ports. The markings should not be removed until the termination of the treatments. More than one area of the body may be used as a portal of entry for x-rays. (The lung may be treated through the back and the chest.)

5. Although reactions to x-ray therapy occur frequently, the nurse should not suggest or imply that reactions are to be expected. Whether a reaction is experienced may depend upon the general physical condition of the patient, the dosage of roentgens administered, and the size of the area being treated. Also with the newer high- and supervoltage machines, skin reactions are negligible.

The undesirable reactions to x-ray therapy may be either systemic or local or both. The systemic reaction is known as radiation sickness. Symptoms may vary from mild symptoms such as headache, fatigue, loss of appetite and mental depression to more severe symptoms such as nausea and vomiting. With large doses of radiation, a local reaction may occur on the skin depending upon the sensitivity of the skin (the face is extremely sensitive) and the amount of friction from motion of the part (the axillae). Skin reaction is noticeable by a gradually increasing erythema which can become a vivid scarlet coloration within 5 to 7 days. If large doses of radiation are being given, a period of moist desquamation follows during which the superficial layer of epidermis is shed. The reaction then recedes through a stage of reepithelialization—usually with much crusting—then the erythema fades, and the skin returns to normal. The entire cycle may last several weeks. To lessen the severity of skin reactions, the patient should be given the following instructions:

1. The part of skin exposed to the treatment should not be washed with soap and water during the treatment and for two weeks thereafter.

2. Affected skin should not be massaged, and friction from clothes or bed linens should be prevented.

3. If a man's jaw is being treated, he should not shave.

4. The daily liquid intake should be increased.

5. When the reaction is severe enough to warrant the use of dressings, a thin layer of ointment such as vitamin A and D ointment should be placed on the lesion to prevent the dressing from adhering to the skin. Apply the ointment by spreading it on the dressing, not on the skin. Thick layers of ointment should be discouraged, since this prevents serous oozing, thus causing infection. No powders or metallic ointments should be used because the presence of metal in them will further irritate the skin.

6. If there is a skin breakdown, a 1 per cent gentian violet solution may also be prescribed for itching or pain.

7. By all means, nothing should be applied to the skin unless ordered by the doctor.

8. Outpatients should be instructed not to sunbathe during therapy.

Reactions to x-ray therapy gradually subside after the termination of the treatment.

RADIUM

Radium is a natural radioactive element. During disintegration all radioactive elements emit rays consisting of alpha rays, beta rays, and gamma rays. The alpha ray has no significance therapeutically. The beta ray does not penetrate as deeply into the tissue as the gamma ray. The beta ray is also more easily obstructed than the gamma ray. The gamma ray, similar in character to the x-ray, moves at a high speed and penetrates deeply. The gaseous product of the disintegration of radium is called radon. Radium and radon are both used therapeutically.

Radium is applied in plaques, tubes, and needles. *The radium plaque* is a small, flat, square brass container in which a certain amount of radium is embedded.

The plaque is used principally in the treatment of skin and other superficial lesions. *The radium tube* is made of silver, platinum, or brass. Inside the metal tube is a glass tube containing the radium. The size of the tube depends upon the amount of contained radium, larger quantities of radium obviously requiring larger containers. Here are two types of radium tubes.

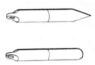

This diagram shows how several tubes are prepared for application. See illustration at bottom of page.
The radium needle is made of gold, platinum, or steel alloy containing varying amounts of radium. Sometimes needles are grouped together and used as a tube type applicator. Here is a single radium needle threaded for use.

Radon is applied in small seeds which are small gold or glass ovals several millimeters in length. The seeds are introduced into the tissue to be irradiated and are left there to slough out with the necrotic tissue. If the seeds are not discharged from the body, they remain permanently and lose all radioactivity in approximately 28 days. The process of placing a solid medication in tissue is called implantation. Radon seeds are sometimes referred to as implants.

When the effect of both the beta ray and the gamma ray is desired, glass seeds are used because the beta ray will not pass through metal. When the effect of the gamma ray only is desired, the metal seeds are used.

Radium and radon treatments are used mostly for carcinoma of the uterine corpus and cervix and for carcinoma in the cavities of the head, especially the tongue. The tubes, needles, and seeds are put in place in the operating room. Radium tubes are held in place with gauze packings. Needles are placed inside a tumor mass, and each needle is sutured in place. When several needles are used, the threads from all the needles are collected and fastened to a convenient area with adhesive tape. See illustration on opposite page.

The dose of radium and the length of time for irradiation are calculated by the physician. The dosage of radium is calculated in milligrams, usually 10 to 100 mg. The dosage of

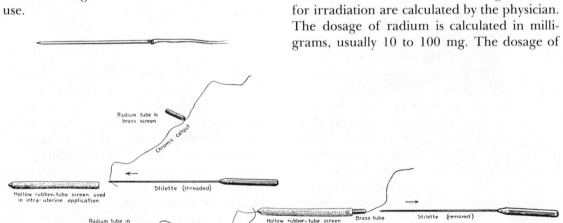

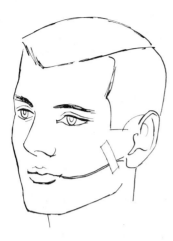

radon is calculated in millicuries. The location of the radium and the exact time for its removal must be noted on the patient's chart. *While the patient is receiving radium therapy, the nurse should adhere to the following rules:*

1. Any shifting of the radium applicator, whether seen or suspected, should be reported to the physician at once. Do not try to replace applicators which have shifted or fallen out.
2. Patients are not permitted out of bed during the administration of the treatment.
3. Patients are allowed visitors according to the usual hospital rules. Visitors should sit about three feet away from the patient.
4. Nurses should spend no more than the adequate amount of time near the patient required for nursing care. Good planning for nursing care is essential to prevent overexposure of the nurse. Undue haste should be avoided so as not to give the patient a hurried feeling.
5. Private duty nurses should receive special instructions from the physician as to the distance to maintain when not administering actual nursing care.
6. Special precautions for handling bodily excretions, dishes, instruments, dressings, and bedding are not needed.
7. Instruments and containers used in handling the radium sources do not become radioactive.
8. Dressings should be changed only as directed by the physician.
9. Perineal pads may be changed when necessary, making certain the radium con-tainers are not loosened. Perineal care is not given during treatment.
10. Radium applicators are always handled with long-handled instruments kept at arm's length. Working behind a lead shield is preferable, as shown here.

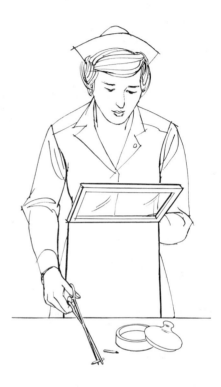

11. Portable lead carriers are used to transport radium applicators to and from the treatment area. There are several sizes of lead carriers. The larger size is sometimes transported on a special pushcart shown here.

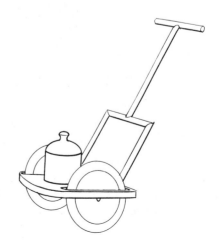

12. A Geiger-Müller counter is used when there is a question of contamination, especially whether or not radium may be misplaced within bedding or dressings. The Geiger-Müller counter is an instrument which detects beta and gamma rays and indicates the quantitative estimate of radioactivity present and is operated by personnel from the physics or radiotherapy department. Here is one type of counter.

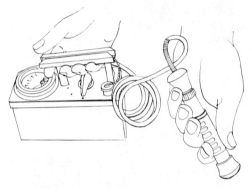

13. Nurses who regularly care for patients receiving radium therapy and those who assist with the implantation and removal of radium applicators should wear a film badge. A film badge is a device which contains photographic film. The film indicates any exposure to radiation rays in degrees proportionate to the amount of exposure. Exposure to both beta and gamma rays can be measured on the film badge. These badges are supplied and read by several commercial companies. Film badges are usually worn on the left breast pocket. Those whose hands receive exposure while handling radium applicators may wear a film badge on the wrist. The pocket and wrist badges look like this:

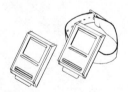

The badge should be worn during all working hours. Film badges should be removed if a diagnostic x-ray examination (chest or dental) is made of the nurse. Film badges are usually worn for one month, after which they are sent to a commercial laboratory to be read.

14. A placard reading "Radium" should be hung on the door or on the head of the bed while the patient is being treated. This will alert all personnel to the precautions needed.

RADIOACTIVE ISOTOPES

WHAT IS A RADIOACTIVE ISOTOPE?

All elements are composed of atoms. Each atom has a nucleus which is built up of two types of particles, protons and neutrons. The number of neutrons within the nuclei of different atoms of a given element is not always the same. Atoms of the same element with differing numbers of neutrons are called isotopes. Most atoms found in nature are stable and never change unless attacked from the outside. The unstable atoms, or those in which the number of neutrons change, give off radioactive particles, a process known as disintegration. During disintegration the nucleus of the atom does not fall apart but rearranges itself. Many radioactive isotopes are artificially created by placing a given element within a nuclear reactor where it is bombarded with neutrons.

As can be remembered from the study of chemistry, there are 92 basic elements occurring in nature. Each element has a chemical symbol, an atomic number, and an atomic weight. The atomic number defines the element. There is only one natural element for every number from 1 to 92 (examples: 1 hydrogen, 2 helium, 3 lithium). The atomic weight of an element refers to the number of protons and neutrons in the atomic nucleus. An atom with few neutrons and protons will be light; one with many neutrons and protons will be heavy. When chemical symbols are written, the atomic number appears at the lower left and the atomic weight appears at the upper right, like this:

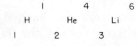

$$_1H^1 \qquad _2He^4 \qquad _3Li^6$$

Here is a table containing the elements commonly used in nuclear medicine, showing the symbol, atomic number and atomic weight of each.

ELEMENT	SYMBOL	ATOMIC NUMBER	ATOMIC WEIGHT
Bromine	Br	35	80
Copper	Cu	29	64
Chromium	Cr	24	52
Carbon	C	6	12
Cobalt	Co	27	59
Calcium	Ca	20	40
Gold	Au	79	197
Hydrogen	H	1	1
Iron	Fe	26	56
Iridium	Ir	77	192
Iodine	I	53	127
Phosphorus	P	15	31
Potassium	K	19	39
Rubidium	Rb	37	85
Sodium	Na	11	23
Sulfur	S	16	32
Yttrium	Y	39	89
Zinc	Zn	30	65

Because the atomic number is always the same for each element, it is usually omitted when referring to the isotopes of the element. The atomic weight is used because this number actually describes the isotope. The atomic weight of some isotopes may be altered in numerous ways. Take iodine, for instance, which may be converted in the nuclear reactor to an atomic weight of 119 to 139. (Note that natural iodine has an atomic weight of 127.) When referring to radioactive isotopes in nuclear medicine, they are written as follows: iodine-131, phosphorus-32 or I^{131}, P^{32}.

Radioactive isotopes emit both beta and gamma rays. An advantage in the use of the artificially made radioactive isotopes is that they emit mostly beta rays and very few gamma rays. Some isotopes emit no gamma rays. Obviously this is a distinct advantage over the use of radium, which emits gamma rays. (Remember, gamma rays penetrate deeply, affecting the entire body; whereas beta rays can penetrate no more than a few millimeters of tissue.) For instance, the beta rays from iodine-131 are able to destory thyroid tissue without harming the parathyroids.

Another characteristic of the radioactive isotopes is the rapid rate of disintegration, ranging from several minutes to several years. The length of time required for 50 per cent of the radioactivity to disintegrate from an isotope is called a half life. In other words, if it takes two days for one half of gold-198 to disintegrate, the half life of gold is considered to be two days. Each particular radioactive isotope will always disintegrate at the same rate of speed. The half life of each radioactive isotope commonly used in medicine will be noted when each isotope is discussed separately later in this chapter. As a point of interest, it may be noted that the half life of radium (previously discussed) is 1590 years, and the half life of radon is 3.83 days. When the first half life of a given isotope is known, the remaining half lives can be calculated, thus determining the exact time of disintegration.

USES OF RADIOACTIVE ISOTOPES

Radioactive isotopes are used diagnostically and therapeutically.

For diagnostic purposes the radioisotopes are administered in liquid form, either intravenously or orally. The oral solution is a clear, tasteless liquid.

The therapeutic dose is implanted in a specific area. There are several implantation methods currently being tried. One method includes the insertion of a small plastic catheter around the lesion to be treated. The plastic catheter is circled in and around the lesion; then the isotope liquid is injected into the catheter. Another method uses nylon tape and plastic envelope implants.

RADIOISOTOPE DOSAGE

The dosage administered for diagnostic purposes is usually small in comparison to the amount used for therapeutic purposes. The physician calculates the isotope dosage in curies. A curie is a quantity of radioactive substance in which 37 billion atoms disintegrate per second. A millicurie (mc.) is a thousandth part of a curie, and a microcurie (μc.) is a millionth part of a curie. Radioactive isotopes are usually ordered in microcuries for diagnostic purposes and in millicuries for therapeutic purposes.

The amount of energy transferred from the radioactive isotope to the body cells is measured in roentgens or rads. The roentgen is a large unit. Usually a therapeutic dosage of an isotope will transfer amounts of roentgens measured in units of milliroentgens (millirads). A milliroentgen is one-thousandth of a roentgen, abbreviated as mr. To illustrate further the use of the terms millicuries and milliroentgens, one may say that a bottle containing 100 millicuries (mc.) of a radioactive isotope may give off 16 milliroentgens (mr.) at a distance of 2 inches from the surface.

EFFECTS OF RADIATION

The effects of radiation and the approximate doses of rads (roentgens) which cause these effects are tabulated below. It should be understood that the response of individuals to the same dose of radiation may vary. Also, the doses listed in the table shown below refer to amounts administered within short periods of time, either single doses or doses given within several days. The same doses administered over a period of several years would have little or no effect. Reactions to exposure to radiation never occur immediately at the time of exposure. A period of from several hours to several weeks or longer passes before any reaction becomes visible. Often the first symptoms of a reaction completely disappear and do not reappear again until years later. If repeated very small doses are kept up for a long time, the reaction usually appears years

later. In order for the reader to visualize the size of a rad, it should be mentioned that during a routine chest x-ray, the lungs receive a dose of 1/10 rad.

SAFETY MEASURES

Obviously, the radiation hazards with the use of the artificially produced radioactive isotopes are much less than those with the use of radium. Although precautions in using the radioactive isotopes vary with each isotope, there are some general precautions which apply to the use of all isotopes. These considerations do not apply to patients undergoing diagnostic tests because of the minute quantities involved.

1. The room door of the patient who has received therapeutic amounts of any radioisotope should be suitably marked with a card containing the amount administered, and special instructions for nursing care.
2. One patient per room is desirable but not essential.
3. Brief visits from relatives are not restricted except for children and pregnant women.
4. After the room is vacated, it must be thoroughly monitored.
5. Under no circumstances should a nurse care for a patient being treated unless she has received adequate instruction.
6. A film badge and/or pocket meter must be worn at all times (see p. 22).
7. A gown and rubber gloves are worn during the handling of contaminated excreta and utensils. Both help to reduce penetration of beta rays. All alpha and low-energy

BODY AREA	DOSAGE OF RADS	EFFECTS
Entire body	25	Reduction in white cell production
	50	Malaise; nausea, vomiting; diarrhea
	100	Leukemia (leukemia can also result from long continuous exposure to a few rads a week)
	500	Permanent sterility
	1000	Miscarriage or stillbirth during pregnancy
Skin	1000	Temporary tanning; hair may fall out but regrows
	2000	Permanent tanning; permanent hair loss; destruction of sweat glands

beta particles emanating from radioactive isotopes are blocked completely by a thin layer of rubber or a few layers of cloth.

8. The nurse's complete blood count should be checked at three-month intervals. Overexposure to radioactivity tends to lower the white blood cell count.

9. Linens contaminated by excreta or during administration must be put in a closed can until monitored to determine whether they should be stored to allow for disintegration of radioactivity or whether they should be sent to the laundry.

10. The nurse should not be responsible for quantitative measurement (monitoring) of contamination. This is the responsibility of the radiologist or "safety officer."

11. The exposure to radioactivity should never exceed 300 mr. per week. This permitted limit is based on facts secured from studies made on individuals who work around radioactivity continuously, as might be the case for the radiologist. The nurse would automatically be considered a great deal safer.

Needless to say, the mental attitude of the nurse plays an important part in promoting safety. It is not hard to be careful when first working with new developments. Many nurses, however, become careless as procedures become more familiar. Every nurse must realize that radiation injury may not become apparent for many years, and by this time it is too late.

MONITORING DEVICES

With the increased use of radioactive isotopes, many types of monitoring instruments have been developed for the safety of the worker. Since the nurse is not permitted to conduct general monitoring, a detailed discussion of monitoring instruments need not be included in this topic. Various types of monitoring instruments will be described briefly to aid the nurse in identifying them.

1. The film badge is worn by the worker for personal monitoring. (See description and instructions on page 22.)

2. A pocket dosimeter is an instrument about the size of a fountain pen and is worn for personal monitoring. This instrument is frequently called the pocket meter.

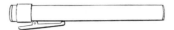

The pocket dosimeter is charged by insertion into a dosimeter charger which contains a battery and looks like this:

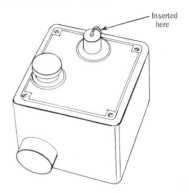

Inserted here

The charge gradually decreases as the instrument is exposed to radiation. The pocket dosimeter measures exposures up to 200 mr. Some types are available that measure exposures up to 100 r. The pocket dosimeter is designed to be read by the wearer, simply by holding it toward light. The reading looks like this:

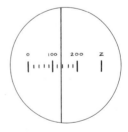

3. Portable survey meters like the one shown on page 22 are used for measuring instantaneous dosages. The survey meters are lightweight and battery operated. They are used for monitoring external areas of exposure on the body, areas of possible spillage of isotopes during administration, linens and excreta, and the patient's room following discharge. Nurses do not operate these meters.

4. Instruments used for monitoring internal exposure include the scintillation probes. These are used for diagnostic purposes

and are somewhat larger than the portable meters. A scintillation probe looks like this:

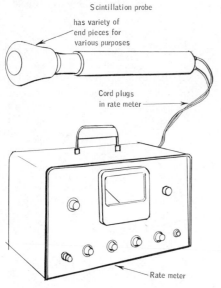

Scintillation probe has variety of end pieces for various purposes

Cord plugs in rate meter

Rate meter

In some clinics the probe and rate meter are placed on a special stand with a movable arm like this:

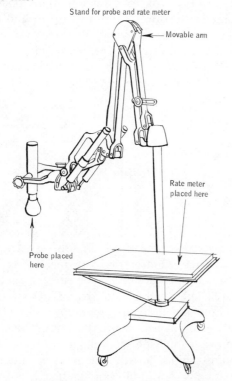

Stand for probe and rate meter

Movable arm

Rate meter placed here

Probe placed here

SPECIFIC RADIOACTIVE ISOTOPES

The diagnostic tests, therapeutic uses, and some specific precautions to be taken with each radioactive isotope are listed here.

Iodine-131

Half life 8 days; beta and gamma radiations.

Diagnostic Tests

Thyroid Uptake. Two to 50 μc. of I[131] are administered orally or intravenously. Twenty-four hours later the amount of radioactive isotope which had accumulated in the thyroid is measured with a scintillation probe. *Results:* 0 to 15 per cent radioactivity present indicates hypothyroidism; 15 to 35 per cent indicates a normal thyroid; 35 to 100 per cent indicates hyperthyroidism. This test is usually performed on an outpatient basis. (See also page 99.)

Excretion Studies for Thyroid Function. Two to 50 μc. of I[131] are administered orally or intravenously. The rate at which radioactive iodine clears from the blood stream, is excreted in the urine, and is utilized in the formation of thyroxine, and the amount contained in the saliva, may be measured by monitoring. These tests may also be performed on an outpatient basis. (See also page 99.)

Blood Volume Studies. I[131] is combined with serum albumin and administered intravenously in dosages of 5 to 50 μc. This solution mixes only with the plasma in the blood stream.

Liver Function Studies. I[131] is combined with rose bengal and administered intravenously in doses of 5 to 15 μc. Rose bengal should accumulate in the liver within the first 10 minutes. A scintillating detector can determine the rate of absorption in the liver and the rate of elimination through the bile duct.

Thyroid Scanning. I[131] is needed in doses of 20 to 300 μc. A point-by-point diagram is obtained (scintigram), which reveals any part of the thyroid that may be functioning. Here is a scintigram of a normal thyroid:

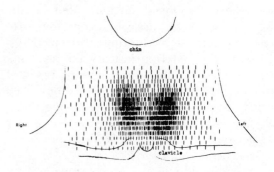

chin

Right   Left

clavicle

Kidney Function. This is performed by administering 10 to 20 μc. of I^{131} combined with Diodrast.

Therapeutic Uses

Hyperthyroidism: 3-15 mc.
Cardiac dysfunction: 3-15 mc.
Some thyroid tumors: 10-150 mc.

Precautions with Therapeutic Doses

1. All precautions should be observed during the first 48 hours following the administration of the isotope.
2. Protect the entire pillow and mattress with a plastic or rubber covering during hot weather because iodine is excreted in perspiration.
3. No precautions with linen need be used unless the patient vomits, has urinary incontinence, or perspires.
4. If the patient vomits within 6 hours following the administration of up to 25 mc. and within 24 hours with doses above 25 mc., the vomitus is cleaned up from furniture, etc., with cloths held in forceps, by a person wearing rubber gloves and a protective gown. Do not allow personnel to walk over contaminated areas on the floor until the areas have been monitored. If the patient became contaminated from vomitus, either request him to take a bath or give him a bath while he lies on a rubber sheet. The same nurse should not both bathe the patient and clean up the vomitus from the floor or furniture. Nurses involved in cleaning up a contaminated patient should be carefully monitored for contamination and should be removed from isotope responsibility for a suitable time.
5. An ambulatory patient may takes baths and use the bathroom. The bathtub should be thoroughly rinsed after use, and the toilet should be flushed an extra time.
6. If the patient is not ambulatory, the nurse must wear gloves and a gown while giving a bath and handling the bedpan or urinal. Excreta may be emptied into the toilet. Utensils are rinsed well. The patient should use the same utensils throughout the treatment.
7. Rubber gloves are worn when dressings are changed.

8. All gloves, gowns, dressings, linens, etc., must be monitored before being processed in the usual manner.
9. There need be no restrictions on visitors except for children and pregnant women. Visitors should sit at least 3 feet away.
10. Ambulatory patients should be encouraged to collect their own urine specimens. When the nurse collects a urine specimen, she must wear rubber gloves and use a lead protection shield around the specimen bottle. If urine is spilled, the same precautions for cleaning it up are used as when cleaning up vomitus. (See 4.)
11. Private duty nurses should remain 2 feet away from the patient when not performing nursing procedures.
12. Special nursing precautions may be discontinued 48 hours after the initial dose or, when large doses are used, after the radioactive iodine content of the body is less than 30 mc.

Phosphorus-32

Half life 14.3 days; beta radiations only.

Diagnostic Tests

Brain Tumor Localization. One-half to 1 mc. is injected intravenously 12 to 24 hours before surgery. During surgery the location of the tumor is discerned by means of a scintillation probe.

Localization of Intraocular Tumors. Five hundred millicuries are administered intravenously. Counts are taken over both eyes one hour and 24 hours later. Concentrations 30 to 40 per cent greater than in the surrounding tissues indicate a pathologic lesion. This test may be performed on an outpatient basis.

Therapeutic Uses

Polycythemia vera: 2.5-5 mc.
Chronic leukemia: 1-2 mc.

Precautions with Therapeutic Doses

1. There are no time or distance restrictions.
2. No special precautions are needed for handling excreta and utensils.
3. If the phosphorus is given intravenously, no precautions are needed for handling vomitus.
4. If the phosphorus is given orally and the patient vomits within the first 24 hours, the same precautions are needed as when

dealing with the vomitus from radioactive iodine (see p. 27).

Gold-198
Half life 2.7 days; beta and gamma radiations.

Therapeutic Uses
Pleural effusion: 35-75 mc. (intracavitary)
Ascites: 100-150 mc. (intracavitary)
Prophylactic against the spread of tumor cells following surgical removal from closed serous cavities: amounts corresponding to the above intracavitary doses

Precautions with Therapeutic Doses
1. Whatever time is necessary for ordinary nursing care may be spent with the patient.
2. During the first 48 hours after administration, private duty nurses should remain about 6 feet away from the patient except during actual nursing procedures.
3. Patients are allowed visitors. During the first few days, visitors should sit at least 3 feet away from the patient.
4. No special precautions are needed for the handling of excreta and utensils.
5. Dressings should be changed only as directed by the physician.
6. Dressings over the puncture wound which become stained from radioactive gold should be sent to the radioisotope laboratory. Gold stains linen red or purple.
7. If there is any serous fluid or other drainage from the puncture wound, do not touch the dressing. Call the physician.

Chromium-51
Half life 27.8 days; gamma and x-ray radiations.

Diagnostic Tests
1. Determination of red cell volume   } Done by testing
2. Study of red cell survival times   } samples of blood
3. Evaluation of blood loss by bleeding: If at least 200 μc. of chromium-51 tagged cells are injected into the blood stream, active bleeding—as into the digestive tract—can be followed both through the decrease of activity in the blood and through the amount of activity in the stools.

No hazards are involved with the use of chromium-51.

Iron-59
Half life 45.1 days; beta and gamma radiations.

Diagnostic Test
Iron Turnover Rates. Doses of 10 to 30 μc. are administered, and repeated blood samples are tested. These tests may be conducted on an outpatient basis.

No hazards are involved with the use of Iron-59.

Cobalt-60
Half life 5.27 years; beta and gamma radiations.

Diagnostic Test
Pernicious Anemia. 0.5 μc. is administered. The test may be performed on an outpatient basis.

Therapeutic Uses
1. Cobalt-60 seeds or needles are used to take the place of radium and radon in intracavitary or intrastitial treatments. For this type of treatment with cobalt-60, wires containing cobalt-60 are placed inside special stainless steel refillable capsules. Doses of 50 to 75 mc. are used. The cobalt applicator capsule looks like this. The exterior is shown on the left, and a cross section of the capsule is shown on the right.

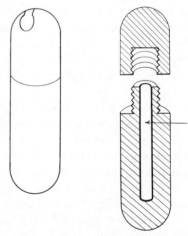

2. Cobalt is also used for external irradiation, as are high-voltage x-rays (see p. 18). This type of therapy is called teletherapy. The machine which houses the cobalt is large and similar in size to the x-ray machine.

The cobalt irradiator is located in the radiation department and presents no radiation hazards. When the treatment is over, no radioactivity remains on the patient.

Precautions. Precautions with the use of cobalt-60 needles and seed implants are the same as those for radium and radon implants (see p. 21).

Iridium- 192

Half life 74.4 days; beta and gamma rays.

Therapeutic Uses. Administered in permanent implants in doses around 30 mc.

Precautions. The precautions are the same as those for radium implants.

Thorium X

Half life 2.64 days; alpha radiation.

Therapeutic Uses

Dermatological disorders: 50-100 μc.

The patient is usually treated in the clinic or in the doctor's office.

Precautions. A gas called thoron is given off from thorium X during the disintegration process. The gas emits gamma rays. Therefore:

1. Thorium solution should be kept in a tightly capped bottle.
2. Thorium is usually applied to the skin with a brush or cotton swab. Rubber gloves should be worn during the application.
3. Do not inhale the gas emitted from thorium during the application.
4. Cotton swabs and waste from the application should be put in a paper bag inside a closed garbage can. The garbage can should be turned over to a radiation safety officer.

EMERGENCY SITUATIONS WITH THE USE OF RADIOACTIVE ISOTOPES

The nurse who is ready to begin work with patients receiving radioactive isotopes may feel more secure if she knows that the Atomic Energy Commission, under the direction of Congress, has a law stating that any laboratory storing and handling radioactive isotopes must have a license to do so, and in order to secure a license, the isotope unit must have a radiation protection officer. It is the responsibility of the radiation protection officer to see that no one working with radioactivity receives more than the permitted dose of radiation. He must provide instructions for maintaining safety and make certain that procedures are carried out without hazards. If situations involving radiation hazards arise which cannot be coped with by the nursing personnel, the radiation protection officer should be contacted.

BIBLIOGRAPHY

Best, N.: Radiotherapy and the Nurse. Am. J. Nurs., *50*:140, 1950.

Brown, A. F.: Medical Nursing. 3rd ed. Philadelphia, W. B. Saunders Co., 1957, pp. 97-103.

Brucer, M.: Levels of Radiation. J.A.M.A., *175*:36, 1961.

Duffy, B. J., Jr.: Atomic Energy in the Diagnosis and Treatment of Malignant Diseases. Am. J. Nurs., *55*: 434, 1955.

Handbooks of the National Bureau of Standards, Superintendent of Documents, Government Printing Office, Washington 25, D.C.:

No. 38. Protection of Radium during Air Raids.

No. 41. Medical X-ray Protection up to Two Million Volts.

No. 42. Safe Handling of Radioactive Isotopes.

No. 51. Radiological Monitoring Methods and Instruments.

No. 52. Maximum Permissible Amounts of Radioisotopes in the Human Body and Maximum Permissible Concentrations in Air and Water.

Kautz, H. D., Storey, R. H., and Zimmerman, A. J.: Radioactive Drugs. J. Nurs., *64*:124, 1964.

Luros, G. O., and Towne, J. C.: Essentials of Chemistry. 7th ed. Philadelphia, J. B. Lippincott Co., 1966.

Martin, E. R.: Technique for Handling Radioactive Isotopes. AORN J., Jan. & Feb., 1966.

Murphy, W. T.: Radiation Therapy. 2nd ed. Philadelphia, W. B. Saunders Co., 1967.

Quimby, E. H.: Safe Handling of Radioactive Isotopes in Medical Practice. New York, The Macmillan Co., 1960.

Skaggs, L. S., and Haughey, R.: Radioactive Isotope Therapy. Nurs. Outl. *4*:214, 1956.

Tabern, D. L., and Gleason, G. I.: What Nurses Should Know about Isotopes. Compliments of Abbott Laboratories. Reprinted from The Modern Hospital, August, 1955.

Welsh, M. S.: Comfort Measures during Radiation Therapy. Am. J. Nurs., *67*:1880, 1967.

Administration of Oxygen

Oxygen is administered to treat anoxia, the term for oxygen deprivation. Oxygen is added to inhaled air so that blood can be oxygenated more readily. In an abnormality of the lungs such as pneumonia, additional oxygen is required because the total functional lung surface is reduced. In an abnormality of blood circulation, such as with heart failure, lung congestion also produces anoxia. Oxygen is also used for conditions such as anemia, when anoxia results from an insufficient amount of hemoglobin needed to carry oxygen to the tissues. Oxygen occasionally is given to conserve energy during respiration, when strict bed rest is essential.

The nursing responsibilities in the administration of oxygen vary somewhat in each institution. Some hospitals have an inhalation therapist who supervises all oxygen therapy. The duties of the inhalation therapist also vary with each institution. In smaller institutions the duties of the inhalation therapist may include setting up the oxygen equipment when the patient is started on oxygen therapy. For the benefit of the do-it-yourself nurse, we are including the complete methods of oxygen therapy from start to finish.

OXYGEN SUPPLY

Oxygen is supplied either in individual cylinders or through pipes. Piped oxygen comes from a central source to outlets in rooms throughout the hospital. Nearly all hospitals built recently have piped oxygen. A number of older hospitals also have installed piped oxygen during remodeling programs. Both types of supply are described here.

OXYGEN CYLINDERS

These are made of stainless steel built to withstand pressures in excess of 2200 lbs. per

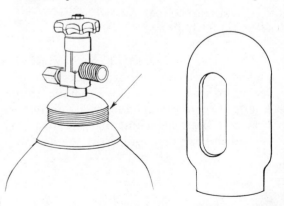

square inch, which is the usual pressure in a full oxygen cylinder. A valve at the top of the cylinder turns the oxygen on and off and is designed to withstand the high pressures to which it is subjected during the shut-off. Every cylinder has a steel cap that screws onto the top of the cylinder to protect the valve from damage while the cylinder is not in use.

Safe Handling of the Cylinders

There is no reason to fear an oxygen cylinder, but it should be handled with care and respect. In the hands of a careless person, it can be a hazard.

The following safety rules should be observed:

1. Never permit oil or grease to come in contact with oxygen, oxygen cylinders, valves, regulators, or other fittings.
2. Never drop cylinders or permit them to strike each other.
3. Never tamper with safety devices or attempt to repair cylinders or valves.
4. Close all oxygen cylinder valves when the cylinders are empty.
5. Store cylinders of oxygen in a cool place, away from radiators, etc. When the temperature inside the cylinder rises, the pressure of a full oxygen cylinder will increase about 25 pounds for each five degrees above 70° F.
6. Always look at the cylinder label before administering any gas.
7. Where caps are provided for valve protection, they should be kept on the valves when cylinders are not in use.
8. If fire breaks out in the hospital, close all cylinders in use.
9. While in use, the cylinder should be strapped to the bed or wall.
10. "NO SMOKING" signs should be placed in all areas where oxygen is being used.

Cylinder Regulator

When using oxygen from a cylinder, an oxygen regulator must be used to change the pressure at which the oxygen leaves the cylinder to the pressure needed for administration. The regulator is adjusted to deliver the desired rate of flow required for the patient. The regulator has two gauges. One tells the rate of flow; the other tells how much gas is in the cylinder. Here are several differently designed regulators; on this one the contents gauge is on the left, and the flowmeter is on the right:

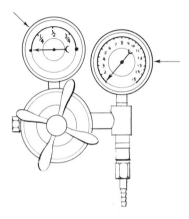

On this one the flowmeter is on the left and the contents gauge is on the right.

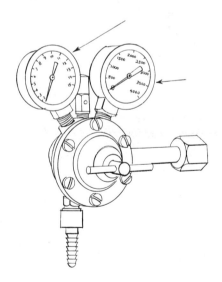

This one has a ball float flowmeter. As the oxygen is turned on, the ball in the flowmeter rises.

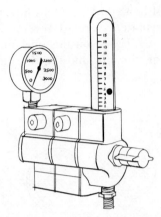

A regulator should be attached to the cylinder before it is brought into the patient's room so that the patient will not be disturbed by the noise.

To attach a regulator to a cylinder, follow these steps: Before attaching a regulator to a cylinder, open the cylinder valve slightly, then quickly close it. This is called "cracking" the valve. It prevents any dust that may have lodged in the valve opening from entering the regulator and causing a leak.

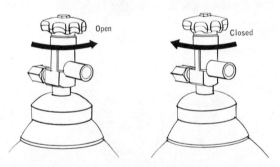

Connect the regulator to the cylinder by inserting the regulator inlet in the cylinder valve outlet as shown.

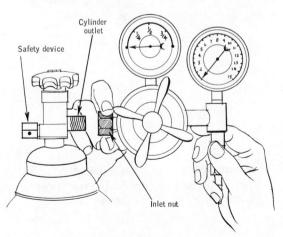

Then tighten the inlet nut with a wrench like this:

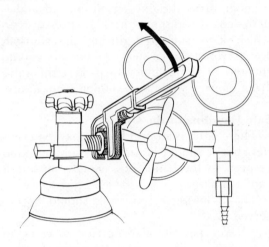

Turn the flow-adjusting valve to "off" position. The location of the flow-adjusting valve on the three designs of regulators is shown here:

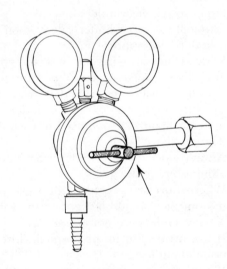

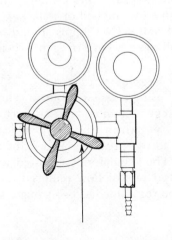

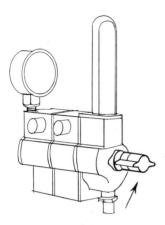

The direction of turn differs with the type regulator used. It is important for this step to be taken before the cylinder valve is opened.

Connect the hose to the regulator like this:

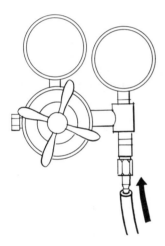

Next, open the cylinder valve very slowly — the slower the better — until the needle on the cylinder contents gauge stops moving.

If the valve is opened too rapidly, the sudden inrush of high pressure gas may damage the regulator. If a regulator with a ball float is used, the ball float will rise in the tube for a moment, then quickly return to zero. This indicates that oxygen has entered the flow indicator tube.

Now turn the regulator-adjusting valve slowly to the "open" position. Again the direction of the turn depends upon the design of regulator used. Continue turning the handle until the flow gauge registers the number of liters desired.

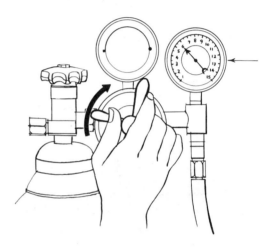

The cylinder and regulator are now ready for use. To stop the flow for short periods, simply close the flow-adjusting valve.

When the flow of oxygen is to be stopped for half an hour or more or when the regulator is to be disconnected from the cylinder:

Close the cylinder valve tightly. Do NOT touch the flow-adjusting valve yet.

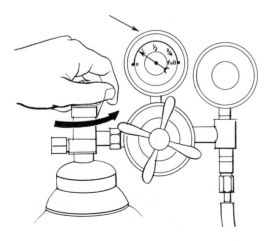

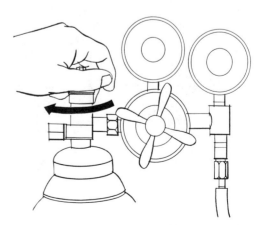

Wait until both the liter-flow gauge and the cylinder-contents gauge have returned to zero.

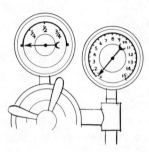

Close the flow-adjusting valve.

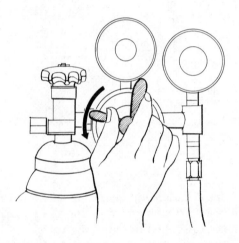

To disconnect the regulator, unscrew the inlet nut.

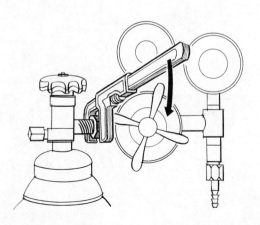

Where oxygen is to be obtained from a piped supply, a station valve is located on the wall. Two general types of station outlet valves are currently in use: One is a manually operated valve with which the oxygen is turned on and off with a knob like this:

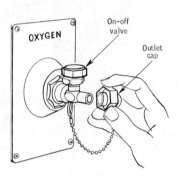

The other is the "quick-connect" coupler to which a flowmeter can be connected simply by plugging it into the valve. Two types are shown here.

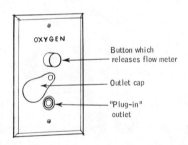

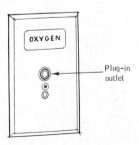

Other piping outlets such as vacuum or nitrous oxide may be located in the same area with the oxygen outlet. In this event the wall outlet looks similar to this:

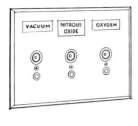

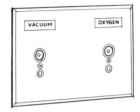

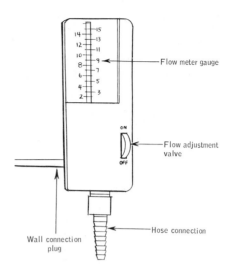

Oxygen flows through the pipeline at a low pressure, usually 50 to 60 lbs. per square inch. To control the flow to the patient, the operator must attach a flowmeter to the wall outlet. Here are several types of flowmeters used with the wall outlets:

The wall outlet is keyed so that only oxygen equipment can be plugged into an oxygen valve and only vacuum equipment can be plugged into a vacuum valve.

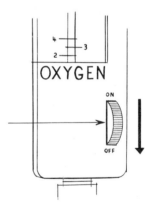

To attach a flowmeter to a wall outlet: Close the flow-adjusting valve of the flowmeter.

Insert the flowmeter adapter into the open-

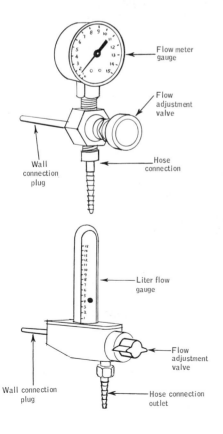

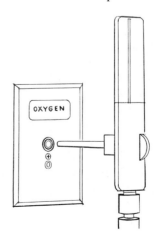

ing of the outlet, and press until a firm connection is made.

Slowly open the liter flow-adjusting valve on the flowmeter until the desired flow is obtained.

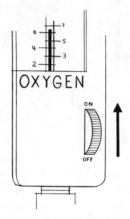

To administer oxygen, attach the administering apparatus to the outlet on the flowmeter.

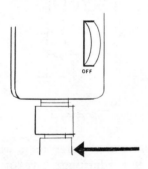

When disconnecting the flowmeter, first close the flow-adjusting valve. When the gauge has dropped to zero, gently pull the flowmeter from the wall outlet. If there is a dust cap for the outlet, replace it.

To attach a flowmeter to a manually operated wall outlet valve (shown on p. 34), follow the same steps as are taken attaching a regulator to an oxygen cylinder (see p. 32).

METHODS OF ADMINISTRATION

Oxygen is administered by way of a nasal catheter, nasal inhaler, face mask, or tent.

The advantages and disadvantages of each method are discussed under the separate headings which follow.

NASAL CATHETERS

Where concentrations up to 50 per cent are required, the nasal catheter is usually the method of choice. The administration of oxygen by catheter makes it easier to examine the patient and give nursing care and treatments. Another advantage of this method is that the patient is able to move about freely in bed. One of the disadvantages is that the catheter is likely to produce some irritation to the mucous membranes.

Oxygen catheters are made of plastic. They are about 16 inches long and come in several sizes in diameter. A No. 14 French is the size usually used for adult patients. An ordinary rubber catheter with extra holes (six to eight) cut in the end may also be used.

There are two methods for administering oxygen by catheter: the "shallow" technique, in which the tip of the catheter is placed in the nasopharynx, and the "deep" technique, in which the tip of the catheter is placed into the oropharynx.

To insert a nasal catheter into the oropharynx: Determine the approximate depth to which the catheter is to be inserted by measuring the distance from the tip of the nose to the ear lobe as shown. Mark this point on the catheter with a small piece of adhesive tape.

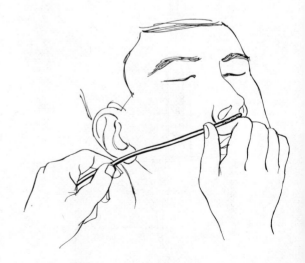

Next connect the apparatus, and start the flow of oxygen at about 3 liters. A humidifier (see p. 49) is always used with nasal oxygen. The setup looks like this:

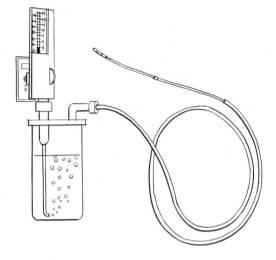

Hold the tip of the catheter in a glass of water to make certain that the holes are not plugged.

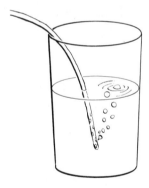

Then, with the oxygen flowing, lubricate the catheter sparingly. A water-soluble lubricant such as surgical jelly is used. Never use

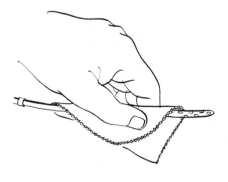

mineral oil or petroleum jelly, as this irritates the respiratory tract. Spread the lubricant with a piece of gauze as shown.

Determine the natural droop of the catheter by holding the taped part with the thumb and forefinger and slowly rotating it until the tip hangs at the lowest level like this:

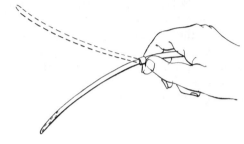

With the oxygen flowing at 3 liters, slowly insert the catheter to the measured depth. It is easier to insert the catheter if the tip of the patient's nose is elevated like this:

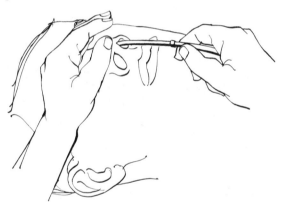

Then use a tongue depressor and light to check the position of the tip of the catheter through the patient's open mouth. The tip should rest approximately opposite the uvula like this:

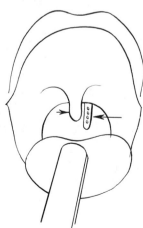

Adjust the liter flow to the desired concentration, as ordered by the physician. To be completely certain that the catheter tip is in the correct position, you may insert the catheter tip slightly beyond the measured depth until the patient swallows oxygen; then withdraw the catheter very slowly to a point where swallowing stops. This last procedure cannot be done on an unconscious patient.

To hold the catheter in place, split a 3-inch length of adhesive tape halfway down its length. Wrap one split end around the catheter like this, and use the other two ends to fasten the catheter to the face.

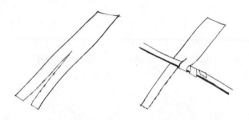

The catheter may be taped to the face either along the bridge of the nose or to the side of the nose as shown at the bottom of this page. Make sure that the catheter is never kinked. Clip the tubing to the bedclothes. Do not puncture the tube. Leave enough slack to allow the patient to move his head freely.

A freshly lubricated catheter must be inserted every eight hours or more often during the treatment. The opposite nostril should be used each time a fresh catheter is put in place. Other points to observe during the treatment are:

1. Examine the position of the tip of the catheter at least every hour.
2. Make sure that the humidifier is not leaking around the gasket and that it is filled to the water level mark (see p. 50).
3. Make certain that the flow of oxygen is at the correct level.
4. Check the tubing to make sure that it is not pinched or kinked.
5. Check all connections for leaks.

Some physicians recommend that the flow of oxygen be discontinued when the patient is being fed in order to prevent swallowing of oxygen.

Inserting a Catheter into the Nasopharynx. In the shallow technique the catheter is inserted about 3 inches beyond the nostril. The tip of the catheter should not go beyond the nasopharynx. The equipment, procedure, and precautions are the same as with the deep technique.

Cleaning and Sterilizing the Oxygen Catheter

Rubber Catheters. Wash in warm sudsy water, rinse, and sterilize by boiling, autoclaving, or by immersion in 1:1000 mercury bichloride solution. Zephiran Chloride solution should not be used, as it has been found to be irritating to the mucous membranes.

Plastic Catheters. These are usually dis-

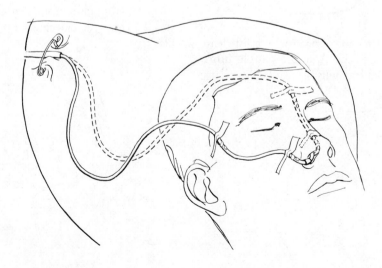

carded but may be sterilized in a disinfectant solution.

After sterilization, dry and store the catheters in a clean container.

NASOINHALERS

The nasoinhaler, sometimes referred to as a nasal cannula, is used when oxygen concentrations up to 35 per cent are needed. Nasoinhalers consist of either plastic or metal tubes, the ends of which are inserted about $\frac{1}{4}$ to $\frac{1}{2}$ inch into the nostrils. The metal type like the one shown here

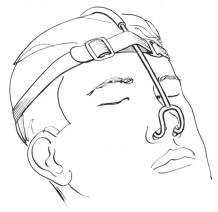

is usually malleable and can be bent to fit faces of various shapes. Some operators prefer to use short pieces of rubber tubing on the ends of the metal prongs. The tubing should be about $\frac{3}{4}$ inch long and should not block the nostrils, or the patient will be forced to breathe through the mouth in order to receive the necessary volume of air. The plastic nasoinhalers are disposable and look similar to this:

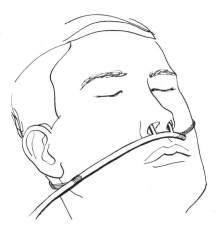

Oxygen administered in this manner must also pass through a humidifier (see p. 49).

The same points are observed during the treatment as in the administration of oxygen through the nasal catheter (see p. 36).

FACE MASKS

The face mask is used when oxygen concentrations around 100 per cent are needed. The face mask is the quickest and one of the most effective methods of administering high oxygen concentrations. Concentrations of oxygen can be attained almost immediately, and high percentages may be maintained over a long period of time. The mask is an efficient apparatus for emergency treatment and is usually found in areas of the hospital where emergency situations may arise.

There are four basic types of face masks:
1. The face tent or open-top mask
2. Partial rebreathing mask
3. Positive pressure mask
4. Meter or nonrebreathing mask

Face Tent

The face tent operates on the principle that oxygen is slightly heavier than air and will remain within the mask providing a proper flow is maintained. Since carbon dioxide is still heavier than oxygen, a flow of 6 to 8 liters of oxygen is recommended to prevent an excess accumulation of carbon dioxide. The face tent looks like this:

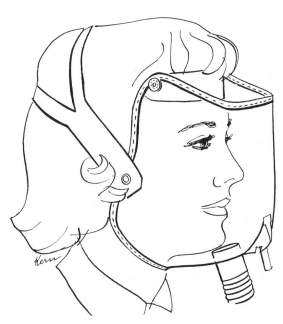

Partial Rebreathing Mask

This type of mask is probably the one with which most nurses are familiar. In this mask the exhaled air is caught in a bag below the facepiece of the mask. Before each act of exhalation is complete, the oxygen flowing from the supply goes into the bag and fills it to capacity. The oxygen flowing into the bag forces part of the exhaled carbon dioxide out through valves purposely located in the facepiece. The next inhalation then consists of air drawn from the rebreathing bag. Consequently, this air is a mixture of both the previously exhaled air and some of the fresh oxygen. The parts of a partial rebreathing mask are shown here:

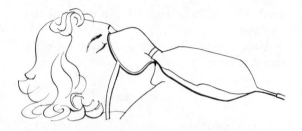

The nasal mask permits the patient to take medication and food while receiving the therapy. When wearing the nasal style, the patient must keep his mouth closed and breathe through his nose. If the patient does not cooperate, oxygen will become diluted by atmospheric air, and it will be impossible to maintain a known concentration.

There are also several varieties of both the nasal and oronasal style. The new lightweight plastic masks are tolerated well by most patients. The facepiece of these masks is framed by lightweight flexible metal bent to fit the contour of the face. Plastic masks are economical and are discarded after use. The plastic mask looks like this:

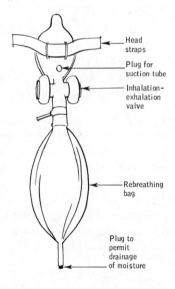

Head straps

Plug for suction tube

Inhalation-exhalation valve

Rebreathing bag

Plug to permit drainage of moisture

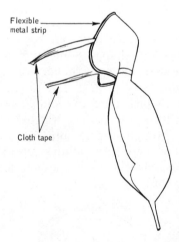

Flexible metal strip

Cloth tape

There are two styles of partial rebreathing masks. The nasal style covers the nose only, as shown:

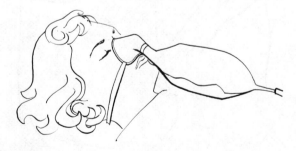

The oronasal style covers the nose and the mouth, as shown:

The B.L.B. mask (named for its designers— Boothby, Lovelace, and Bulbulian) is the most commonly used rebreathing mask. On either side of the facepiece of the B.L.B. mask are rubber turrets containing sponge rubber discs which are about the size of a half-dollar. These are the inhalation-exhalation valves. If these discs become moist or obstructed, air will not move freely through them, and the mask will not function properly. When the mask is not functioning properly, the patient usually complains of increased difficulty in breathing. When this happens, remove the sponge discs and replace them with dry ones, or rinse them thoroughly, dry well by squeezing in a towel, then reinsert. The B.L.B. mask has two plugs: one in the facepiece to permit the insertion of a suction tube, the other at the bottom of the breathing bag to permit drainage of accumulated moisture. These plugs must not be removed except for the purposes mentioned and for washing the mask.

When therapy with a mask is begun, 20 to 30 minutes must be spent with the patient, instructing him in the use of the mask. Allow the patient to take a few breaths first with the mask, then without the mask until he becomes accustomed to the feel of the mask. With the proper instructions a conscious, cooperative patient can usually adjust the facepiece and head straps to the position most comfortable to him and at the same time most leakproof. Answer all the patient's questions before applying the mask.

To start the treatment with the partial rebreathing mask:

1. Select a mask of the correct size (small or large).
2. Attach the rubber tubing from the mask to the oxygen flowmeter outlet.
3. Start the oxygen flow at a high rate (14 to 15 liters per minute) because most patients breathe more deeply and rapidly when the mask is first applied. If the oxygen flow is not high enough, the patient may have difficulty in completing the first inhalation and become apprehensive.
4. Carefully adjust the facepiece of the mask to the patient's face. Have the patient exhale during the application. Adjust the head straps so that the mask fits snugly. In order for the mask to function properly, there should be no leakage of oxygen between the mask and the face. On extremely thin or oddly shaped faces, it may be necessary to place a piece of dampened cotton or gauze over the bridge of the nose or under the chin to maintain a leakproof fit. Safeguard against making the head straps too tight, as this causes abrasions of the skin.

5. Readjust the flow of the oxygen to the number of liters needed for continuation of the treatment (usually 8 to 10 liters). Whether or not the patient is receiving a sufficient supply of oxygen is best noted by watching the rebreathing bag. The bag should collapse only one third to one half its capacity on each inhalation and should fill to capacity on each exhalation. After the beginning of the treatment, it may take 10 to 15 minutes to partially alleviate severe symptoms of anoxia. After this period it will be necessary to adjust the flow of oxygen further.

As a rule, a humidifier is not used when administering oxygen by mask. The moisture that collects within the mask from the patient's exhalations usually provides enough humidification for the oxygen. If the patient complains of dryness of the throat, a humidifier is used. To use the humidifier, assemble the apparatus as shown on page 49.

Procedures to be followed during the administration of oxygen by mask are:

1. Remove the mask to sponge and dry the patient's face and the interior part of the mask every 2 hours. Put a slight application of powder on his face and replace the mask. Perform any necessary nursing procedures such as mouth care while the mask is removed.
2. Check the entire apparatus for leaks every hour. Check the tubing to make certain it is not kinked or pinched.
3. Frequently check the action of the rebreathing bag and make any necessary adjustments to the liter flow.
4. Do not leave the patient unattended for long periods of time.

Positive Pressure Mask

The positive pressure mask exerts force during the breathing cycle. Depending upon the apparatus used, force may be exerted during inhalations, exhalations, or intermittently against both inhalations and exhalations. Positive pressure mask therapy is used to prevent an accumulation of exudation in the alveoli, to retard blood circulation, and to maintain a patent lumen in the bronchi. The type of positive pressure mask discussed here will be that which exerts pressure against exhalations. This type of mask is most frequently used for treatment of pulmonary edema.

The positive pressure mask looks exactly like a simple rebreathing mask except that it has a meter valve built in over the exhalation valve like this:

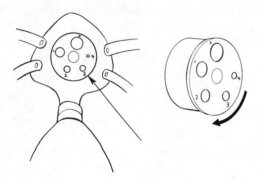

Because this type of mask is a nonbreathing mask, the exhalation valve is needed to permit the escape of the previously inhaled gases. The meter valve built in over the exhalation valve contains small holes. The exhalation gases being forced through these small orifices create a back pressure against exhalation called positive pressure. The holes on the pressure valve range in size from about $1/2$ to $1/16$ inch in diameter. The largest hole is labeled "0," which means that when the pressure disk is adjusted at this reading, there is no positive pressure, and the mask functions as a simple oxygen mask. The remaining numbers on the pressure disc (1 through 4) each refer to the amount of pressure created by exhaling through a tube immersed an equal number of centimeters under water. (If the pressure valve is set at number 1, the same amount of pressure is created by exhaling through a tube immersed 1 cm. under water.) The actual pressure created, then, depends upon the setting of the valve and upon the rate and volume of the patient's respirations. *The rate of oxygen flow does not affect the amount of pressure exerted.*

The methods used in applying the positive pressure mask and in starting the oxygen are the same as those used in applying the B.L.B. mask. Additional points to be observed in using the positive pressure mask are as follows:

1. Set the positive pressure meter at the largest opening to start (the 0 reading upward).
2. Wait several minutes (5 to 10 minutes) before turning the meter to the number 1 reading, then several minutes again before turning the meter to the number 2 reading, and so on to the number 3 or 4 reading. The physician prescribes the amount of pressure desired and the length of time this pressure is to be maintained.
3. While the patient is receiving oxygen with the positive pressure mask, the blood pressure must be checked frequently. Any sudden extreme drop in blood pressure must be reported immediately to the physician.
4. When removing the positive pressure mask the pressure valve must be turned to the 0 reading before removing the mask. Again, turn the meter one number at a time, and wait several minutes between each number setting.

Meter Mask

The meter or nonrebreathing type mask has the same functions as the rebreathing mask. With the meter type mask the oxygen flow is regulated by an attached concentration meter, NOT by the oxygen liter flow. The concentration meter is a small drum-shaped device which mixes the oxygen from the cylinder with the room air to produce the desired percentage of oxygen concentration to be administered to the patient. Around the front rim of the meter are stamped the percentage concentrations.

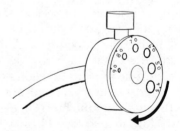

To use the meter mask, first remove the hose nipple and nut shown here from the outlet of the flowmeter and put them in a safe place.

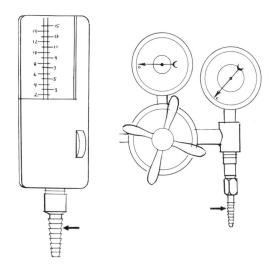

Then attach the concentration meter to the flowmeter outlet like this:

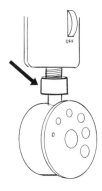

Then attach one end of a large-diameter rubber tubing to the outlet of the concentration meter.

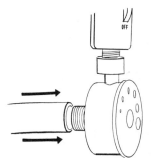

The diameter of the rubber tubing for this type mask is larger than that for the rebreathing mask. Substitution of a tube with a smaller diameter will prevent proper functioning of the concentration meter.

Next attach the other end of the rubber tubing to the mask like this:

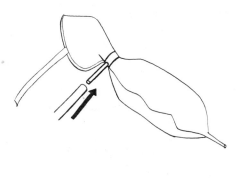

The mask must be assembled so that the inlet connection points slightly downward.

Set the meter disc by turning it until the hole corresponding to the desired oxygen concentration is at the top:

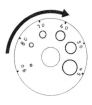

then turn the oxygen flow on high and proceed to apply the mask to the patient's face as when applying the rebreathing mask (p. 41).

Since the meter mask is a nonrebreathing mask, all exhaled gases are expelled from the mask through the exhalation valve.

The bag at the base of the mask is a reservoir bag for the continuous flow of oxygen. During each inhalation, then, the bag should remain partially inflated. As long as the bag remains partially inflated, the patient is receiving the percentage of oxygen concentration preset on the meter. When the concentration meter is reset, the oxygen flow must be readjusted. During the treatment, the same procedures are to be followed as when administering oxygen through the nonrebreathing mask.

Cleaning Masks

After use, all nondisposable masks are soaked in a detergent-disinfectant solution until sterilized, then rinsed thoroughly. Dry and lightly powder each part, assemble, and store in a sealed package.

OXYGEN TENT

There are several reasons for oxygen to be administered by tent in preference to other methods.

1. The air circulating within the tent is cooled. This cooling effect promotes the comfort of the patient.
2. The tent provides humidification.
3. The patient is more comfortable than when wearing a mask or catheter attached to the face.

One disadvantage of administering oxygen by tent is that it is the most difficult method with which to regulate the concentration of oxygen. Every time the canopy is opened, a large amount of oxygen is lost. Oxygen is also lost when the canopy is not properly tucked under the mattress. The highest oxygen concentration possible with the tent is 50 to 55 per cent.

The advantages, however, are usually sufficient to offset the disadvantages.

Setting Up the Tent

Most of the oxygen tents now in use are the electrically refrigerated models similar to this:

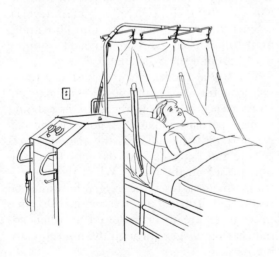

The tents manufactured by various companies look slightly different in design, but all tents have the same basic mechanics. When the orderly brings the tent to the department for use, the tent should be completely assembled. The overhead arm which holds the canopy is usually folded down and must be braced in the horizontal position. The nurse puts the arm up and folds the canopy like this:

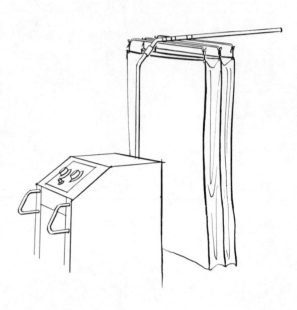

The tent is then placed next to the patient's bed and plugged in. The motor is turned on, and the controls are set. The control panel looks like this:

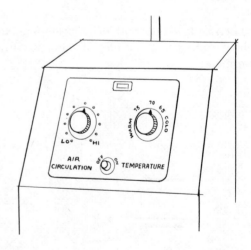

Note the air circulation knob, the temperature dial, and the "on-off" knob. The ideal temperature is 70° F., but the temperature should never be set more than 10 to 15° F. below room temperature even in very hot weather. Unless otherwise indicated, the air circulation is set about halfway between low and high.

Next, connect the oxygen outlet tube to the oxygen flowmeter, and start the oxygen flow at 15 liters per minute.

In some models of oxygen tents, air deflectors must be adjusted so that the air entering the canopy does not blow directly on the patient's face like this:

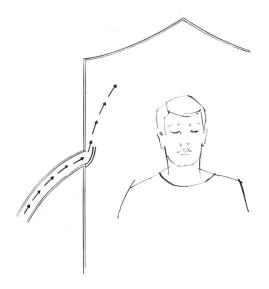

The canopy is then arranged over the patient. Hold the canopy high so that it does not touch the patient's face.

The cabinet should be placed at a position in relation to the patient's head like this:

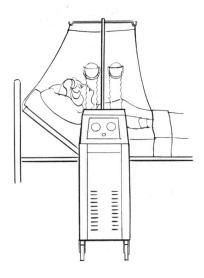

The canopy should be molded loosely over the patient's body and/or his top covers, then covered with a drawsheet or cotton blanket tucked in on both ends. Many nurses believe that the tighter this covering is stretched across the patient, the lesser the amount of oxygen lost. As a matter of fact, just the opposite is true. The top covers should fit around the contours of the body like this:

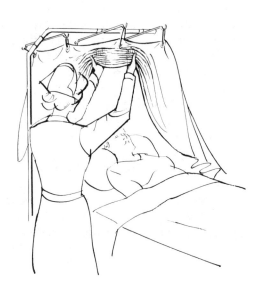

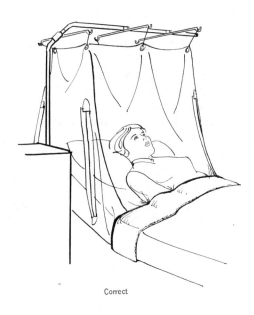

Correct

and should NOT be stretched tightly like this:

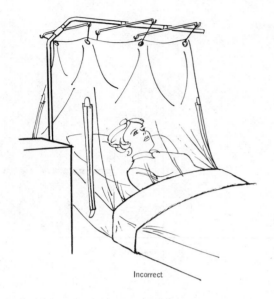

Incorrect

In order to obtain a therapeutic level of oxygen in the canopy as quickly as possible, flood the tent with oxygen by pressing the flush valve for 2 minutes or by allowing the oxygen to flow at 15 liters for at least 30 minutes. Pressing the flush valve causes a large amount of oxygen to rush into the tent. This makes a loud noise and should be explained to the patient.

Unless otherwise prescribed, the oxygen flow is set at 10 to 12 liters per minute. (Ten liters is usually sufficient to maintain the desired 50 per cent oxygen concentration.)

Maintenance of Oxygen Tent Therapy

Important points to be noted while the patient is under the tent are these:

1. The only way of knowing whether or not the oxygen concentration within the canopy is being maintained is to check the air within the canopy with an oxygen analyzer (see p. 48). An analysis should be made every 4 hours and whenever the tent has been open for an extensive period of time.

2. Regardless of the liter flow, if the canopy is not tucked in properly, the oxygen concentration will decrease until it has no therapeutic value.

3. Maintain the liter flow at at least 10 liters per minute.

4. When an intravenous or drainage tube is present, the liter flow should be raised to 13 to 14 liters per minute.

5. To reduce oxygen loss, plan nursing care so that as much as possible can be done at one time while the tent is open.

6. Open the tent no wider than necessary.

7. For baths and examinations, slide rather than lift the canopy up to the patient's neck.

8. To reduce oxygen waste, always turn off the blower before opening the tent.

9. When closing the canopy, restart the motor and flood the tent with oxygen.

10. The temperature within the tent should be regulated at the level most comfortable to the patient. Elderly patients may require a slightly higher temperature.

11. If the patient complains of extreme warmth or if the inside of the canopy becomes cloudy, the tent should be removed immediately. This is usually a sign that the circulation motor has stopped. When this happens, the carbon dioxide level within the canopy becomes dangerously high. If the circulation motor has stopped, check the electric plug to see if it has become disconnected, as this is usually the difficulty.

12. The height of the canopy should be adjusted so that the space within the canopy is just large enough to prevent claustrophobia. The smaller the space, the less oxygen is needed to maintain the percentage concentration.

13. Some oxygen tents are equipped with a drip pan located under the cabinet. The pan catches water that may form on the exterior of the cooling coils and should be emptied according to the manufacturer's instructions (usually once daily).

14. Most elderly patients prefer a head and shoulder wrap, as the air entering the tent is usually quite cool to them. The head wrap can be made from a folded face towel like this:

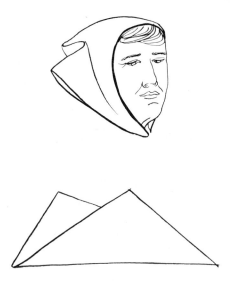

Use a cotton bath blanket folded in a triangle for the shoulder wrap.

15. The temperature of the patient must be taken rectally while the patient is in the oxygen tent.
16. Charting during the treatment should include the amount of oxygen being administered, the length of time the patient is in the tent, and the patient's general physical and mental reaction to the treatment.

Safety Rules during Tent Therapy

Since oxygen supports combustion, there are several safety rules which must be adhered to during tent therapy. These rules should be explained to the patient and also to the patient's visitors. The rules are as follows:

1. No electrical devices should be placed in an oxygen tent. This includes electric call bells, electric heating pads, radios, electric razors, hearing aids, or x-ray machines.
2. Oil or alcohol rubs should not be given to the patient in an oxygen tent.
3. Do not use wool blankets.
4. No smoking should be allowed inside the tent or anywhere in the patient's room. Place "NO SMOKING" signs where other patients and visitors can see them.

When the tent therapy has been discontinued, the patient is gradually removed from the high concentration of oxygen. The usual procedure is to remove the tent for 15- to 20-minute periods several times daily before totally discontinuing the treatment. During the brief periods when the patient has been removed from the tent, the nurse should be on the alert for signs of anoxia.

Care of Tent after Use

In institutions where this is a nursing procedure, the nurse proceeds like this:

1. Wash the outside of the cabinet with a detergent-disinfectant solution, using a brush on the ventilation louvres; rinse with clear water, and wipe dry.
2. Soak the canopy with a detergent-disinfectant solution, rinse thoroughly, and sponge dry. Torn canopies can be mended with plastic tape or transparent plastic material.
3. Remove metal filters, rubber ventilation ducts, and all rubber tubing, and wash in a detergent-disinfectant solution, rinse with clear water, and dry.
4. If the tent was used for an infectious case, the entire system through which oxygen passes must be sterilized. To do this, plug the drain and vents, and with a funnel pour a disinfectant solution into the oxygen inlet, and let stand until sterilization is complete; then drain off and flush the system with clear hot water.

After the unit has been cleaned, assemble all the parts, and store in complete readiness in a clean place.

The Open-top Tent

A variation of the oxygen tent is the open-top tent shown here:

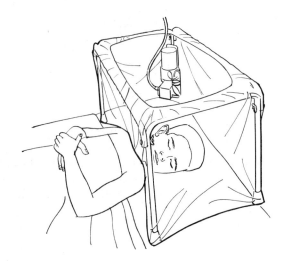

This tent has a small canopy with an opening in one side through which the patient's head is placed. The opening is closed around the patient's neck with a drawstring, sheet, or specially designed sleeve, depending on the manufacturer. The open-top tent operates on the principle that oxygen is heavier than air and will seep out through the top at a rate much slower than the rate of the oxygen flowing in from the supply source. A concentration of 50 to 60 per cent can be maintained at an oxygen flow of 10 liters providing there is no draft in the room. Any increased movement of air over the canopy causes rapid escape of oxygen through the canopy top.

The open-top tent cannot be used for patients who are restless. This type tent is used most frequently for children; however, it may be used effectively for adults.

The air within the open-top tents may be either kept at room temperature or cooled with the use of an ice tray.

THE OXYGEN ANALYZER

The concentration of oxygen with the mask and catheter is satisfactorily determined by regulation of the liter flow. However, with the oxygen tent and with apparatus used for children such as the oxygen hood and incubator, the only certain way of knowing the amount of oxygen present is by analysis. An analysis of the atmosphere of the tent, etc., can be made with an oxygen analyzer. When an oxygen analyzer is used in tent therapy, the doctor prescribes the liter flow and/or the percentage of oxygen concentration desired. Modern oxygen analyzers are simple to use and require little or no maintenance. They are now standard equipment in many hospitals.

There are several different types of oxygen analyzers which operate on either of two principles, magnetic or electrical balance. The analyzer shown here operates on the principle of electric balance. These illustrations are adapted from the oxygen analyzer manufactured by the National Cylinder Gas Co., Chicago, Ill.

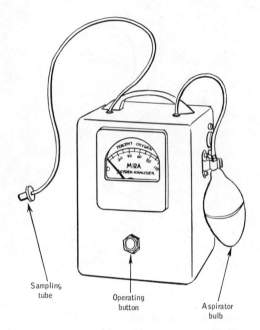

The operation of all types of analyzers is basically the same. Proceed like this:

1. Squeeze five or six times on the aspirator bulb so that room air is drawn into the analyzer. This is done to test the accuracy of the analyzer.

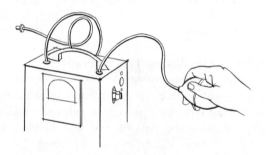

2. Then press the button, and while the button is depressed, read the concentration on the dial. If the instrument is accurate, the concentration of oxygen in the room air should be around 21 per cent.

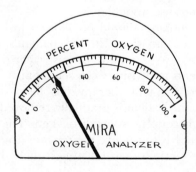

Next insert the sampling tube into the tent (or other apparatus) so that it lies near the same depth as the patient's nose, and repeat Steps 1 and 2 to get the concentration reading inside the tent.

When using the analyzer, always stand it on a level surface. Results of the analyses should be recorded on the patient's chart.

Never use the analyzer to test the oxygen concentration in mixtures of gases other than oxygen-nitrogen unless the manufacturer's instructions state otherwise.

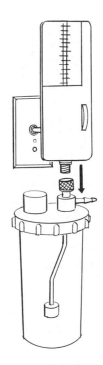

HUMIDIFIERS

When oxygen is administered in high concentrations by mask for long periods of time and when it is administered by a catheter or nasoinhaler, it must pass through a humidifier to provide moisture. Since oxygen is a dry gas, it causes local irritation to the mucous membranes.

A humidifier consists of a glass or plastic bottle with a cap which can be connected to an oxygen regulator. A metal tube extends from the cap down into the bottle.

3. Attach the tubing from the nasal catheter or other apparatus to the outlet on the cap like this:

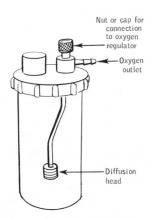

Nut or cap for connection to oxygen regulator

Oxygen outlet

Diffusion head

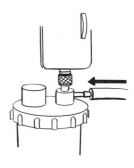

To use the humidifier, proceed as follows:

1. Unscrew the bottle cap, and fill the bottle with distilled water to the indicated water level. If there is no level mark, fill the bottle only half full. When indicated by the manufacturer, tap water may be used. Replace the cap.

2. Attach the top of the humidifier to the oxygen regulator or flowmeter like this:

4. Start the flow of oxygen as prescribed. Oxygen enters the bottle through the metal tube and causes bubbles to form in the water. As the bubbles of oxygen rise in the water, they gather moisture. The moistened oxygen then passes upward and out through the tubing to the administering apparatus.

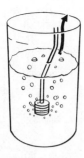

When one understands how the humidifier functions, one can easily see that in order for the humidifier to function efficiently, (1) the metal tube must always be inserted at least an inch under water, and (2) the bottle must never be filled to the top.

When water is to be added to the humidifier, first turn off the oxygen, then unscrew the jar, and add the water quickly so that the patient is without oxygen for a minimal period.

A humidifier with a diffusion head such as the one just shown can produce a relative humidity of 60 to 70 per cent.

NEBULIZERS OR JET HUMIDIFIERS

Nebulizers or jet humidifiers are special devices designed for the purpose of aerosol therapy. The nebulizer or jet humidifier produces a higher percentage of humidity than a humidifier. With these devices the water is blown from a nozzle in the form of a fine misty spray like this:

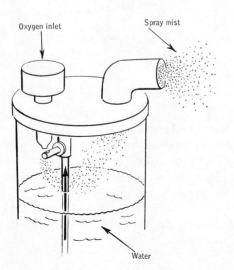

Nebulizers are available in several sizes and can be used in a variety of ways. The spray may be obtained by hooking a suitably styled nebulizer to an oxygen supply, to a compressed air machine, or to a rubber hand bulb. The large nebulizers, which hold up to 500 cc. of solution, are used for continued aerosol therapy. They may be used to administer water in aerosol form for the purpose of high humidity or to administer certain liquid drugs such as antibiotics, bronchodilators, and wetting agents (example: Alevaire).

Some of the larger nebulizers are designed for use with a face mask and are hooked up to oxygen as is a humidifier. The smaller nebulizers hold up to 25 cc. and are usually used to administer drugs in aerosol form intermittently.

HYPERBARIC OXYGEN THERAPY

Recently there has been an increased interest in hyperbaric oxygen (OHP) therapy, which is the administration of oxygen in an environment of increased atmospheric pressure. In hyperbaric oxygen therapy, the patient is placed in a specially designed hyperbaric chamber in which the atmospheric pressure can be increased to several times the normal pressure at sea level. While the atmospheric pressure is increased, 100 per cent oxygen is administered by mask to the patient. This procedure permits more oxygen to be dissolved in body fluids.

During normal respiration the amount of oxygen in 100 cc. arterial blood is about 20 cc.; of this 2.5 per cent or 0.5 cc. is dissolved in the plasma and 97.5 per cent or 19.5 cc. is carried by the hemoglobin. When 100 per cent oxygen is administered under normal atmospheric pressure, there is little change in the amount of oxygen carried by hemoglobin; however, the amount of oxygen dissolved by plasma increases from 0.5 cc. to about 2 cc. per 100 cc. of blood or two volumes per cent.

When the atmospheric pressure is doubled or tripled, while 100 per cent oxygen is administered, the amount of oxygen dissolved in the plasma also doubles, triples, and so forth, with no additional increase in oxygen carried by the hemoglobin. This increase of plasma oxygen can then provide most, if not all, of the oxygen needed by the brain, visceral organs, kidneys, myocardium, and muscles, without the use of hemoglobin.

The increase in plasma oxygen then facilitates the oxygenation and healing of anaerobic body tissues (as in gas gangrene, some malignant tumors, and tetanus) and of ischemic tissues (as in frostbite, varicose ulcerations, and trauma).

Design of the Hyperbaric Chamber

The hyperbaric chamber is a large cylinder with airtight doors called locks. The size of the chamber depends upon the purpose for which it was built. A chamber can hold from one to six patients and several attendants. In some institutions one chamber is built to serve several purposes such as for medical therapy, a surgical operating suite, and experimentation; another institution may have three separate chambers for the same three purposes. The actual size inside the chamber may range from 10 to 12 feet in diameter to 20 to 40 feet in length.

All controls are housed in a separate unit outside the chamber. Specially trained men operate the controls, which include regulation of pressure, temperature, and humidity. Each chamber is equipped with a two-way communication system between the control operator and the chamber occupant.

The equipment needed to set up the inside of the chamber again depends upon the purpose of use and could include anything from a stretcher to complete operating room equipment.

Patient Care

Since a select nursing staff is trained to care for a patient exposed to hyperbaric oxygen therapy, only a generalized description will be included here.

When it has been decided that the patient requires hyperbaric oxygen therapy, the procedure is explained to the patient and his family, and he is given a consent form to sign. He is then transferred to the chamber for a specific prescribed time under a prescribed amount of pressure. For therapeutic purposes

hyperbaric oxygen therapy may be given for periods of 1 to 2 hours, two or three times daily (every 8 to 12 hours), until marked improvement is achieved. For most therapeutic purposes, 2 to 3 atmospheres absolute pressure (ATA) or 14 to 29 pounds per square inch gauge pressure (PSIG) are prescribed. The chamber is pressurized within about 20 minutes. During this time there is some pain and blocking of the ear; these may be relieved by swallowing. The noise within the chamber can be compared to that of an airplane. The fact that the nurse and other attendants with the patient share similar feelings in this situation can give comfort and security to the patient.

The patient is given 100 per cent oxygen by mask during the entire treatment. Fire-resistant clothes are worn by the patient and the attendants. During pressurization the patient's vital signs are recorded, and he is observed for symptoms of oxygen toxicity, air embolus, spontaneous pneumothorax, and claustrophobia. The decompression procedure is carried out slowly, and all staff and patients remain in the area for at least 1 hour after decompression, in case the "bends" should appear. Detailed records of the patient's condition during therapy are kept by the nurse and are attached to the patient's chart.

Currently, hyperbaric oxygen therapy is used successfully to treat gas gangrene, tetanus, chronic osteomyelitis, trauma (when many small blood vessels are damaged), frostbite, carbon monoxide poisoning, varicose ulcerations, and burns. Hyperbaric oxygen therapy is also used surgically in resection of abdominal aneurysms and during correction of renal, carotid, and peripheral occlusive artery disease.

Additional Procedures. Nurses working in the hyperbaric chamber are required to know the following procedures:

Use of defibrillator and external pacemaker (see pp. 242 and 243)

Use of respirator (see Chapter 5)

Venipuncture (see p. 85)

Tracheal suction (see p. 354)

External cardiac massage (see p. 242)

Inflation of cuffed tracheostomy tube (see p. 66)

Use of hypothermia (p. 10)

Blood transfusion and intravenous administration (p. 93)

Collection of blood specimens via artery (p. 93)

Insertion of nasogastric tube (p. 150)

Use of oral airways (p. 135)

Organizing and assisting in surgical operations

As noted, nurses may be taught to carry out some procedures ordinarily performed by the doctor. In this case, these procedures are lifesaving measures carried out by the nurse when there is no doctor in the chamber.

THE ADMINISTRATION OF OTHER GASES

HELIUM

Helium is a light, colorless, odorless, and tasteless gas. Because helium is lighter than air, inhalation of an 80 per cent helium – 20 per cent oxygen proportion, is much easier than inhalation of a mixture of the same proportions of nitrogen and oxygen (the usual components of the atmosphere we inhale). Under ordinary circumstances the energy expended in the act of inhalation need not be reduced. However, when inhalations are labored because of an obstructed or constricted airway, inhalation of an oxygen-helium mixture aids in relieving dyspnea.

The helium-oxygen mixture in therapeutic proportions is commercially prepared in cylinders. Helium is administered most commonly through a face mask (B.L.B. or meter). The techniques are the same as in the administration of oxygen. The following rules apply to the administration of helium-oxygen mixtures:

1. A special regulator calculated for helium should be used.
2. Never use a regulator used for helium in the administration of oxygen.
3. Tents, catheters, and nasoinhalers are not suitable for helium-oxygen therapy because helium diffuses rapidly.
4. If for any reason a tent is used, the canopy must be made of a special helium-proof fabric.

5. The administration of helium and oxygen is usually begun by the physician or specially trained technician. The nurse may maintain the treatment after it has been successfully inititated.
6. When higher concentrations of oxygen are needed, the helium-oxygen mixture is connected with a pure oxygen flow like this:

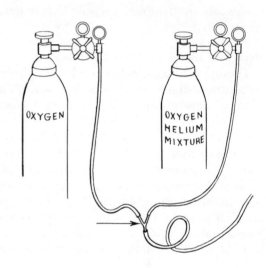

CARBON DIOXIDE

Carbon dioxide is a colorless gas with a slightly acid taste and a slight pungent odor. Carbon dioxide is used as a respiratory stimulant in the resuscitation of the newborn, the drowned, the victims of drug poisoning, and to stimulate deep breathing in the postoperative patient.

Carbon dioxide is administered with oxygen in proportions of carbon dioxide 3 to 10 per cent to 97 to 90 per cent oxygen. Mixtures of these proportions can be obtained in commercially prepared cylinders.

Carbon dioxide may be administered with an anesthesia mask, a B.L.B., or a meter mask (the oronasal type). The methods for the use of the B.L.B. and meter masks are the same as in the administration of oxygen (see p. 42) except for the following:

1. For treatment of asphyxiation, the physician usually performs the procedure.
2. The nurse usually performs the procedure when ordered to be given postoperatively to prevent pulmonary complications.

3. A physician or well trained nurse must remain with the patient during the entire treatment.

4. The patient must be watched for signs of carbon dioxide toxicity: vomiting, unbearable dyspnea, disorientation, elevated systolic blood pressure, a weak pulse, irregular pulse, and an increase in pulse rate of more than ten beats per minute.

5. The treatment must be immediately terminated if the patient does not respond by increased breathing after six inhalations and/or if the patient shows any signs of approaching toxicity.

6. Before starting the treatment, explain to the patient that the gas is not an anesthetic.

7. When the treatment is included in the postoperative orders, apply the mask for a few minutes only, then allow the patient to breathe normally several times before re-applying the mask. Repeat this procedure for as long as the physician has ordered. For example: When the physician has requested the use of the carbon dioxide mask for 15 minutes, the nurse would allow the patient to breathe with the mask for several minutes, then without the mask for several respirations, then again with the mask for several minutes, etc., for the entire 15-minute period.

8. Note and record the rate and depth of the respirations before, during, and at the termination of the treatment. Record the time of termination of the treatment and the patient's general reaction to the treatment.

BIBLIOGRAPHY

Burgess, A. M.: A Comparison of Common Methods of Oxygen Therapy for Bed Patients. Am. J. Nurs., *65*:96, 1965.

Campbell, D.: Oxygen Therapy at Home. Nurs. Mir., *123*:12, 1967.

Catterall, M.: Oxygen Therapy. Nurs. Mir., *124*:5, 1967.

Clark, T. J.: Respiratory Failure. Nurs. Mir., *124*:5, 1967.

Cockerill, G.: Hyperbaric Oxygenation, a New Field Opened for Nurses. Nurs. Times, *63*:216, 1967.

Hanson, G. C.: Hyperbaric Oxygenation. Nurs. Times, *63*:213, 1967.

Ludwig, W. D.: Precision, Safety Keynote Design for Hyperbaric Oxygen Facilities. Heating, Piping & Air Conditioning, May, 1964.

Pascale, L. R., and Wallyn, R. J.: Surgical Application of Hyperbaric Chamber. Surg. Clin. N. Amer., *48(1)*: 63, 1967.

Trippel, O., Ruggie, A., Staley, C., and Van Elk, J.: Hyperbaric Oxygenation in Management of Gas Gangrene. Surg. Clin. N. Amer., *47(1)*:17, 1967.

Venger, M. J.: Hyperbaric Oxygenation: Nursing Responsibility in Planning for a New Clinical Service. Nurs. Clin. N. Amer., *1(1)*:131, 1966.

The Use of Respirators

The increase in knowledge of pulmonary physiology has also brought about the development of new and improved respirators. The newer models most commonly used as well as the older types will be discussed here.

PHYSIOLOGY OF RESPIRATION

Since all respirators either assist the patient with respirations or completely control respirations when the patient is unable to breathe by himself, it is imperative that the nurse have some basic understanding of the mechanics of breathing.

Respiration involves perfusion, diffusion, and ventilation.

Perfusion. This is the supplying of blood to the lungs from the heart. When the patient is immobile for periods of time, an imbalance between ventilation and perfusion occurs. This is one of the reasons for the "stir-up" regimen postoperatively.

Diffusion. This is the exchange of oxygen and carbon dioxide between the alveoli and the capillaries.

Diffusion and perfusion occur simultaneously with ventilation. Although the use of respirators effects all three phases of respiration, it is the mechanics of ventilation which must be thoroughly understood.

Ventilation. This aspect of normal respiration includes the cycle of inspiration and expiration followed by a brief pause. The brief pause after expiration is mentioned here because most patients do not realize this pause exists and because of its importance for the nurse in adjusting some types of respirators. During inspiration air flows into the lungs until the pressure within the lungs equals that of the atmosphere. At this point expiration begins. During expiration air is expelled from the lungs, and the pressure within the lungs rises above atmospheric pressure. As a summary, intrapulmonic pressure is below atmospheric pressure during inspiration, equal to atmospheric pressure at the end of inspiration, above atmospheric pressure during expiration, and again equal to atmospheric pressure at the end of expiration. This series of changes is repeated with each respiratory cycle.

Another aspect of ventilation includes the volume of air taken into the lungs during inspiration and expelled during expiration. The average adult inhales about 400 to 500 cc. of air during each inspiration (called tidal volume) with a minute volume of 6 liters per minute (total minute ventilation).

TYPES OF RESPIRATORS

The choice of respirator depends upon the physician's personal preference and the type available. Respirators are either external or airway applied. The external respirator includes the older types which are now used less frequently (discussed later in this chapter). The airway-applied respirators are of two types: volume-cycled and pressure-cycled. With the volume-cycled respirator, the respiratory cycle is regulated according to the volume of air inhaled; with the pressure-cycled respirator, the respiratory cycle is regulated according to the variations in pressure which occur during inhalation and exhalation. Because the airway applied respirators have many uses, the nurse will encounter these respirators frequently. The airway-applied respirator is called the intermittent positive pressure-breathing apparatus or simply the IPPB unit.

IPPB THERAPY (INTERMITTENT AND CONTINUOUS)

EFFECTS

IPPB therapy is used for the following effects:

1. As a mechanical aid to ventilation

2. As a vehicle for the maximum effect in aerosol therapy
3. To aid expectoration
4. Cardiovascular effects, in that it increases arterial and tissue-oxygen tension

INDICATIONS

The following conditions may be indications for IPPB therapy:

Physiologic

Obstruction in airway due to bronchospasm, secretions, and edema; inadequate alveolar ventilation; respiratory acidosis, and respiratory arrest.

Specific Conditions

Acute and chronic bronchitis and asthma, pneumonia, pulmonary edema, atelectasis, pulmonary infarction, respiratory center depression by drug intoxication, cerebrovascular accident, cardiac resuscitation, emphysema, congestive heart failure, pulmonary fibrosis, bronchiectasis, "flail chest," paralyzed diaphragm, and any neuromuscular or skeletal disease with acute or chronic respiratory complications. IPPB therapy is also used in surgery to treat acute respiratory complications and postoperatively as a prophylaxis complementary to (not a substitute for) frequent changing of position, deep breathing, suctioning, coughing, and so forth. When IPPB therapy is anticipated after surgery, it is also used preoperatively to prepare the patient for its use.

DOCTOR'S ORDERS

When the physician prescribes IPPB therapy, he will specify the following:

Frequency and Duration

In most cases IPPB therapy will be ordered three or four times daily for periods of 15 to 20 minutes. Continuous therapy is used during respiratory arrest. Therapy ordered every hour or two may be required in conditions associated with marked airway obstruction such as status asthmaticus and respiratory acidosis.

Inspiratory Pressure or Volume

This would deal with the amount or pressure of air to be inhaled and would require specific settings on the IPPB unit. Usually new patients are started at a low pressure range (12 to 15 cm.), which is then gradually increased 1 to 2 cm. per treatment to the desirable range of 20 cm.

Air Mixtures

With use of the different IPPB units available, the following variations in inhaled air are possible:
1. 40 per cent oxygen
2. 100 per cent oxygen
3. 40 per cent oxygen and 60 per cent helium
4. Compressed air

Aerosol Therapy

All IPPB units contain parts to which either nebulizers or humidifiers can be attached. In many instances drugs are ordered to be administered. The commonly used drugs are as follows:

Bronchodilators. Bronchodilators are usually given in doses of 4 to 8 drops four times daily or less. Bronchodilators are NEVER given without dilution and are NEVER USED IN CONTINUOUS THERAPY. Commonly used bronchodilators include: Isuprel 1:200 (isoproterenol hydrochloride; asthmanefrin); vaponephrine (racemic epinephrine hydrochloride); Dylephrin (2.5 per cent epinephrine HC1, 0.5 per cent atropine); Aerolone Compound (cyclopentamine hydrochloride 0.5 per cent and isoproterenol hydrochloride 0.25 per cent with propylene glycol and water); NebuPrel (isoproterenol sulfate 0.4 per cent, phenylephrine hydrochloride 2 per cent, propylene glycol 10 per cent).

Diluents, Detergents, and Mucolytic Agents. The following drugs are usually given in doses of 15 to 30 drops: Tergemist (sodium 2 ethylhexyl sulfate, potassium iodide); Alevaire (Superinone, sodium bicarbonate, glycerine); ethyl alcohol (50 per cent); Mucomyst (acetylcysteine, usual dose 1 to 3 cc.); Dornavac (pancreatic dornase, usual dose 50,000 to 100,000 U.).

Antibiotics. These include tetracycline, neomycin, kanamycin, oxytetracycline and polymyxin, all in usual doses of 25 to 50 mg. Penicillin (50,000 to 100,000 U.) may also be used.

All the preceding dosages are those administered when the IPPB therapy is used for 20-minute periods several times daily. In more frequent treatment the dosage would be altered.

USING AN IPPB UNIT FOR INTERMITTENT THERAPY

When intermittent therapy is prescribed, the patient may be transferred to an IPPB therapy unit for each treatment if such a facility is available in the hospital. If not, it would be a bedside nursing procedure. When giving intermittent therapy, the respirator is used expressly for therapeutic treatment. The therapeutic effect is achieved by controlled inflation of the lungs while simultaneously delivering medication or humidification to the respiratory system.

There are at least 50 models of respirators developed by a number of manufacturers. Some models are designed exclusively for home use. Only two makes will be dealt with in this text, the Bird and the Bennett. Both respirators are pressure-cycled (see p. 57).

The operation of the respirator for intermittent therapy is relatively simple and entails only four main steps: (1) Connecting the machine to an air pressure source; (2) setting the pressure control gauge; (3) adjusting the dilution control for the prescribed percentage of oxygen/air mixture; (4) filling the nebulizer and adding medications if prescribed.

AIR PRESSURE SOURCE

The air pressure source may be obtained from an oxygen wall outlet, cylinder oxygen, or an air compressor machine.

When attaching the unit to an oxygen source, all the precautions used in connection with the administration of oxygen are used (see p. 36). No matter which source of oxygen is used, *a flowmeter is not used.* The location of the air pressure hose to be connected to the oxygen source is shown as follows: on the

Bennett respirator Model PV-3P and PR-2, the pressure hose is here:

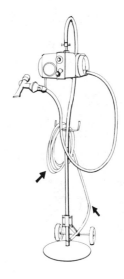

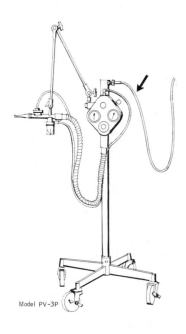

Model PV-3P

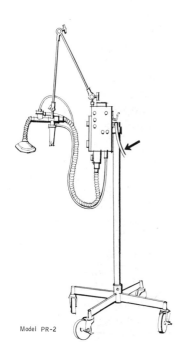

Model PR-2

On the Bird respirator the pressure connecting hose is here:

When the pressure hose is connected to the oxygen wall outlet, it is simply plugged in as shown:

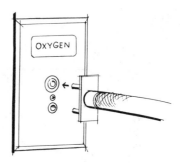

When the pressure hose is connected to cylinder oxygen, a specially designed screw connector must be used. It is screwed to the regulator as shown:

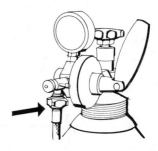

Note also the type of regulator which must be used. This regulator contains only a contents gauge, not a flowmeter. To turn on the oxygen with this type of regulator, first open the cylinder valve all the way:

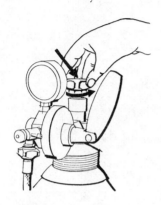

Then pull the shut-off lever to the right and all the way down:

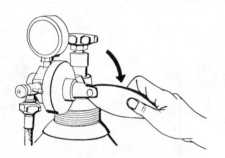

In the event oxygen is not required in therapy, the pressure hose is connected to an air pressure machine (compressor). The compressors are also available in a variety of designs. All types deliver air at approximately 50 to 60 pounds per square inch. The compressors operate by electric motors.

SETTING THE PRESSURE CONTROL GAUGE

The physician usually prescribes a pressure setting of 12 to 20 (cm. H_2O). To adjust the proper pressure on the Bird respirator (Mark 7 or 8 model), the pressure control, sensitivity control, and flow rate dial are all adjusted at the same setting as shown:

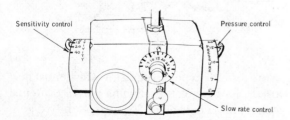

Sensitivity control   Pressure control

Slow rate control

To adjust the pressure setting on the Bennett, the pressure dial is turned to the right until the pressure gauge reads the desired setting:

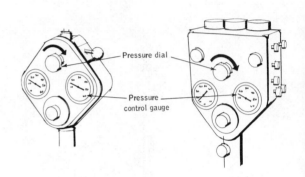

Pressure dial

Pressure control gauge

On the Bennett Model PR-2 shown on the right, make certain all additional dials are in the "off" position.

ADJUSTING THE DILUTION CONTROL

The dilution control setting regulates the oxygen/air mixture when the respirator is connected to oxygen. Two settings are possible—40 per cent oxygen and 100 per cent oxygen. The need for 100 per cent oxygen is rare and is used only on doctor's orders. For 40 per cent oxygen concentration and for use with an air compressor, the dilution control on the Bird is pulled out:

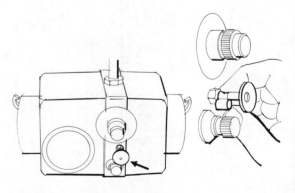

On the Bennett, the dilution control is pushed all the way in:

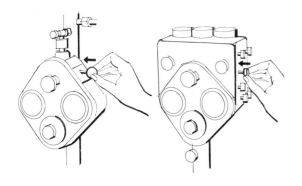

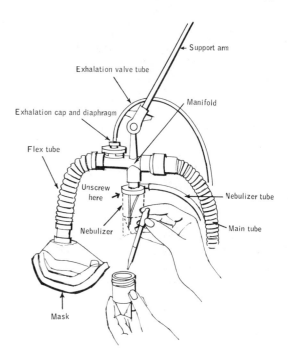

FILLING THE NEBULIZER

If a medication is prescribed, the medication is added to the nebulizer (see p. 56 for medications used and precautions). If no medication is prescribed, place distilled water in the nebulizer.

Details of the nebulizer assembly on the Bird model are shown here:

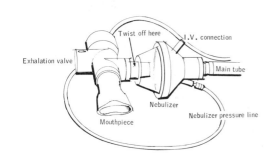

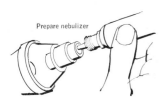

When using distilled water in the Bird model, 4 to 5 cc. is used. This model nebulizer is ready for use after filling.

The nebulizer assembly of the Bennett is shown here:

Before using the respirator, the nebulizer flow must be checked to make certain it is functioning properly. To check the nebulizer flow on the Bird respirator, push inward the small pin located in the center of the sensitivity control:

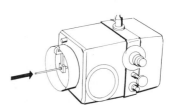

This will manually turn on the machine. As the machine cycles, check to see if a light fog is coming from the mouthpiece. If so, the nebulizer is functioning properly. After checking, pull the manual control pin out.

On the Bennett machine the nebulizer flow is adjusted as follows: On Model PV-3P open the nebulizer control until a light fog is produced from the mouthpiece. The nebulizer control on the Bennett Model PV-3P is shown here:

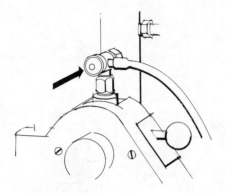

To adjust the nebulizer flow on the Bennett Model PR-2, after filling the nebulizer and screwing it back in place, remove the entire nebulizer attachment from the nebulizer manifold as shown:

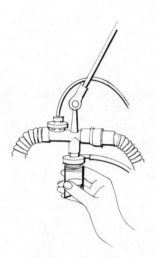

Adjust the nebulization-expiration control for a light fog (coming from top of nebulizer attachment):

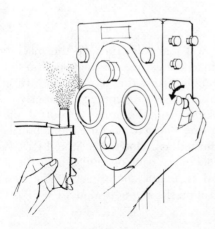

Remove the dust cap from the valve, and lift the drum pin up with the finger tip:

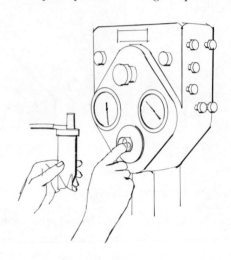

Adjust the nebulization-inspiration control for a light fog:

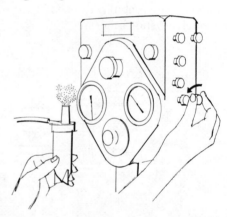

Lower the drum pin and replace the dust cap on the valve; then attach the nebulizer to the nebulizer manifold.

After checking and adjusting the nebulizer flow, the respirator is prepared for patient use. To recapitulate, four steps should have been carried out in this order.

1. Place all respirator controls in off position and connect respirator to pressure source
2. Adjust pressure control
3. Adjust dilution control
4. Fill nebulizer and adjust flow

ATTACHING THE RESPIRATOR TO THE PATIENT

IPPB therapy is most effective when the patient is sitting up, preferably in a straight-backed chair. Regardless of whether the patient is in an upright position or slightly reclining position, the mouthpiece and nebulizer attachment must be in a horizontal position. (In the Bird model the arrow on the nebulizer points toward the floor.) Before attaching the respirator to the patient, check the respiratory rate of the patient as a basis for determining whether the treatment is effective. During therapy the respiration rate should decrease.

The patient breathes into the respirator by means of a mask or a mouthpiece. Before attaching the face mask to the patient, remove facial oils from the face with a tissue. First, place the top of the mask high on the bridge of the nose as shown:

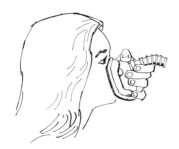

Then, slide the mask downward and place the lower portion against the cheeks:

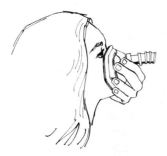

Press the lower portion firmly against the cheeks; then, fasten the mask straps—top straps first, lower straps second:

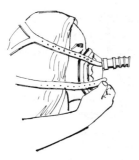

The lower strap should be tighter than the upper strap. If the mask leaks around the nose, tighten the *lower* straps to pull the mask farther down on the face. The upper strap should not be too tight. Care should be taken to fit the mask properly because leakage will make expiration difficult.

With the use of a mask the patient can breathe through the nose or mouth during therapy.

With the use of a mouthpiece, the patient must breathe only through the mouth. To use the mouthpiece, the patient is instructed to bite lightly on the tube, then seal the lips tightly around the mouthpiece:

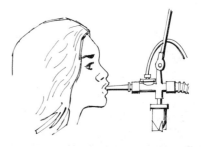

The mouthpiece is more comfortable and more convenient than the mask. Tell the patient not to breathe through his nose. If he has difficulty with this, there is a nose clip available which can be used until mouth breathing is mastered.

To teach the patient how to breathe with the respirator, either by mask or by mouthpiece, tell him to inhale slowly and deeply. A slight inspiratory effort on his part will switch the respirator on. The patient should be told that as soon as the respirator turns on, he should relax and allow the unit to fill his lungs with air. When the lungs are filled, the machine will turn off. During the off period the patient exhales completely, then takes a brief pause before the next inhalation. During exhalation coach the patient to squeeze all the air from his lungs. Some practice is required for the most effective use of the respirator.

To further assist the patient in breathing with specific models of respirators, the following can be done:

With the Bennett Model PV-3P, tell the

patient to watch the mask pressure gauge as
he inhales,

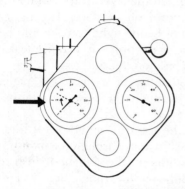

and to try to keep the needle of this gauge at
pressure longer by breathing in more deeply.

With the Bennett Model PR-2 and the Bird
Mark 7 and 8, the nurse watches the breathing
pressure gauge;

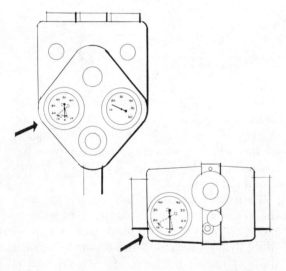

As the patient begins inhalation through the
mouthpiece, the needle, which has been resting at zero, makes a swift movement about one
point to the right of the dial (negative pressure
side); then, as the machine is triggered "on,"
the needle moves to the left of the dial (positive pressure side) to the pressure desired.
This is the needle pattern which it is hoped
will be achieved.

If the needle does not deflect at all and the
unit does not turn "on," the patient is not inhaling air from the machine. If using a mouthpiece, he is either inhaling air from around
the mouthpiece or through his nose.

If the needle deflects up to 4 or 5 on the
negative side before going to the positive side,
the patient is inhaling too hard and too
rapidly. In this event, tell him to relax and to
breathe naturally.

If the needle deflects 3 or 4 units to the left
side of the dial before the unit switches "on,"
the sensitivity control needs readjusting. The
sensitivity control setting is that which controls the amount of exertion on inhalation
needed to trigger the unit "on." The sensitivity control should be turned very slightly,
as too much adjustment will cause the unit to
turn "on" before the patient is ready:

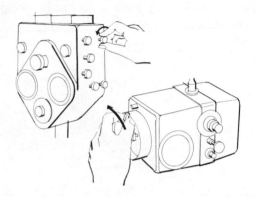

Note that, normally, on the Bennett PR-2
this setting would be on OFF or normal, and
on the Bird the setting would correspond with
the pressure setting (see p. 58).

With any type of respirator, if the unit
turns "off" before the patient has completed
inhalation, the patient is blowing into the
machine before the lungs are filled with air.
Again, coach the patient to relax and allow the
machine to fill his lungs with air.

CONTINUATION OF THERAPY

After it is felt that the patient understands
how to breathe with the respirator, the nurse
directs her attention to continued close observation of both the patient and the respirator.

The nurse should realize that not every
patient will be able to achieve the utmost in
therapy during the first treatment. Patients
with severe bronchospasm, congestion, and
dyspnea, for example, cannot be expected to

achieve full ventilation until after several days of therapy.

During and after IPPB therapy, expectoration of secretions is normal. When therapy first begins, secretions are usually dark colored. After several days they become clear. If the patient is receiving a racemic epinephrine drug via nebulization, he should be told that his secretions will be colored pink, so that he does not imagine he is coughing up blood. Close observation and recording of the patient's respiration rate and effort during therapy are essential to effectual therapy.

In observation of the respirator during therapy, the nurse should make certain the dials, as discussed previously, continue to register properly. An alert patient can be instructed to do this. The nebulizer must also be watched to make certain the patient is receiving continual moisture as well as any prescribed medication. When plastic nebulizers are used initially, medication tends to cling to the sides in small droplets. To remedy this, merely tap the nebulizer. The solution in the nebulizer should last throughout the entire treatment. If not, add more distilled water, as breathing dry air prevents loosening of bronchial secretions. Make certain the nebulizer is not leaking. Leakage is due to a worn gasket (get a new one) or a loose connection. The nebulizer will also not function if it is not cleaned properly between uses.

USING AN IPPB UNIT FOR CONTINUAL THERAPY

Continuous IPPB therapy is used when there is respiratory arrest, severe respiratory acidosis, or any other condition which renders the ventilation inadequate. Continuous therapy may be employed for a period of hours, days, or weeks, depending upon the patient's condition.

In continuous IPPB therapy the respirator is used either to completely *control* respirations for the patient who cannot breathe on his own or to *assist* the patient who is breathing erratically and who may stop breathing. Because of these two functions of the respirator, the terms "controlled ventilation" and "assisted ventilation" are commonly referred to.

In continuous IPPB therapy a special adjustment is made on the respirator so that the machine turns itself on without any inspiratory effort on the patient's part. (You will recall that in the previous discussion of IPPB therapy, the patient's inhalation triggered the machine to turn on.) All the models of respirators discussed previously can be used for controlled respiration except the Bennett PV-3P.

In using the Benett PR-2 and the Bird Mark 7 or 8 for controlled ventilation, all controls are turned off and the unit is set up using the same steps as discussed previously for intermittent therapy. Additional adjustments required on the IPPB unit are as follows (again all respirator adjustments are made only under doctor's orders):

AUTOMATIC CYCLING CONTROL

This control sets the rate of respirations. It is used to turn the machine "on" automatically without any inspiratory effort on the patient's part. If the patient begins breathing on his own while the machine is on automatic operation, his breathing pattern will override the machine. The machine works with the patient, not the patient with the machine. On the Bennett PR-2 the automatic cycling control, termed "rate control," is located here:

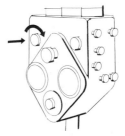

This control is turned slightly until the desired respiration rate is achieved.

On the Bird Mark 7 and 8, the rate control is located here:

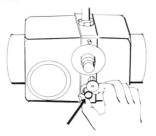

The setting on this model is made to correspond with the pressure control setting. This is a trial setting which may be too fast or too slow.

Regardless of which type respirator is used, the respiration rate must be adjusted so that enough time is allowed for complete exhalation and for the pause that follows exhalation.

For the patient who is breathing on his own and who may stop breathing, the rate control is set slightly slower than the patient's rate. With this setting, if the patient does not turn on the machine by his inspiratory effort, the unit will automatically take over that function.

ADDITIONAL CONTROLS

Additional controls on the Bennett PR-2 (not explained previously) which the physician may wish to use in controlled ventilation are these:

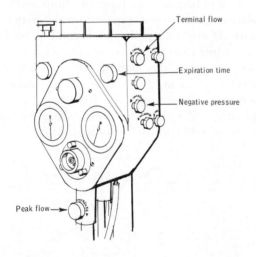

Expiration Time

This control may be used to lengthen the time of exhalation. When the rate control is turned on and the expiration time control is on "normal," the expiration time is normally 1½ times longer than inspiration. Regardless of the rate of respiration, this ratio remains the same, unless of course the expiration time control is used to increase the length of exhalation.

When the Bennett PR-2 is in operation, the length of the inspiration-expiration cycle can

be observed by watching the pistons located here:

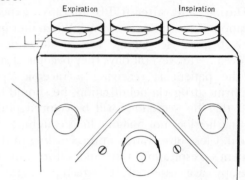

The expiration piston moves downward during exhalation, and the inspiration piston moves downward during inhalation. The middle piston rephases the other two pistons.

During automatic cycling the movement of these three pistons up and down with the breathing cycle indicates that the automatic cycling mechanism is functioning properly.

Terminal Flow

This control regulates the liters per minute of air flow into the lungs and is used to compensate for leaks in the unit. If the unit does not turn "off" at the prescribed pressure reading on inhalation, the terminal flow is turned slightly to the left.

Peak Flow

This allows a slower filling of the lungs and a slower rise in pressure.

Negative Pressure

The use of this control creates a negative pressure during expiration. When this control is used, the nebulization-expiration control must be turned off to conserve medication. This control is used primarily to augment filling of the right heart or for immediate handling of an airway obstruction.

It should also be noted at this point that the Bird Mark 8 model also contains a negative pressure control. In fact, the only difference between the Bird Mark 7 and Mark 8 is that the Mark 7 does not have a negative pressure control setting. On the Bird Mark 8 the negative pressure control is turned on, and the sensitivity indicator is rotated to the negative scale to match the pressure reading on the gauge.

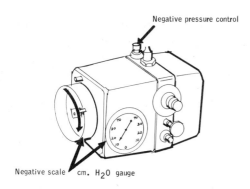

Negative pressure control

Negative scale   cm. H$_2$O gauge

HUMIDIFICATION

On continuous IPPB therapy, adequate humidification of inspired air is a necessity. Because of the small size of the nebulizers shown previously, a larger humidification reservoir is usually added to the respirator as shown:

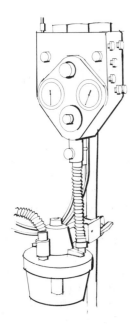

Humidifiers should be filled with water only (preferably distilled water). Some humidifiers, as the one shown, contain a heating element which delivers warm moisture to the patient. Warm moisture is especially recommended for use with a tracheotomy because the body's mechanism for warming and moistening inhaled air is by-passed. When aerosol medications are ordered for administration, they are added to the nebulizer (see p. 59), not the humidifier. The physician may prescribe medication to be administered every three or four hours.

MAINTAINING AN ADEQUATE AIRWAY

The Endotracheal Tube

In assisted ventilation for a short period of time, an adequate airway is maintained by means of an inflatable endotracheal tube inserted either through the nose or mouth. The tube looks like this:

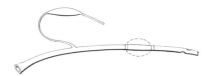

The Tracheotomy Tube

When the IPPB unit must be used continuously for periods longer than a day, a tracheotomy tube is put in place. Several new types of tracheotomy tubes have been designed for use with the IPPB unit. These are made of metal, rubber, and plastic. One popular design metal tracheotomy tube is shown here:

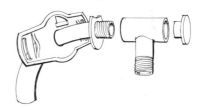

Note the screw top on this inner cannula. A T-connector screws into the inner cannula. The flexible tubing of the respirator attaches to one part of the T-connector, whereas the other opening is plugged and opened for aspiration of secretions. If a specially designed tracheotomy tube is not available, an ordinary tracheotomy tube is used and special adaptors are used to connect to the respirator as shown:

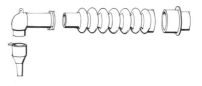

The same type of adaptor is also used to connect the respirator to the inflatable endotracheal tube.

The Tracheotomy Tube Cuff

For use with an IPPB unit, an inflatable rubber cuff is first placed around the outer cannula before insertion to prevent air leakage between the tracheotomy tube and the trachea. Two types of tracheotomy cuffs, the single cuff and double cuff, are shown here:

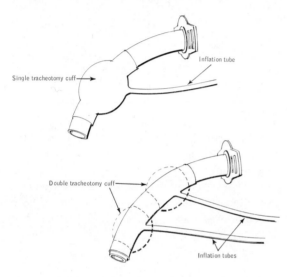

With the double cuff each balloon is inflated alternately to prevent pressure necrosis on the walls of the trachea. The inflation tube to the cuff contains a small balloon which also inflates when the cuff is inflated:

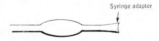

The physician places the cuff over the end of the tracheotomy tube before insertion. If this is done at the bedside, the physician needs in addition to the tracheotomy tray (see p. 353) the following:
1. A long-bladed nasal speculum or Kelly clamp
2. A 10-cc. syringe
3. A metal cup with water to lubricate the cuff and tracheotomy tube

After the tracheotomy tube is in place, the respirator is connected and turned on. The tracheotomy cuff is then inflated with 2 to 10 cc. of air by means of a 10-cc. syringe (as prescribed by a physician). The inflation tube is then clamped with a hemostat, the ends of which are covered with 1-inch strips of rubber tubing. The hemostat is then pinned to the patient's gown, leaving enough slack to prevent its weight from pulling on the cuff and causing pressure on the tracheotomy wound:

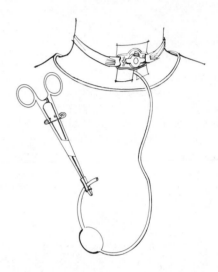

Note the inflation of the small balloon in the inflation tube, indicating that the tracheotomy cuff is inflated (this same procedure for inflation also applies to the inflatable endotracheal tube shown previously).

The amount of air used to inflate the cuff must be recorded on the patient's chart.

The cuff is inflated properly if there is no appreciable leakage of air around the tracheotomy tube and if the respirator cycles properly. With the Bird and the Bennett respirators, a small amount of leakage is permissible as well as advisable because a cuff that is too tight causes tracheal necrosis; also, overdistention of the cuff has a tendency to force it down over the end of the tracheotomy tube, causing airway obstruction. A small leak also allows secretions to be swept past the inflated tracheotomy cuff into the pharynx, thus causing obstruction distal to the cuff. Any difficulty in inflation of the cuff should be reported to the physician.

The physician will write orders for the cuff to be deflated for periods of 5 to 15 minutes every 2 to 4 hours to prevent pressure necrosis of the trachea. While the cuff is inflated, there is a tendency for secretions to accumulate in the trachea above the cuff. Because of this, the pharynx and trachea should be suctioned immediately prior to deflating the cuff. Each time the cuff is reinflated, the amount of air used should be recorded. Any appreciable increase in the amount needed must be reported to the physician, as this may indicate dilatation of the trachea.

Tracheotomy Suctioning Procedure

With tracheotomy tubes that have no separate outlet for suctioning, the patient is "sighed," following which the respirator adapter is removed from the tracheotomy tube, and the suctioning is done briefly as described on page 354. The respirator adapter is then attached, and the patient resumes the usual breathing cycle.

MAINTAINING ADEQUATE VENTILATION

Constant close observation of the patient and the respirator must again be emphasized. The patient's chest should be expanding properly, and he should not be fighting the machine. If the patient is restless, he is not being ventilated properly. Additional symptoms of hypoventilation include cyanosis and rapid pulse. The signs of hyperventilation that one must also look for are head or chest pain, tingling or numbness of the fingers and toes, and dizziness.

It is possible to accidentally brush against the respirator and change the control setting; therefore, the nurse in attendance must also inspect the controls as well as listen to the sounds of the machine. Ordinarily the physician sets up the respirator, and the nurse is not to change the controls unless she is specifically instructed to do so.

X-rays and laboratory studies are taken periodically of PO_2, pCO_2, and pH in order to assess adequate ventilation. A bronchoscopy may be done 3 or 4 days after the insertion of the tracheostomy tube and periodically thereafter, if warranted because of excessive secretion.

Vital capacity may be measured by means of a specially designed respirometer for use with IPPB equipment.

In order to prevent atelectasis, the patient is sighed as prescribed, every half-hour to every few hours. Sighing is a method of providing for two or three extra deep breaths. To do this, the pressure control of the machine is increased for two or three inhalations. The frequency of sighing and the pressure settings during sighing are recorded.

A manually operated ventilator should be kept nearby in the event the respirator fails to operate.

PREVENTION OF INFECTION

The occurrence of infection is a constant threat when the patient is on continuous IPPB therapy. In order to prevent infection, the following precautions are adhered to by the nurse:
1. Absolute sterility in tracheal suctioning is essential (see p. 354).
2. Respirators are cleaned and sterilized between use.
3. Fresh sterile breathing hoses should be used daily for a patient on respirators more than 24 hours.
4. The level of the nebulizer should be slightly lower than the trachea so that particles of moisture do not collect in the tubing. This is a frequent source of infection.
5. Daily cultures of tracheal secretions are done. The nurse obtains the specimen.

NUTRITION

The patient on continual IPPB therapy may be too ill to eat or may find eating too difficult. High caloric intravenous infusions and/or gastrostomy feedings through a small nasal tube are given. If gastrostomy feedings are given, check for abdominal distention, as this interferes with respiration. (See also p. 162.)

PHYSIOTHERAPY

Depending upon the patient's condition, the foot of the bed may be elevated about 12 inches to facilitate drainage of secretions. For this same reason the patient should be turned from side to side every half hour to every hour.

When the conditions permit, the head of the bed should be elevated during gastrostomy feeding.

WEANING FROM THE RESPIRATOR

This is done gradually by taking the patient off the respirator for increasing periods of time. During the trial period off the respirator, oxygen is usually administered by the use of a tracheotomy mask (see p. 357).

When the patient no longer needs the respirator, it is removed from his room, is semi-disassembled and washed, and is then returned to the central supply department for sterilization. Consult the manufacturer's manuals as well as your hospital procedure manual for the disassembly procedure.

USING A TANK RESPIRATOR

Tank respirators are used rather infrequently especially since the advent of the IPPB unit; however, occasions do arise from time to time when every nurse feels the need to review the mechanics of the respirator. For this reason we are including a detailed guide on how to use this type of respirator.

The tank respirator is used for the same reasons that the IPPB unit would be used for controlled respiration.

Several companies manufacture tank respirators; all are similar in design, and all operate on the same principle, the principle being that air pressure within the body tends to be equal to the pressure of air outside the body. In the respirator the pressure of the air surrounding the body is periodically reduced to less than atmospheric pressure. This reduced pressure is called negative pressure. When negative pressure surrounds the body, it causes the chest to expand and pull the air into the lungs as shown in this illustration:

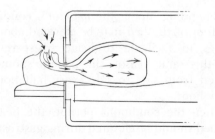

When the pressure surrounding the body is returned to normal, the chest walls contract and force air out of the lungs as shown here:

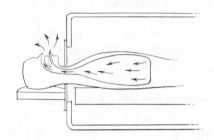

The respirator then is an airtight chamber from which air is alternately removed and replaced. If the nurse keeps in mind that there are two distinct periods of alternating pressure within the respirator chamber (one when the pressure is less than the atmospheric pressure outside the chamber and one when the pressure inside the chamber is the same as that outside the chamber), she will be able to understand the use of the respirator.

The respirator itself is a large apparatus which tends to look complicated. Once the principle of its operation, as just outlined, is understood, the actual use of the respirator is fairly simple. Here is a simplified sketch of a respirator.

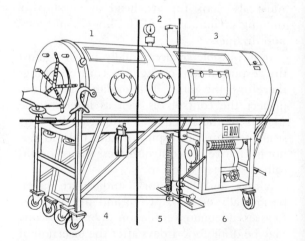

You will notice that the sketch is mapped into six sections. We have done this so that subsequent illustrations of parts of the respirator may be located on the machine. All illustrations in this chapter are adapted from the

Emerson respirator, courtesy of the J. H. Emerson Company, Cambridge, Massachusetts.

PREPARATION OF THE RESPIRATOR FOR USE

A team of four or five persons is needed to place a patient in the respirator. Several persons can prepare the machine for use as follows:

Plug the cord into an outlet, and turn on the motor to test the machine. The motor switch looks like this (see section 6).

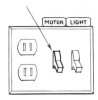

Open the respirator by unlocking the clamp on the front of the machine, and pull the carriage out as far as possible (see sections 1 and 4).

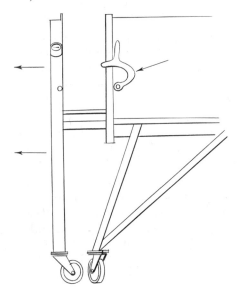

Make up the cot with two sheets as shown here.

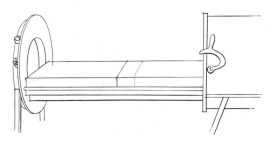

The sheet over the lower half should be placed last and should overlap far enough over the top half sheets so that it will fit under the patient's buttocks. The sheet over the bottom half will be changed most frequently.

PLACING THE PATIENT IN THE RESPIRATOR

Place the patient's stretcher or bed at a right angle to the respirator and lift as shown here:

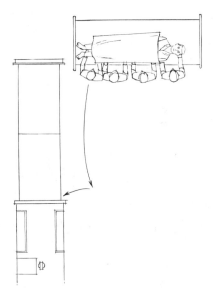

The patient is placed, feet foremost, on the cot.

One person then moves immediately to the head end of the cot and opens the sponge rubber collar by pulling out on each collar strap and snapping it in place like this:

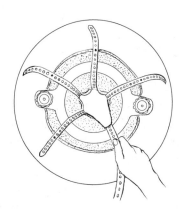

A recent model of respirator may have a plastic collar which opens and closes by turning a ring like this:

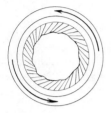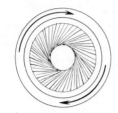

During this time another person places a stockinette cap and neck padding on the patient. The cap is placed on the patient's head to protect the ears and keep long hair in place. The neck padding may be a strip of cotton flannel, a thin piece of sponge rubber inside stockinette, or several layers of cotton wadding. The stockinette and neck padding are not needed when the respirator with a plastic collar is used.

The patient's head is then moved upward through the collar. Four persons lift, and the fifth person supports, guides, and protects the head as it is moved through the collar opening as shown here.

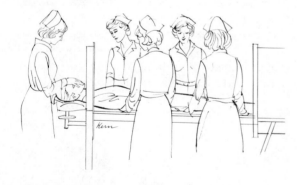

Note how the nurse's hand protects the patient's nose as it passes through the collar.

The person at the head then adjusts the height of the cot and the head rest on the same level so that the patient's neck rests in the center of the collar. The headrest is adjusted by turning the wheel at its base (section 1).

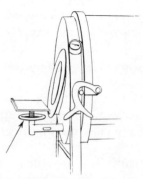

The cot is adjusted by turning both levers at the bottom of the head end in the same direction (section 4, p. 68).

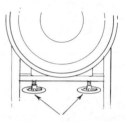

The collar straps are then slowly loosened, and the collar is closed until it just touches the neck.

While the person at the head end is performing, other persons should check to make certain that the cot mattress and the patient's shoulders are both up against the head plate. Cover the patient with a cotton bath blanket, and make certain that the patient's arms do not extend over the edge of the cot; then slide the cot into the respirator and lock the headplate in place.

Turn on the motor, and adjust the respirator rate and the negative pressure. The wheel at the base of the motor is turned clockwise to increase the rate of respiration and turned counterclockwise to decrease the rate (section 6, p. 68).

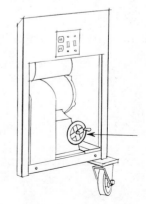

The rate of the respirator is adjusted to synchronize with the patient's breathing. The rate of respirations is usually rapid at first, then becomes slower as the patient becomes accustomed to the machine. A rate of 16 to 30 respirations per minute is usually possible with the adult respirator. To arrive at the prescribed rate, the nurse must time the respirator rate with a watch, then increase or decrease the speed as necessary.

Meanwhile the person standing at the patient's head instructs the patient how to breathe with the machine. For the first few minutes, instruct the patient when to inhale and exhale by saying "inhale" when the collar moves in and "exhale" when the collar moves out. (The pressure changes inside the respirator cylinder cause the flexible collar to maintain this inward-outward motion. The pressure changes may also be observed on the pressure gauge, discussed later.) The patient is also taught (later) to speak and swallow on expiration only.

The negative pressure is adjusted by turning the handwheel at the left of the control panel either clockwise to increase the pressure or counterclockwise to decrease it (section 6, p. 68).

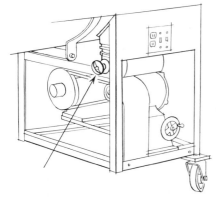

After turning the negative pressure regulator, the pressure gauge on the top of the respirator must be watched to make certain that the correct setting has been made. The needle on the pressure gauge intermittently fluctuates from "0" to the prescribed amount of negative pressure. In most instances the negative pressure is set at 15 (correlated as 15 centimeters underwater). At a setting of 15 then, the pressure gauge needle would fluctuate from "0" to "15" (section 2, p. 68)

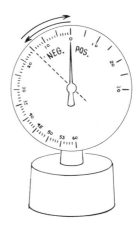

While the needle registers "0," the pressure within the respirator is the same as the atmospheric pressure (the peak of the patient's expiration). While the pressure gauge needle registers "15," reduced or negative pressure exists within the respirator (the peak of the patient's inspiration).

CONTINUATION OF CARE

The patient may remain in the respirator for a period of days, weeks, months, and in rare cases years. In the continuation of the treatment of artificial respiration, the following points should be observed:

1. Aspiration of the nose, mouth, and throat is usually necessary to keep the air passages open. A suction apparatus is attached to the respirator, and is always ready for use when the respirator is in operation. Suction is used only when the patient exhales. The tubing for suction must be attached at the place shown (section 4, p. 68).

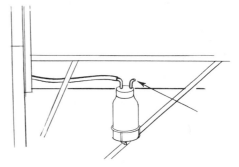

2. The patient is taught to talk and swallow during expiration. Talking or swallowing during inhalation causes insufflation.

3. If the motor of the respirator stops, push down on the emergency lever at the foot of the respirator, grasp the emergency handle with both hands, and pull alternately backward and forward at the same rate the patient had been breathing previously. On recent models there is a foot pedal that is pushed with one foot while pulling with the hands as shown here.

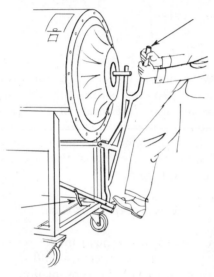

To revert to motor operations, raise the emergency lever to its original position, and move the emergency handle until the catch engages.

4. Frequent changes of position are important to avoid pneumonia, bedsores, and circulatory complications. Light patients can be turned to a side-lying or prone position. To turn extremely heavy patients, it is easier to tilt the entire cot sideways. To tilt the cot sideways, turn the handwheels at the head end of the respirator in opposite directions as shown here.

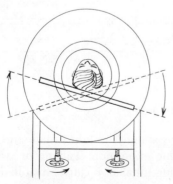

Both wheels should be turned correspondingly so that as one side of the cot is raised, the other is lowered. This will keep the patient's neck centered in the collar.

5. In the event that the patient is to be placed in Trendelenburg position, pump the jack handle located under the respirator (section 6, p. 68).

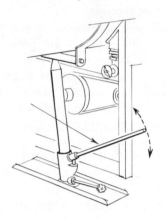

This raises the foot end of the entire respirator. Padding between the patient's shoulders and the head plate is necessary when the foot end of the respirator is raised. To lower the respirator to a horizontal plane, open the hydraulic air valve by gradually turning it counterclockwise. Do not jar the patient by too rapid a descent.

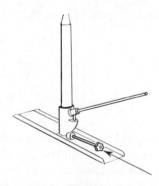

Note: It is impossible to jack up the respirator when this air valve is open.

6. The temperature within the respirator may be raised by the use of electric lights located within the cylinder.

7. Neck care is essential in preventing irritation to the skin. Two persons are needed

to perform neck care; one holds the head and retracts the collar while the other one washes the neck with soap and water. The neck should be dried thoroughly. Powder and ointment should not be used because they cake and cause irritation from the neckband.

8. All nursing care to the part of the body inside the respirator is given through the portholes located on both sides of the respirator. The portholes are opened by turning a latch as shown here:

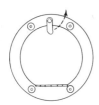

An opened porthole looks like this:

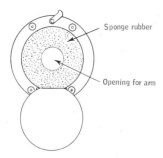

9. Portholes are opened only when the pressure gauge registers zero. When two persons (one on each side) wish to enter the portholes, the person facing the pressure gauge must inform the other person when to enter the respirator. When the pressure gauge registers zero, the portholes are opened and the arms are immediately extended into the porthole opening far enough to seal the ports. The entire process of opening the ports and putting the arms inside the respirator must be done within one or two seconds. Removal of the arms from the respirator is also performed as quickly while the

pressure gauge registers zero. All articles such as linens, basin of water, hypodermic syringes, bedpan, catheterization tray, etc., which are needed in performing treatments are placed inside the respirator through the large porthole shown here (section 3, p. 68):

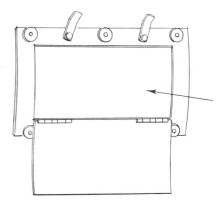

The entire procedure of opening the large porthole, placing the article inside the respirator, and closing the porthole is done while the pressure gauge registers zero. Removal of equipment is done in the same manner.

10. Tubing for the administration of enemas or intravenous fluids is passed through a plugged opening. The plugged opening is located at the top of the headplate. The holder for an I.V. pole is located at the side of the headplate. Both are shown here:

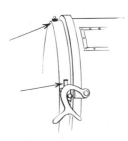

11. Observations of the patient inside the cylinder are made through the four observation windows. There are two windows on each side of the respirator as shown here:

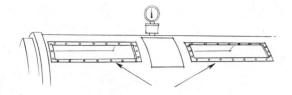

12. Personal hygiene should be the same as for any patient who is critically ill.
13. Emergency equipment such as oxygen, tracheotomy set, tongue depressor, and an airway should be kept close by at all times.
14. Some form of diversion to prevent mental depression is essential for the patient in the respirator. A mirror placed above the patient's head enables him to watch activities through the doorway. A bookrack similarly placed will hold a book, the pages of which may be turned by the nurse. This diagram shows the location of the holders for the bookrack and head mirror.

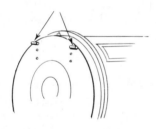

15. Charting is especially important for the patient in the respirator. Observance of the respiratory rate, the temporal pulse, mental attitudes, ability to swallow, presence of mucus, amount of sleep, and any deviations from normal are to be recorded.

VARIATIONS WITH THE USE OF THE CYLINDER RESPIRATOR

Positive Pressure

In some cases positive pressure is used in addition to negative pressure within the respirator cylinder. Positive pressure or increased pressure within the respirator aids chest movements of expiration. Conditions in which there is circulatory depression usually indicate the use of the combination of negative and positive pressure. The physician prescribes the amount of positive pressure desired.

To obtain positive pressure, the positive pressure valve shown here (section 3, p. 68)

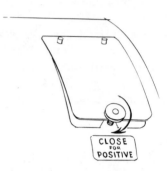

is gradually turned shut until the desired amount of positive pressure is reached. Refer also to the pressure gauge shown on page 71.

The Dome

There is a plastic dome available that fits over the head end of the respirator. The plastic dome is used to give artificial respiration to the patient while the cylinder of the respirator is open. The air pressure inside the dome increases, causing inhalation. During inhalation, then, the pressure within the dome is greater than atmospheric pressure. During exhalation the pressure within the dome is the same as atmospheric pressure. The increased pressure within the dome is called positive pressure. The dome functions on the same principle as the cylinder—i.e., to create inhalation, the pressure of the air around the mouth and nose must be greater than the pressure of the air around the chest.

All nursing procedures can be carried out more easily and safely with the use of the dome. The dome is generally used after the first few days of artificial respiration.

To Use the Dome

1. The patient should be told that although respirations with the dome will feel somewhat different from respirations produced by the cylinder, the rate and depth of respirations will be the same. The patient can hear and be heard through the dome.
2. Unclamp the head end of the respirator, and pull the bed out; then clamp the dome over the patient's head as shown here:

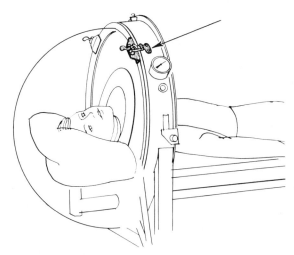

3. Adjust the pressure within the dome by means of a valve on the inside of the head plate (dotted line) while watching the dome pressure gauge indicated by arrow here:

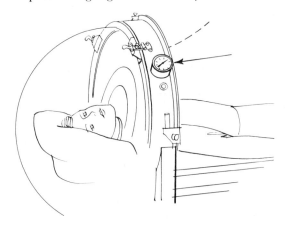

The positive pressure setting should be the same as the negative pressure setting within the cylinder. It is best to set the pressure gradually so that the patient can first have a few breaths at a minimum pressure.

4. When discontinuing the use of the dome, first unclamp the dome, then close the respirator.

DISCONTINUING THE USE OF THE RESPIRATOR

When the respirator is to be discontinued, the portholes are usually left open for short periods of time to determine whether the patient can breathe on his own. If the patient cannot tolerate this, the respirator is usually left open briefly, once or twice daily. Until the nurse is certain how the patient will tolerate the periods during which the respirator is left open, the motor should remain on while the respirator is open. The portable respirator and the oscillating bed (see Chap. 13) may also be used to help wean the patient from the respirator.

ADDITIONAL PROCEDURES TO REVIEW

Tracheostomy care (p. 353)
Aseptic technique (p. 354)
Gastrostomy feeding (p. 162)
Gastric suction (p. 158)
Administration of oxygen (p. 30)
Intravenous infusion (p. 83)
Artificial respiration (p. 217)
Pulmonary function tests (p. 210)
Bronchoscopy (p. 211)
Examination of sputum (p. 212)
Therapeutic and rehabilitative procedures in diseases of the nervous system (Chapter 17)
Breathing exercises (p. 227)

BIBLIOGRAPHY

Cherniak, R. M.: Tracheostomy and Its Management. Can. Anesth. Soc. J., 12:386, 1965.
De Meyer, J.: Emphysema: Effective Positive-pressure Breathing Therapy. R N, 31:46, 1968.
Manual of Intermittent Positive Pressure Breathing Therapy. Hospital of the Good Samaritan Medical Center. 1st ed. May, 1965.
McArdle, K. H.: The Patient and the Bennett. Nurs. Clin. North America, 1(1):143, 1966.
McCallum, H. P.: The Nurse and the Respirator. Nurs. Clin. North America, 1(4):597, 1966.
Nett, I. M., and Petty, T. L.: Acute Respiratory Failure. Am. J. Nurs., 67:1847, 1967.
Shulman, M., M.D.: Use of Respirators in the Surgical Patient. Surg. Clin. North America, 48:37, 1968.
Sovie, M. D., and Israel, J. S.: Use of the Cuffed Tracheostomy Tube. Am. J. Nurs., 67:1854, 1967.
Staub, E. W., and Beattie, E. J.: Respiratory Support in the Postoperative Period. Surg. Clin. North America, 44:227, 1964.

6

Injection, Infusion, and Transfusion

INTRAMUSCULAR INJECTIONS

Some may question the inclusion of a discussion on intramuscular injections. Not too many years ago this procedure was done only by the physician because of the risk of striking a blood vessel and a nerve. The nurse is now the one who gives most of these injections; therefore, it is essential that she understand the subject thoroughly in order to reduce the many risks involved.

Drugs are administered intramuscularly in quantities of 2-10 cc. A 2-, 5-, or 10-cc. syringe may be used, depending on the amount of solution being administered. The nurse should check the policies of her hospital regarding the amount. Some hospitals permit nurses to give amounts no larger than 5 cc. The size of needle may range from No. 19 to 22 gauge. Select a heavy needle for thick solutions and a thin needle for thin liquids. Use a short needle (1 to 1½ inches) when the patient is thin and a long needle when the patient is obese.

The intramuscular route is used in preference to the subcutaneous route because (1) some substances are irritating to the subcutaneous tissues; (2) there is more rapid absorption in muscular tissue; and (3) the muscle can more readily absorb larger quantities of certain fluids.

The common sites for the intramuscular injection are the buttocks, the thigh, and the upper arm.

The Buttocks. The buttocks are preferred because the gluteal muscles are thick and because these muscles are utilized frequently in daily activities, thus causing complete absorption of drugs. Two injection sites may be used in the buttocks: the dorsogluteal and the ventrolateral gluteal.

Using the dorsogluteal site, the injection is placed in the gluteus maximus muscle. In using the ventrolateral gluteal site, the gluteus medius and minimus muscles are involved as shown:

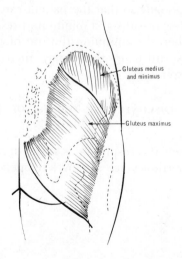

Gluteus medius and minimus

Gluteus maximus

In the dorsogluteal site the area in which there is the least possibility of hitting a bone, large blood vessel and nerve is the middle or outer aspect of the upper outer quadrant as indicated in the following diagram. Note also the related bones, large blood vessels and sciatic nerve.

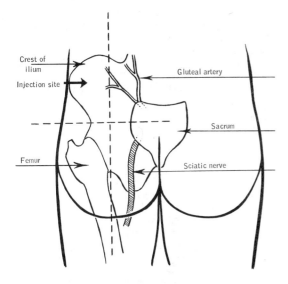

It is now recommended that the inner angle of the upper outer quadrant should not be used because in some individuals the sciatic nerve may lie in this area. Also, if the inner angle is used, there is particular danger to the sciatic nerve if the needle is slanted downward and inward.

In order to relax the buttocks, ask the patient to lie in the prone position with the head turned sideways (preferably away from you so that he cannot witness the injection), the arms resting at the side, and the toes turned inward like this:

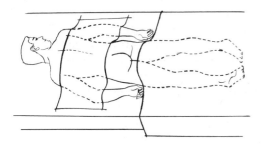

Note that the buttocks are the only part of the body exposed. The patient should not lie on

his side while receiving an intramuscular injection in the dorsogluteal area because the side-lying position distorts the shape of the buttocks, thus resulting in the injection being given lower than it should be.

To locate the ventrolateral gluteal site on the right hip, place the palm of the left hand on the greater trochanter of the patient's right femur. Place the index finger on the antero-superior iliac spine and the middle finger toward the crest of the ilium as shown:

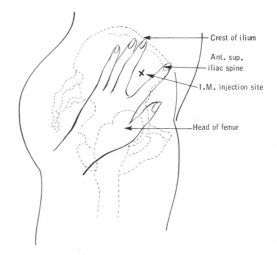

To locate the ventrolateral gluteal site on the left hip, place the middle finger on the anterior crest of the ilium, then spread the index finger to form a V, as shown:

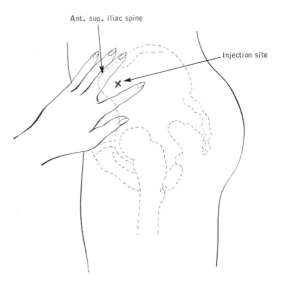

After cleansing the area with a disinfectant,

the cotton ball containing the disinfectant is held in the left hand (providing the operator is right-handed) like this:

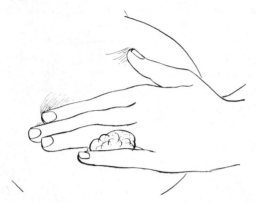

When inserting the needle at this site, direct it toward the iliac crest. In this area the needle may be inserted to a depth of 3 inches with no danger to important structures. This is due to the fact that the muscles involved lie one beneath the other in the hollow of the iliac ala. If a nerve is accidentally injured, it would be a branch of the superior gluteal nerve rather than a main trunk.

To give the injection in the ventrolateral gluteal site, the patient should be placed on his side and facing you.

The Thigh. Intramuscular injections are given in the vastus lateralis muscle located on the lateral thigh. The vastus lateralis is about 3 inches in width and extends the entire length of the thigh as shown:

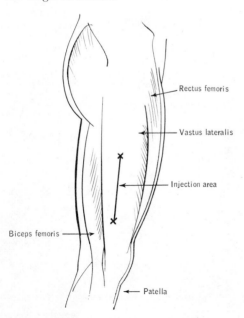

Intramuscular injections may be given in any part of this muscle from about a hand's width above the knee to a hand's width below the hip joint. Do not inject into the areas close to the knee and hip joint.

There are no main blood vessels or nerve trunks in the lateral thigh injection site. The branches of the lateral femoral cutaneous nerve, however, are superficially located, and a few cases of damage to these branches have been reported.

The Arm. Intramuscular injections can be given in the deltoid muscle located on the lateral side of the humerus. The injection site in the deltoid is located about three fingers' width below the acromion process as shown:

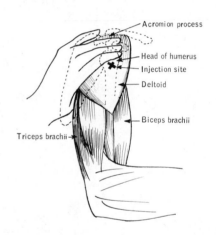

Intramuscular injections should never be made in an area lower or more posterior than the one shown because there is great danger of injury to the radial nerve. To give the injection, the patient's gown must be removed from the shoulder.

If the patient is receiving a number of intramuscular injections over a prolonged period of time, the site of injection should be rotated. A record of injection sites must be kept on the chart for this purpose. The arm and leg are used for intramuscular injections only when the amount given is small (under 2 cc.) or if the buttocks are irritated, inflamed, or injured. If amounts larger than 2 cc. must be given in the arm or thigh, the medication must be given in a divided dose.

Giving the Injection

When giving an intramuscular injection, an aseptic technique is used. That is, the syringe, needle, and fluid being injected must remain sterile. The skin must be cleansed with a disinfectant. The skin is stretched and held taut with the thumb and middle finger of the left hand. (When giving an injection in the arm, it may be necessary to pinch the skin if the patient's arm is small.)

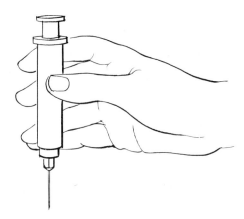

In the right hand, hold the syringe like this at a right angle to the skin and insert the needle by exerting a quick, firm, bold pressure. When the needle is inserted the entire depth, hold the syringe with the left hand and pull gently upward on the piston with the right hand as shown:

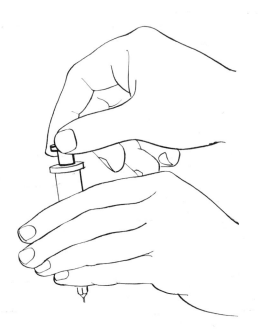

If blood is drawn up into the syringe, withdraw the needle immediately, and reinsert it about ½ inch from the original site. (A new needle must be used when this occurs. Some authorities also advocate using a new syringe and fresh medication. Check your hospital's policies.) If blood is not aspirated, inject the solution slowly. While removing the needle with the right hand, support the surrounding skin by lightly pressing on the area with the disinfectant cotton ball in the left hand as shown:

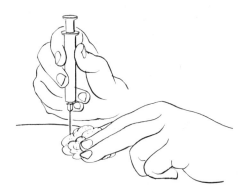

After removing the needle, gently massage the area to aid absorption, unless contraindicated by the nature and action of the drug being used.

Variations in Technique

Slight variations in the technique of intramuscular injection may be encountered in some hospitals. These may be as follows:

Use of Air Bubble in Syringe. A small bubble of air is drawn into the syringe. When the syringe and needle are inverted during the injection, the bubble rises as shown:

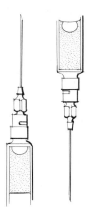

When administering the medication, the air clears the needle of medication, thus reducing the dripping of medication through the subcutaneous tissues upon withdrawal of the needle.

Zigzag Line of Injection. With this method the needle is inserted on a zigzag line rather than on a straight line. That is, the needle is first injected through the subcutaneous tissue. The insertion is then stopped, and the needle is removed slightly to the side, then inserted the remainder of the way; the nurse continues, of course, to hold the syringe at a right angle to the patient. This method is used because it prevents leakage of medication from the muscle area into the subcutaneous tissue and then onto the skin.

FLUIDS AND ELECTROLYTES

Since the techniques of intravenous injection, hypodermoclysis, and transfusion will be dealt with later in this chapter, it seems appropriate at this point to offer a brief discussion on fluids and electrolytes. Actually, this subject could in itself include several volumes. An attempt will be made here to concisely review the basic principles of fluid balance within the body and to show the relationship to therapy.

Electrolytes

An electrolyte is a compound whose solution will conduct an electrical current. Pure water does not conduct electricity, but put a pinch of salt into it and it will. This is because salt is composed of sodium and chloride held together by electrostatic forces. Placed into water, the sodium and chloride crystals break apart into positively charged ions (cations) and negatively charged ions (anions) and thus can conduct electricity.

Sodium chloride is an electrolyte. This and other inorganic salts commonly used in therapy are shown here broken into cations (positive) and anions (negative):

Cations		Anions	
Na^+	Sodium	SO_4^{--}	Sulfate
K^+	Potassium	Cl^-	Chloride
Ca^{++}	Calcium	HCO_3^-	Bicarbonate
Mg^{++}	Magnesium	HPO_4^{--}	Phosphate
		Proteins, lactate and citrate	

Substances such as glucose and urea are not electrolytes because they have no electrical charge.

The quantities of cations and anions in a solution always equal each other. Quantities of these ions are expressed in milliequivalents (mEq.). A milliequivalent measures the POWER of an ion, not its weight. Thus one mEq. of one ion would equal the power of one mEq. of any other ion.

The proper distribution of the inorganic salts or electrolytes within the body is called electrolyte balance.

Acid-base Balance

At this point one may wonder what is meant by acid-base balance. Years ago it was thought that all anions were acids and all cations were bases. In view of our present scientific knowledge, this can no longer be correct. A substance is either acid or base, depending upon whether it gives or receives hydrogen ion (H). Sodium, for example, when added to water could be neither acid nor base because sodium does not receive or give hydrogen. Chloride, on the other hand, when combined with water accepts the hydrogen ion, thus becoming a base or alkaline. The important feature of acid-base balance is the concentration of H^+ in the solution. It is this concentration which determines the degree of acidity of a solution. This is measured as pH. Electrolytes are thus important also in maintaining the body's acid-base balance.

Body Fluids

Approximately 60 per cent of body weight is composed of fluids. Fluids within the body are located either within the cells (intracellular) or outside the cells (extracellular). The extracellular portion includes the intravascular fluid (plasma) and the interstitial fluid (that which bathes the tissue cells). Two thirds of the body fluid is intracellular fluid; one third is extracellular. There is a difference in electrolyte composition of the intracellular and extracellular fluid. The principal cation in the extracellular fluid is sodium. The principal cation in the intracellular fluid is potassium. An electrolyte balance between the plasma and the fluid within and surrounding the cells is maintained by (1) diffusion of water between all three, (2) diffusion of electrolytes between the plasma and the fluid surrounding tissue cells, and (3) the transport of sodium and potassium into and out of the cells.

Normal Fluid and Electrolyte Requirements

The amount of water and electrolyte within the body is regulated by the kidneys, skin, and lungs. From a normal daily intake of 2500 cc. of fluid, about 1000 cc. is lost in breath and perspiration and about 1400 in urine. During the same time, about 500 cc. of water is produced in the body by the process of oxidation of food within the cells.

As far as electrolyte requirements are concerned, none are lost via the lungs, and the loss via normal perspiration is very low. Normal kidney function eliminates small amounts of electrolytes; therefore, the required intake of electrolytes is normally negligible.

It can then be concluded that anything which causes an upset in fluid and electrolyte intake and output could also result in an electrolyte imbalance. Some factors that upset the electrolyte balance are as follows:

1. Absence of food by mouth (reduces amount of water derived from food metabolism)
2. Excess loss of extracellular fluid (hemorrhage and surgery)
3. Increase in output of hormones which cause increased retention of sodium and water in renal tubule (extreme body stresses, i.e., surgery, renal malfunction)
4. Dehydration resulting from lack of intake of fluids or extreme loss of fluids (vomiting, diarrhea, oliguria, extreme perspiration, or hyperventilation)
5. Overhydration caused by body containing too much fluid, as in heart failure (increased peripheral vascular pressure) and kidney failure
6. Retention of losses of electrolytes out of proportion with retention or losses of water (for example, when I.V. solutions containing no sodium or chloride are administered to a patient with impaired ability to excrete water)

Parenteral Fluids

Parenteral fluids generally are classified as isotonic (same sodium content as blood), hypotonic (water in excess of salt), and hypertonic (salt in excess of water). Here is a list of the common fluids administered:

Sodium Chloride (0.9 Per Cent; Normal Saline or Physiological Saline Solution [p.s.s.]). It is an isotonic solution that restores extracellular fluid volume and dilutes the cells and other constituents of the blood. It has no effect on the sodium concentration and diffusion of fluid and electrolytes between the cells and the blood.

It does, however, supply chloride in excess of sodium, causing retention of H ions (see p. 80) and thus having a tendency to cause acidosis. Where indicated, it may be given at the rate of 500 cc. to 2000 cc. per hour.

Saline Solution (0.45 Per Cent, 1/2 Strength p.s.s.). It is a hypotonic solution making water immediately available for excretory needs and supplying the necessary amount of sodium. It is useful for daily maintenance but of less value for replacing deficits.

Sodium Chloride (2 Per Cent to 5 Per Cent). It is a hypertonic saline solution valuable for treatment of hyponatremia (reduction in serum sodium to less than 130 mEq./L.). Rates of administration should not be more than 200 cc. per hour. No more than 400 cc. of the 5 per cent solution should be given at any one time.

Sodium Lactate (1/6 M [Molar]). It is an isotonic solution that supplies sodium but not chloride. The lactate has some caloric value and in the process of metabolism may increase the salt bicarbonate to produce an alkalosis. This solution may be used in the treatment of some forms of acidosis.

Sodium Bicarbonate (5 Per Cent). This fluid has the same final effects as sodium lactate. It is given in intravenous doses of 50 cc. or may be added to other intravenous solutions. It may be given by hypodermoclysis if diluted to a 1.5 per cent solution.

Hartmann's Lactated Ringer's Solution. This fluid most nearly resembles the electrolyte structure of normal blood serum. It contains a small amount of potassium, calcium chloride, and bicarbonate, none in amounts large enough to replace deficits or cause changes in reaction of the blood.

Darrow's "K" Lactate Solution. This solution contains sodium and chloride in the normal serum ratio and enough potassium to replace the usual daily loss. The amount of sodium, however, is greater than that required for postoperative use. The solution has been used primarily for diarrhea and diabetic acidosis. It may be given subcutaneously as well as intravenously if the proper precautions for administering potassium solution are used.

Potassium Chloride. Ampuls of 20 mEq. and of 40 mEq. may be added to 5 per cent glucose solutions or other electrolyte solutions for replacement of potassium deficits. No more than 40 mEq. should be given in one liter of solution, and it should be administered at a rate no more rapid than 90 drops per minute. For utilization of administered potassium, adequate amounts of glucose must also be given.

Glucose in Water (5 Per Cent). This is an isotonic solution when administered; however, the metabolism of glucose leaves only water. Thus it may cause some sodium loss in the urine. When given via hypodermoclysis, sodium chloride will diffuse into it from the surrounding tissues and blood, thus aggravating any existing salt depletion. It is apt to cause a rise in spinal fluid pressure in patients with brain injuries.

THAM, TRIS, or Trihydroxymethylaminomethane. This is an organic amine buffer. It is used to buffer or remove the H ion extracellularly and intracellularly. It is also used for acute acidosis. It is administered in doses of 0.33 m. in 0.2 per cent sodium chloride solution at the rate of 300 ml. per hour.

Dextran. This is a carbohydrate with physical properties similar to plasma. It is given in quantities of 500 cc. of 6 per cent solution either with or without normal saline. It causes an increase in blood volume and is especially valuable for the treatment of shock of neurogenic or traumatic origin. It does not replace blood in hemorrhage. The 12 per cent solution is also used for treatment of nephrotic edema because it results in water diuresis.

Mannitol. This is given for its effect as a diuretic, generally administered in quantities of 100 gm. diluted in 500 cc. of solution, administered over a period of 90 minutes. For oliguric or aneuric patients, a test dose of 12.5 gm. is given during a period of 3 minutes. If diuresis is obtained, then it is infused at a rate that maintains urinary flow at 60 to 120 cc. per hour. Mannitol is also used to prevent functional renal failure in aortic resections and in the therapy of acute fluid retention.

Other Solutions. Many additional solutions containing various combinations of electrolytes are available, each having its own field of usefulness. Solutions containing glucose, invert sugar, and amino acids and combined with electrolytes are used for caloric value and protein building. Other solutions are used for gastric, duodenal, and intestinal losses.

The Nurse's Responsibility in Fluid and Electrolytes

Close observation of the patient and proper reporting and recording are of the utmost importance in all postoperative patients and in any other condition which may result in electrolyte imbalance. Especially important are the following:

1. Accurate measurement and recording of fluid intake and output. Not only is it important to record the amount of intake and output, but it is also of extreme importance to record the various channels. For example, in treating the postoperative patient, the surgeon generally treats renal fluid loss and extrarenal fluid loss separately. As a rule, extrarenal fluid and electrolyte losses (through gastric suction, T-tube, intestinal fistula drainages, or diarrhea) must be replaced *as soon as they occur.* Nursing notes should also include comment on nonmeasured fluid losses such as perspiration, hyperventilation, and drainage.

2. Make certain all laboratory tests are done and report abnormal findings to doctor.

3. Make certain that when I.V. fluids are ordered to be given at a certain rate or certain amount over a specific period of time, they are given as such.

INTRAVENOUS THERAPY

Because of the risks involved in administering substances into the veins, an intravenous injection is usually performed by the physician or a specially trained technician. In various hospital situations, however, the staff of physicians and medical technicians is too small to accommodate the increased demands of medical care; consequently, the responsibilities of the procedure are delegated to the nursing staff. Whether or not this should be accepted as a nursing performance is at present a controversial subject among the medical profession, and the pros and cons of the subject will not be dealt with here. Some hospitals have delegated the nursing responsibility of intravenous injection to a specific group of professional nurses. This group is usually called the "I.V. Team," being responsible for all intravenous therapy within the hospital. The intravenous team usually functions under the guidance and supervision of a physician, who in turn is responsible for its activities. In other institutions the bedside nurse is responsible for the intravenous therapy of her patient. Our own opinion is that the majority of bedside nurses who are required to perform this treatment, too often and sometimes too eagerly carry out this procedure, entirely new to them, with little or no knowledge concerning the principles, techniques, or complications involved, thus placing the patient in jeopardy.

Before giving an intravenous injection, the nurse would be doing herself a great favor if she would:

1. Familiarize herself with the state laws regarding the registered nurse's role in intravenous therapy. Some states have specific laws stating whether or not the nurse is permitted to perform venipuncture. In some states the nurse is also restricted in the types of medication she may administer intravenously.
2. To avoid injury, review the anatomy of blood vessels and learn the related position of nerves, bones, and glands.
3. Familiarize herself with the common hypotonic, isotonic, and hypertonic solutions and understand the effects of introducing each into the blood stream.
4. Understand the nature, action, and dosages of substances to be injected.
5. Know the unfavorable reactions to intravenous injections.

Solutions are given intravenously in small or large amounts. When a small amount of solution is administered, the term "intravenous injection" is used. "Intravenous infusion" or "venoclysis" designates the giving of a large amount of fluid. The term "transfusion" designates the administration of blood and its component parts.

Fluids are administered intravenously (1) when a very rapid effect is needed, (2) when the drug is irritating or ineffective given any other way, (3) in treating the blood vessels and blood, (4) in severe disturbance of fluid and electrolyte balance, and (5) when the patient is unable to take and/or retain oral nourishment.

THE INTRAVENOUS INFUSION

The Equipment

There are numerous varieties in the design of intravenous infusion equipment. Infusion sets are either permanent or disposable. A permanent venoclysis set is assembled and sterilized in the sterile supply center of the hospital and returned there for re-use. The disposable unit, commercially prepared by several companies, may be purchased by the hospital, sterile and ready for use, and is to be discarded after use. Disposable units come either with or without needles attached. Check to see which your hospital is using.

When ordering the venoclysis unit from central supply, a separate request must be made for each bottle of solution and for the intravenous set (tubing to be attached to bottle).

The basic venoclysis unit, disposable or permanent, consists of the following:

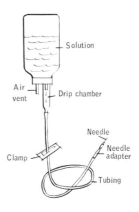

Depending upon the amount of solution to be given or the method and purpose of administering the fluid, the basic venoclysis set may not be desirable. Additional types of sets usually available include these:

"Y"-type Sets. This type of set is used for administereing two solutions alternately or simultaneously:

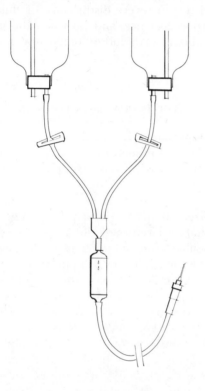

Secondary Set. When a second bottle is added to one which has already been started, or when a series of solutions is to be given in succession, this setup is used:

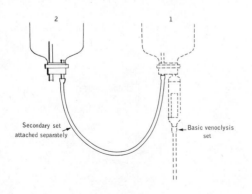

Microdrip Set. This type of set is used when medications that require slow and accurate measurement are administered in intravenous solutions. The microdrip set looks the same as the basic I.V. set, the difference being that in the microdrip set the drip chamber is constructed to deliver 1/50 to 1/60 cc. per drop. (In ordinary sets the drip chamber delivers 1/10 cc. per drop.) In most institutions the physician will specify in his written order that microdrip is to be used.

The Solution. Solution is prepared in bottles in amounts of 500 and 1000 cc. The type and amount of solution is prescribed by the physician. The commonly used solutions were discussed previously in this chapter.

The Needle. Needles vary in size from No. 20 to No. 18 and may be 1½ to 2 inches long. A needle with a medium bevel should be used to prevent injury to the vein. A suitable bevel would be this one:

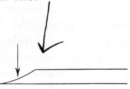

This bevel is not suitable:

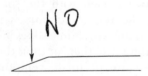

Solutions flow more slowly through a needle with a small opening. Needles with small openings also tend to become clogged with blood clots. If blood is to be given later through the same needle, a needle with a large opening must be used to start the infusion.

Always use a sharp needle and don't wait until inserting the needle into the skin to find out whether or not it is sharp. Pull the needle through a piece of sterile gauze or cotton. If the needle has a hook it will snag the material.

Additional Equipment. In addition to the venoclysis set this equipment is needed:

    Alcohol sponges

Tourniquet
Adhesive tape and sterile gauze
I.V. pole

STARTING THE INFUSION

In preparation for the intravenous infusion, the equipment should be assembled and placed on a cart. When giving several infusions, the equipment for each may be assembled on the same cart. If the physician has ordered a medication to be added to the solution, the medication is prepared and injected into the top of the bottle with a syringe and needle by aseptic technique. The bottle of solution must be labeled with the name and dosage of the drug added. The temperature of the solution at the time of administration is usually room temperature. Solutions colder than room temperature are not considered harmful to the body. If fact, the physician may prescribe a cool infusion for the febrile patient.

Before preparing the patient for the venipuncture, the basic venoclysis unit is properly assembled. Complete instructions for the assembly of commercially prepared units are printed on the outside of each sterile package. The bottle of solution should be inverted and hung on a pole about 3 feet above the bed. Coil the tubing in the hand and squeeze several times to partially fill the drip chamber. Close the clamp on the tubing, and prepare the site for the venipuncture.

VENIPUNCTURE

The site selected for injection depends on several factors. The basilic and cephalic veins located at the inner aspect of the elbow are used for small injections which are not prolonged, because inserting the needle at the bend of the elbow necessitates the use of a splint, and a lengthy immobilization is uncomfortable. For beginners these veins are usually the easiest to locate and manipulate when inserting the needle.

The accessory cephalic or the median antebrachial in the lower forearm are preferred when a prolonged continuous drip is used, because these areas allow more motion of the part:

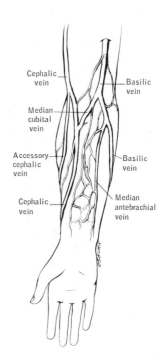

The dorsal metacarpal veins on the back of the hand also provide sites of entry. These are shown here:

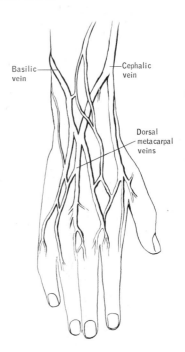

In the legs are the saphenous and femoral veins in the thigh and the saphenous at the ankle. Leg veins should be used only by special written permission of the physician because of the possibility of phlebitis.

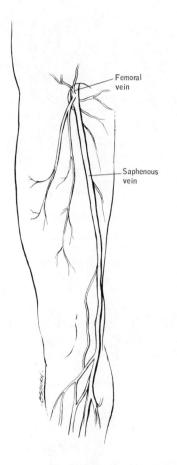

The foot presents the venous plexus of the dorsum, the medial marginal vein, and the lateral marginal vein.

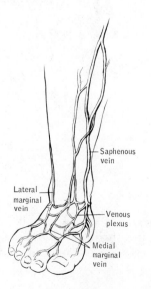

Fluids can be administered more rapidly in larger veins than in smaller veins. When repeated injections are necessary, the site should be rotated because the frequent use of the same vein causes the walls to sclerose, and it is almost impossible to locate a vein that has lost its elasticity. Occasionally one will encounter a patient whose veins are all difficult to locate. In this event the nurse should seek the aid of the physician rather than cause the patient too much discomfort by numerous unsuccessful attempts to enter the vein.

After selecting the vein to be used for the injection, utmost care must be given to the proper distention of the vein. If the veins are prominent, pressure applied by a tourniquet above the site of injection will be sufficient to fill them. A blood pressure cuff may be used in place of a tourniquet. A soft rubber tubing is most commonly used as a tourniquet. The rubber tubing is placed around the limb about 2 inches above the site of the injection. Stretch the tubing slightly, and hold it in place with a hemostat like this:

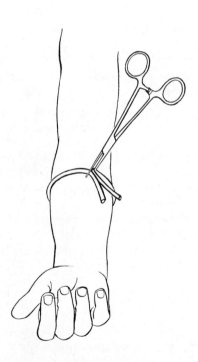

The tourniquet may also be held in place like this: Hold one end longer than the other, forming a loop with the longer end as shown:

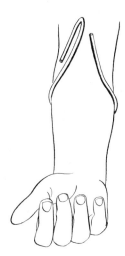

Then pass the looped end under the other end like this:

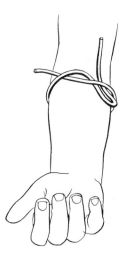

The pressure from the elasticity of the stretched rubber tubing will hold the tourniquet in place. The tourniquet may be loosened with one hand by pulling the looped end.

If a vein at the inner aspect of the elbow is used, tighten the tourniquet until pulsation of the wrist ceases, then slightly release the pressure until the pulse barely reappears. If this is done, the vein will be sufficiently distended, and arterial flow will be maintained. At the same time instruct the patient to open

and close his hand, finally leaving it closed like this:

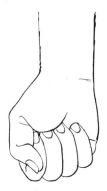

until the needle is inserted.

If the distended vein is too difficult to locate, the following suggestions may help in this sequence:

1. Avoid the use of varicosed veins at or above the point of injection.
2. Allow the selected extremity to hang over the side of the bed for a short time.
3. Apply moist heat to the area for 15 to 20 minutes by wrapping the entire extremity in a warm, moist towel enclosed by a waterproof covering and a turkish towel. Hot water bottles placed around the covering will maintain the heat. If available, a thermostatically controlled electric blanket may be applied directly to the skin for 15 to 20 minutes.

Any or all of these items should be considered before the nurse concludes that it is impossible to locate a vein. If a site near a joint is selected for the venipuncture, a restraint secured comfortably with wide gauze bandage may be necessary to prevent the patient from jerking the part during the insertion of the needle. The restraint should not be secured too tightly, as this will interfere with circulation. For the site at the inner aspect of the elbow, the restraint must extend from the tips of the fingers to above the elbow like this:

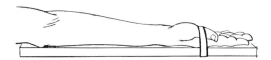

For immobilization of the wrist in using the veins in the back of the hand, the restraint should extend from the point of finger flexion to above the wrist.

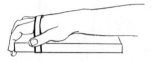

If the fingers are not allowed to remain in the flexed position during the infusion, extreme discomfort will result. A small gauze dressing folded and placed under the palm of the hand allows for the normal cupping of the relaxed hand.

Right angular restraints may be needed to restrain the ankle:

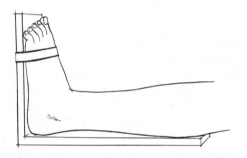

All of these types of restraints are usually kept on hand, padded and ready for use.

After properly positioning the part and distending the vein, cleanse the skin site with an antiseptic solution. It is well to remember that a cold wet sponge may constrict the distended vein.

Before injecting the needle, the air should be removed from the apparatus by allowing a small amount of solution to flow through the needle into a waste receptacle. Secure the regulating clamp tightly, as there should be no seepage of fluid through the needle during the injection. The actual injection of the needle requires two different steps: piercing the skin, and piercing the vein. The entire operation is done as follows:

1. Stretch the skin with the thumb and first finger of the left hand (providing the nurse is right-handed).
2. Hold the needle at a 45° angle, pierce the skin slightly to one side of the vein and about ½ inch below the intended site for

injecting the vein as shown:

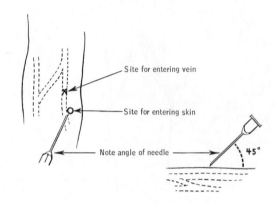

Note the angle of the needle in relationship to the intended site of injection.

3. After piercing the skin, lower the angle of the needle so that it is almost parallel to the skin:

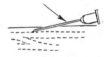

Move the tip of the needle above the vein, and slowly inject the needle into the vein:

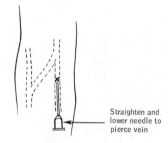

When inserting the needle into a vein considerably larger than the diameter of the needle (as is the usual case), the bevel of the needle should be facing upward, like this:

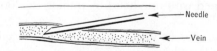

When inserting the needle into a vein that is the approximate size of the diameter of the needle, the bevel should be turned downward. This will prevent collapse of the vein and blockage of the lumen of the needle, which are shown here:

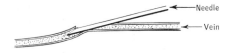

and perforation of the posterior walls of the vein, as shown here:

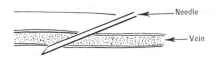

When blood appears, slowly advance the needle by exerting a slight pressure to lift the vein upward with the needle, thus preventing a puncture of the posterior wall. Release the tourniquet, and allow the fluid to flow into the vein. The physician prescribes the rate of flow for the solution. As a rule, the flow should be 60 to 75 drops per minute. The flow may vary with the kind and concentration of solution being administered and the condition of the patient (rapid when the patient is in shock, very slow in cardiac conditions).

Place a small piece of folded sterile gauze under the hub of the needle to protect the skin from irritation, and anchor the needle in place with adhesive tape. Loop the tubing, and tape it to the part to prevent pull on the needle during the patient's movements:

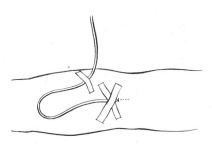

While the infusion is being administered, the patient should be checked frequently to assure comfort, to safeguard the proper rate of flow of the solution, and to prevent infiltration. If the solution is infiltrating (not flowing into the vein but into the surrounding tissues), a swelling will occur. In this event, discontinue the infusion immediately to prevent damage to the tissues. Select a new site for the infusion.

After the patient has received the prescribed amount of fluids, stop the flow, and gently remove the adhesive tape. With one hand hold a small piece of cotton containing disinfectant over the site of injection, and with the other hand slowly remove the needle, keeping the hub flush with the skin to prevent damage to the posterior wall of the vein. Place a small sterile dressing over the injection site. The patient may begin to move the part whenever he wishes.

Variations in Technique

Use of a Separate Syringe in Making the Venipuncture. In this method the venipuncture is made with the needle attached to a 2- or 5-cc. syringe containing sterile normal saline solution. After the needle has been properly injected into the vein, the tourniquet is released, and the syringeful of saline is injected into the vein. The syringe is then removed from the needle, and the infusion tubing (free from air) is attached to the needle.

Use of the Connected Syringe with a Side Arm. In this method the infusion tubing (cleared of air) is connected to a syringe with a side arm after the venipuncture has been made, like this:

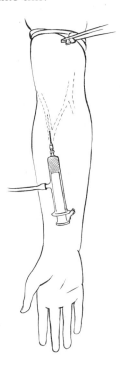

The plunger is then withdrawn past the opening of the side arm like this:

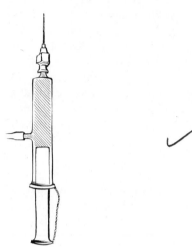

and the tourniquet is released, thus starting the flow of the infusion fluid.

Use of Polyethylene Tubing. Polyethylene tubing is commonly injected into the vein in administering intravenous fluids over prolonged periods of time. A needle is first injected into the vein and then the plastic tubing is inserted through the needle like this:

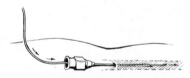

This tubing is calibrated to fit through No. 12 to No. 18 gauge needles. The needle is then removed, leaving the polyethylene tubing in place like this:

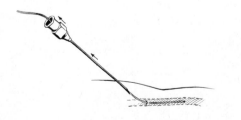

Special adaptors are available to use in connecting the polyethylene tubing to the intravenous tubing. The polyethylene tubing is flexible, allowing some motion of the part during parenteral therapy. It also eliminates the daily search for new veins when prolonged therapy is indicated.

Venous polyethylene catheters may cause complications such as mild local irritation, hematoma, or thrombophlebitis.

When an intravenous catheter is removed, the nurse must make certain that no portion of the tubing remains in the vein. For this reason she should familiarize herself with the various sizes and lengths of polyethylene tubing available. If, on removal, the catheter is found not to be intact, place a tourniquet at the upper part of the extremity and notify the physician.

When the Infusion Has Been Started and the Flow Becomes Too Slow or Stops. An irregularity in the flow of the solution during the venoclysis may be caused by the following:
1. The tubing may have a kink in it.
2. The air filter may be plugged.
3. The bottle of solution may not be high enough.
4. The patient may have shifted his position.
5. The anchoring and/or restraining tape may be too tight.

If none of these conditions seem to exist, there is a possibility that the needle is clogged with a blood clot. If the clot is minute, it may be dislodged by a slight rotation of the needle. If any further difficulty is encountered, stop the infusion, check the equipment thoroughly, and restart the procedure using another sterile needle.

Calculating the Rate of Flow. Here is a shortcut method for calculating the rate of flow for amounts of intravenous fluids to be administered over a specific period of hours:

Amount to be given in 24 hours:

$$\frac{\text{no. of cc. to be given in 24 hours}}{100} = \text{rate of flow plus } 1, 2, \text{ or } 3$$

Divide the total number of cc. to be given in 24 hours by 100. If the answer is less than 11, this is the rate of flow. If the answer is between 11 and 35, add 1. If the answer is between 36 and 59, add 2. If the answer is between 60 and 83, add 3.

Amount to be given in shorter periods:

Eight-hour period:

$$\frac{\text{total no. of cc. to be given}}{100} = \text{rate of flow} \times 3$$

$(24 \div 8 = 3)$, then add 1, 2, or 3 as before.

Twelve-hour period:

$$\frac{\text{total no. of cc. to be given}}{100} = \text{rate of flow} \times 2$$

$(24 \div 12 = 2)$, then add 1, 2, or 3 as before.

To Administer a Medication Intravenously while the Intravenous Infusion Is in Progress.

Before administering medications intravenously, the nurse should first familiarize herself with the hospital policies and state laws regarding the type of medications nurses are permitted to administer intravenously. She should also keep in mind the basic principles of drug administration and make certain that she knows the action of the drug and the dangers of administration. Medications frequently administered include corticoids, antibiotics, vitamins, Levophed, calcium gluconate and aminophylline.

The injection may be made through the gum rubber tubing with a syringe and needle like this:

1. Cleanse the outside of the tube with a disinfectant cotton.
2. Holding the needle at a slant, insert it into the tubing.
3. Slowly inject the medication.
4. Withdraw the needle, and check the tubing for leakage of the solution or for air being drawn into the flowing fluid. Evidence of the drawing of air will be the appearance of tiny air bubbles within the tubing. You can remedy either of these by placing a small piece of sterile adhesive tape over the injection site in the tubing.

HYPODERMOCLYSIS

Hypodermoclysis (commonly called "clysis") is the injection of a large amount of fluid into the subcutaneous tissues by means of a needle. A clysis is given to supply the body with fluid, salts, and nutrients when the intravenous route is necessary but contraindicated or impossible. Subcutaneous infusions are given at room temperature, usually in amounts of 100 to 1000 cc. The physician orders the amount and kind of solution to be given. The solution is usually isotonic or hypotonic (see p. 81). A hypertonic solution is irritating to the subcutaneous tissues.

UNFAVORABLE REACTIONS OCCURRING FROM INTRAVENOUS THERAPY

REACTION	SYMPTOMS	CAUSE
Pyrogenic (Occurs most frequently)	Rise in temperature Severe chills	Elements containing pyrogen present in the fluid Use of improperly sterilized apparatus
Speed shock (Occurs second in frequency)	Headache Flushed skin Nausea and vomiting Irregular pulse Dyspnea	Too rapid administration of fluids, causing circulatory overload
Embolism		Failure to clear apparatus of air before administration of fluid. Infusion should be discontinued with several cc. of solution remaining in the reservoir.
Thrombophlebitis	Hardening of vein Pain in the direction of the flow of the vein	Use of hooked needles Constant use of the same vein
Tissue damage and necrosis	Edema Discoloration of site	Perforation of vein wall Too rapid administration of fluid in too small a vein
Hematoma	Discoloration of site	Posterior puncture of vein wall

For the adult patient the most common site for the injection is the anterior thigh. In many institutions nurses are permitted to make the injection in this area. Other sites used are the area beneath the breast in the female (between the rib cage and the mammary gland) and the abdominal wall just above the crest of the ileum. The nurse would assist the physician with the injection at these two sites.

The Equipment

The hypodermoclysis unit looks like this:

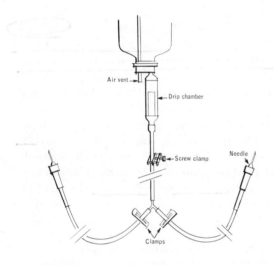

Two needles are used because absorption of fluid in the subcutaneous tissue is slow; thus fluid can be administered in a shorter period of time. 20-gauge needles about 1½ to 2 inches in length are used. Additional equipment that is required is the following:

1. Aseptic skin preparation equipment
2. Skin shaving equipment, especially for male patient
3. Extra bed linen for draping patient (sheet, cotton blanket)
4. I.V. pole
5. Two 2-cc. syringes with 25-gauge needle (one for procaine if used and one for hyaluronidase)
6. Skin desensitizing agent used by some physicians (ethyl chloride spray or procaine)
7. Hyaluronidase
8. Adhesive tape and sterile gauze

Starting the Hypodermoclysis

In preparation for the clysis, the equipment should be assembled and placed on a cart. Before preparing the patient for the injection, the hypodermoclysis unit is assembled and hung on a pole about 3 feet above the bed. Allow the solution to fill the tubing, thus removing air. Close the clamps on the tubing.

Inserting the Needle

As mentioned previously, the nurse may be required to insert the needles if the anterior thigh site is used. Check your hospital's policies. Position and drape the patient; then prepare the skin by shaving, if necessary, on the male and by cleansing each injection site with a disinfectant solution. To insert the needle in the anterior thigh, pinch the skin and insert the needle at a slight angle for 1½ to 2 inches as shown:

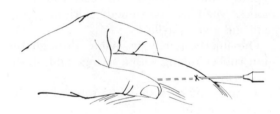

As a guide in knowing how deep the needle should be inserted, it should be remembered that the skin on the anterior thigh is about ½ inch thick. In the elderly and extremely thin individual, it would be slightly thinner and in the obese person slightly thicker. After the needle is inserted, place a piece of gauze between the needle hub and the skin and secure it and the tubing in place with adhesive, as shown for the intravenous needle on p. 89.

The flow of solution can then be started. Hyaluronidase is usually injected as soon as the solution begins to flow. A 2-cc. syringe and a 25-gauge needle are used to inject the prescribed amount into the rubber inserts in the tubing above the needle attachments (see also p. 91). Hyaluronidase (an enzyme) is used because it dissolves cellular protective substances, thus making it possible for the solution to be absorbed into the capillaries more rapidly. Some physicians may prefer to add the dosage of hyaluronidase to the bottle of solution. In this event the written order would specifically be stated. If hyaluronidase is added to the bottle of solution, it is done before assembling the clysis unit, and the bottle must be properly labeled, stating the drug by name and dosage.

Continuation of Care

Flow Adjustment. After the clysis is started, the rate of flow is left to the nurse's judgment. The nurse must adjust the flow to correspond with the rate of absorption. If absorption is occurring too slowly in relationship to the flow, the area around the injection site becomes swollen and the skin becomes taut with a white discoloration. In this event, the rate of flow must be slowed. It may be necessary to readjust either one or both injection sites periodically. A flow that is too rapid for absorption may result in damage to the tissues at the injection site. If the rate of absorption is too slow (that is, a few drops per minute), the physician may want to discontinue the treatment. It usually takes about 1 hour to administer 500 cc. solution. More rapid absorption occurs in thin individuals because the areolar tissue is not packed with fat cells. More rapid absorption also occurs in dehydrated tissue.

Positioning of the Patient. Prior to the injection of the needles, the patient should be made as comfortable as possible and properly draped to eliminate exposure. The patient should be lying on his back. When the injection is given in the thighs, the legs should be slightly flexed and resting on small pillows as shown:

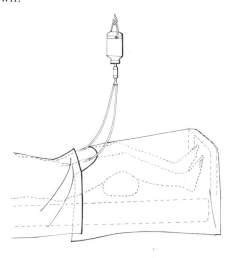

Note also the arrangement of the top bed covers. The top covers must be arranged in two sections as shown, regardless of which one of the three injection sites is used.

The patient's position is changed periodically during the treatment unless contraindicated by his condition. He may be moved slightly toward each side, and the level of the head may be raised or lowered slightly.

Removal of Needles. Withdraw the needles quickly while applying pressure over the injection site with a sterile sponge. Cover the site with sterile gauze (1″ × 1″) and adhesive.

BLOOD TRANSFUSION

The mechanics of administering blood are complex and include a number of important procedures which must be carried out prior to the time the nurse is required either to assist in the administration of blood or to administer it herself. To emphasize the importance of blood compatibility in blood transfusion, a brief background of the preparation of blood will be discussed.

Collection of Blood

In collecting blood from donors, two factors are considered: protection of the donor and protection of the recipient. The first consideration necessitates that donors can be accepted only if they fulfill the requirements as to age, height, weight, and hemoglobin. The second consideration requires the donor to be free of any infections, including tuberculosis, rheumatic fever, and syphilis; and the temperature, pulse, and blood pressure must be within the normal range. Donors who have had malaria or infectious hepatitis should never be accepted. In addition to obtaining the relative information from the donor, adequate records and proper identification are mandatory. In collecting blood, the following precautions are carried out:

1. A sample blood tube is collected simultaneously with the bottle of blood, and both are labeled immediately to prevent mistakes in identity.
2. Aseptic handling is essential to prevent bacterial contamination.

3. Use of proper anticoagulant and preservatives is necessary.
4. Immediate refrigeration is required.
5. Proper storage in a refrigerated area is necessary.

Processing of Blood

Before blood can be released for transfusion, several tests are performed to learn the blood grouping. At present there are 11 independent blood group systems. These are as follows:

1. ABO System: Factors variable in this system include O, A, B, and AB.
2. Rh System: Five main Rh factors include Rh(D), rh'(C), rh''(E), hr'(c), and hr''(e).
3. The MNS System: These factors are MN, M, and N.
4. Additional blood groupings are the P system (P factor), Kell system (K factor), Kidd system (Jk^a and Jk^b factors), Duffy system (Fy^a and Fy^b factors), Lewis system (Le^a and Le^b factors), Lutheran system (Lu^a and Lu^b factors). Other factors found are the Tj^a, Ve, I, Yt^a, Js^a and Di^a.

It should be mentioned that all the previously named factors are completely independent of one another.

Mandatory tests performed on blood prior to release for transfusion include (1) the ABO group; (2) the Rh(D) factor; (3) if the blood is Rh(D) negative, additional tests are rh'(C) and rh''(E); (4) a serologic test for syphilis.

Laboratory Tests for the Patient

Before the patient receives a transfusion, a *type* and a *crossmatch* are performed on the patient's blood. The type determines the ABO grouping and the Rh(D) factor. In the crossmatch a sample of the patient's plasma is mixed with a sample of the donor's red cells (taken from the test tube of blood obtained at the time of collection). If agglutination occurs, the blood is incompatible. The crossmatching of blood determines whether the blood is compatible in the numerous factors other than the ABO group and the Rh(D) factor.

New specimens for crossmatching tests are obtained from the patient whenever more than 24 hours have elapsed since a previous transfusion.

ADMINISTRATION OF BLOOD TRANSFUSION

Proper Identity of Blood

It is hoped that the previous discussion on the meticulous care in the collection and processing of blood has reemphasized the need for an equal amount of care on the nurse's part during the administration of blood transfusion. When administering blood, make certain the label on the blood container is properly identified with the patient. *Most mistakes of blood incompatibility are due to improper identification of blood label and patient.*

Each hospital has some system for double-checking the label on the blood container with the identity of the patient. The system usually requires the signature of both the nurse and the doctor or of two nurses in the event one starts the transfusion. In many cases a form such as the one shown at the bottom of page 94 accompanies the bottle of blood to the patient's unit. This form, containing two copies, is kept on the patient's chart during the transfusion; then the copy is returned to the blood bank with the empty bottle of blood.

The method used for a venipuncture in administering a blood transfusion is the same as for an intravenous infusion.

Blood is administered in units of 500 cc. Blood is given at room temperature or lower; it is never heated. Blood should be administered as soon as it is delivered to the patient's unit and should never be left standing for more than 1 hour prior to transfusion.

The basic blood transfusion setup includes the same components as the intravenous setup, except that a filter is needed to filter the blood as it is being administered. At present there are two types of units used to contain the blood: the glass bottle and the plastic bag. The transfusion setup using the glass bottle looks like this:

The setup using the plastic bag looks like this·

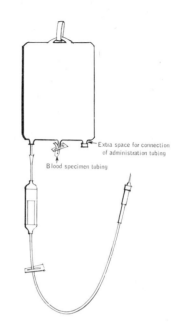

Extra space for connection of administration tubing

Blood specimen tubing

Note that with the plastic bag there are two outlets for use in connecting the transfusion administration set.

The blood specimen tubing as shown contains blood used by the blood bank in cross-matching. This tubing should not be tampered with by the nurse.

Disposable blood administration sets are commercially packaged either with or without needles.

Additional types of setups that may be required in administering blood are as follows:

The Y-type administration set used when blood and intravenous fluids are administered simultaneously:

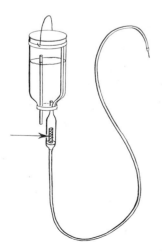

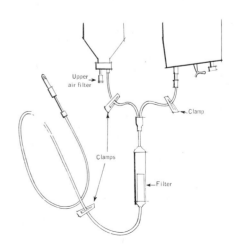

Upper air filter

Clamp

Clamps

Filter

The secondary blood administration set used when blood is ordered to be given after intravenous therapy has been initiated:

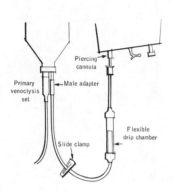

Rate of Flow

The blood unit is hung 3 to 4 feet above the patient's heart level, and needles size 14 to 18 are used in order to allow for an adequate flow. Ordinarily the flow should be adjusted at 20 to 40 drops per minute for the first 10 minutes as a safety measure. If no reaction is observed during this time, the flow may be increased to as much as 120 drops per minute for ordinary purposes when there is no cardiac embarrassment. At this rate it would take approximately 80 minutes to administer one unit of blood.

In elderly persons and when there is cardiovascular embarrassment, the rate of flow must be slower. In this case blood should be administered at 60 to 70 drops per minute. At this rate a unit of blood would transfuse in 2 hours.

Blood cannot be given slower than 60 drops per minute, as at a slower rate the sedimentation causes stoppage.

In treating shock, blood is administered as rapidly as possible. To do so, a No. 14 or a No. 16 needle must be used, and the tubing must be left wide open. In this manner a unit of blood can be given in 20 minutes. This rate, however, is too slow in cases of frank shock; thus the physician would administer the blood more rapidly via use of pressure.

Administering Blood Under Pressure

When blood in a glass bottle is administered by pressure, a blood pump administration set

is used. The setup for this procedure is as shown:

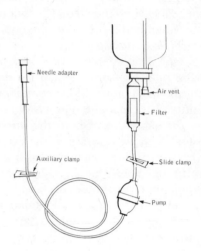

With this setup the rate of flow is increased by a manual pumping action.

To administer blood by pressure in a plastic container, a specially designed pressure cuff is placed around the plastic blood bag. Currently these pressure cuffs are available from several manufacturers. All operate under the same principle. The use of the pressure cuff is shown here:

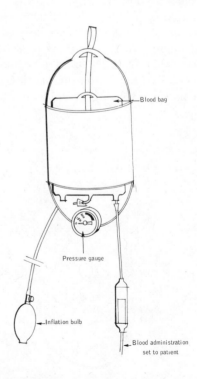

The pressure cuff is operated in the same manner as the cuff placed around the arm when taking the patient's blood pressure. As the cuff is inflated, pressure is exerted against the collapsible plastic blood bag, forcing the blood out of the bag.

Under pressure one unit of blood may be infused in 8 to 12 minutes. During the procedure the transfusion site must be closely observed to make certain blood is not infiltrating into the subcutaneous tissues.

Unfavorable Reactions to Blood Transfusion

All of the unfavorable reactions that may occur during the administration of intravenous fluids may also occur during the administration of blood. In addition to these reactions and their symptoms, a reaction of particular importance to the nurse is that resulting from blood incompatibility. Symptoms of blood incompatibility may appear after the administration of as little as 10 cc. of blood. The patient usually complains of fullness in the head and a generalized tingling sensation. Later he complains of a heaviness in the chest and sudden sharp pain in the lumbar region. The patient's face is flushed, and neck veins are distended; he is dyspneic and restless. A severe reaction may result in rapid coma and death.

The blood transfusion should be terminated immediately upon the first symptom of any unfavorable reaction.

INTRA-ARTERIAL INFUSION OF ANTICANCER AGENTS

The treatment of cancer with anticancer agents is being carried out as an adjunct to surgery and to control effusion of cancer cells. Anticancer drugs are administered orally and intravenously. They are instilled locally in wounds during surgery. They are also given by means of perfusion and infusion.

In perfusion and infusion the anticancer agent (also called chemotherapeutic agent) is injected into the arterial system which leads to the tumor area. In these methods the drug action is concentrated in one area of the body.

Perfusion. This is also called *isolation* and is used for incurable malignant tumors which cannot be treated by other measures. With this technique one catheter is inserted into a major artery leading into a specific organ or anatomic part, and another catheter is inserted into the major vein leading out of the same organ or anatomic part. The catheters are attached to an oxygenator pump. The other chemotherapeutic drug is then instilled into the blood stream of the isolated area and recirculated through the area for a prescribed period of time. This procedure is done in the operating room under general anesthesia; therefore, the nurse has no responsibility for the drug administration

Intra-arterial Infusion. This is a more recent technique than perfusion. With intra-arterial infusion a catheter is simply placed in the artery leading to a malignant tumor. The chemotherapeutic drug is infused into the catheter, a large portion of the drug being absorbed by the tumor before entering the general circulation. The advantage of intra-arterial infusion is that with this method a chemotherapeutic drug can be given over a longer period of time than with perfusion.

In the procedure of intra-arterial infusion the patient is taken to the operating room for insertion of the intra-arterial catheter under general anesthesia. After recovery from anesthesia in the recovery room, he is returned to his own room, and the infusion of the chemotherapeutic agent is continued usually for 5 to 7 days or until toxicity appears.

Placement of Catheter. In the operating room proper placement of the catheter is achieved by the injection of fluorescent dye into the catheter and visualization with an ultraviolet lamp. The catheter is tied into the artery and sutured to the skin.

Frequently used arteries for variously located areas of infusion are as follows:
Head and neck infusions—superficial temporal and superior thyroid:

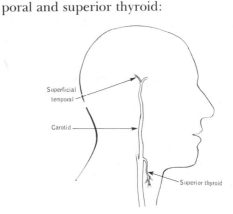

Upper extremity — thyrocervical trunk:

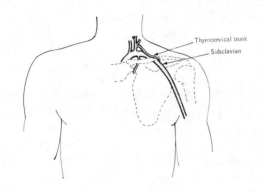

Lower extremity — inferior epigastric artery:

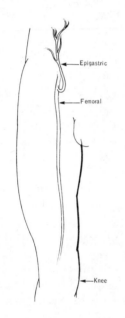

Other arteries that have been used are the gastroepiploic, hepatic, and femoral, all used for the treatment of abdominal tumors.

Chemotherapeutic Drugs. The same group of drugs is used for both perfusion and infusion except that with infusion a combination of several drugs is usually used. Generally used drugs are:

    nitrogen mustard (Mustargen)
    6-mercaptopurine (Puri-nethol)
    5-fluorouracil (5-FU, Fluro Uracil)
    methotrexate
    actinomycin D

    vincaleukoblastine (Velban)
    triethylenethiophosphoramide (thio-
      TEPA, TSPA)
    triethylenemelamine (TEM)
    chlorambucil (Leukeran)
    cyclophosphamide (Cytoxan)
    5-fluoro-2'-deoxyuridine (5-FUDR)
    crystalline penicillin G in 2 per cent
      aluminum monostearate (PAM)

To control toxicity, specific drug neutralizers are administered intramuscularly every 4 to 6 hours during the infusion. Drugs controlling toxicity are leucovorin for methotrexate, thymidine for 5-fluorouracil, and sodium thiosulfate for the mustard drugs.

Signs of toxicity are both local and systemic as follows:

Head and neck infusion: swelling, erythema, stomatitis, pain, headache. Observe for impairment of airway. A tracheostomy (see p. 353) may be done at the time of catheter insertion.

Pelvic infusion: Itching, rash, and breakdown of skin on feet and buttocks. Do not give intramuscular medication in the buttocks of these patients.

Generalized signs of toxicity include low white blood cell count (reverse isolation may be necessary — see p. 110), low platelet count (blood replacement given), diarrhea, nausea, and vomiting.

Administration of Infusion

The physician determines the dosage for a 24-hour period. Dosages are calculated by the patient's weight in kilograms. The drugs are added to bottles of I.V. solution. (These drugs are classified as experimental. Nurses should not administer them unless policies state so.)

The I.V. setup used is either the "Y" type or the secondary type shown on p. 84. The primary bottle usually contains 1000 c.c. 5 per cent glucose in water with 2000 units heparin added. In the secondary bottle is 500 cc. dextrose per cent in ¼ strength normal saline containing also the chemotherapeutic drug plus heparin. The tubes leading from both bottles are left open. The secondary bottle will infuse first because of the higher specific gravity of the solution. In most cases an arterial infusion pump is used to maintain patency of the arterial catheter. The pump is connected to the I.V. setup as shown:

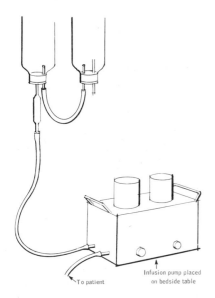

To patient

Infusion pump placed on bedside table

The nurse's responsibilities include:

1. Label bottles of solution properly so that the correct amount of added drugs is visible.
2. Make certain the fluid is flowing at the rate prescribed. Notify the physician if it is not.
3. Make certain that there are no air bubbles in the tubing or that there is no return of blood in the arterial catheter. In either case clamp off the tubing immediately and notify the physician. Return of blood in the catheter could denote hemorrhage.
4. Leakage in the tubing or connections and the presence of blood clots in the tubing must also be called to the physician's attention at once.
5. If the I.V. setup must be discontinued from the intra-arterial catheter for any reason—for example, moving the patient to another department for treatment—it is done by the physician.
6. Give the patient adequate psychological support.
7. Keep accurate intake and output records.
8. Ambulation and mobility are encouraged when the condition permits. Make certain catheters are not dislodged during movement.

9. Encouragement of the patient is necessary with meals to maintain nutrition. Special bland diets are usually prescribed to be given in small feedings every 3 to 4 hours.
10. Special skin care and back care are important when the patient is not ambulatory.

Outpatient Therapy

Intra-arterial infusion therapy can be continued on an outpatient basis with the use of a portable pump as shown:

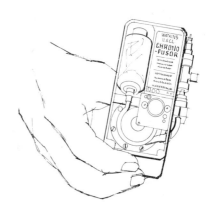

The pump contains a time mechanism which is wound by the patient every 8 hours. The small plastic bag contains the chemotherapeutic drug plus heparin; 5 cc. of the solution is administered by the pump daily. The patient returns to the outpatient department every 4 days for a refill.

A muslin bag can be made to support the portable pump as shown:

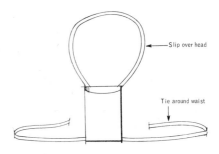

Slip over head

Tie around waist

Instead of the strap that fits over the head, a small tab can be used to pin the bag to the brassière for the female.

BIBLIOGRAPHY

Bergin, M. A.: All Our Nurses Give I.V.'s. RN, *28*:47, 1965.

Burgess, R.: Fluids and Electrolytes. Am. J. Nurs., *65*:10, 1965.

Clack, B.: Intravenous Infusions: Uses and Contraindications. Nurs. Times, *63*:1068, 1967.

Dann, T. C.: Routine Skin Preparation Before Injections— Is It Necessary? Nurs. Times, *62*:1121, 1966.

Davidsohn, I., and Henry, J. B.: Todd-Sanford Clinical Diagnosis By Laboratory Methods. 14th ed. Philadelphia, W. B. Saunders Co., 1969.

Fraser, A. G.: Care of Intravenous Infusion Using Double-Bottle Technique. New Zealand Nurs. J., *58*:13, 1965.

Fream, W. C.: Calculation of Drip Rates. Nurs. Mir., *121*:339, 1965.

Friedrich, H.: Common Sense in Intramuscular Injection. Nurs. Clin. North America, *1*:333, 1966.

Grant, J.: Complications of Blood Transfusion. Nurs. Mir., *124*:60, 1967.

Hershey, N.: The Nurse Wasn't Liable. Am. J. Nurs., *67*: 1875, 1967.

Kernicki, J.: Needle Puncture: Health Asset or Menace. Nurs. Clin. North America, *1*:269, 1966.

Levensteen, B. P.: Intravenous Therapy: A Nursing Specialty. Nurs. Clin. North America, *1*:259, 1966.

McDonald, G. O.: Treatment of Electrolyte Deficiencies in Surgery. Surg. Clin. North America, *44(1)*:125, 1964.

Moore, F. D.: Blood Transfusions: Rates, Routes, and Hazards. Nurs. Clin. North America, *1*:285, 1966.

Mrazek, R. G., Strehl, F. W., and Southwick, H. W.: Chemotherapy for Cancer. Surg. Clin. North America *44(1)*:113, 1964.

Pitel, W.: The Intramuscular Infection. Am. J. Nurs., *64*:1044, 1964.

Reddin, M.: Blood Transfusion Unit. Nurs. Times, *63*: 952, 1967.

Salsbury, A. J.: Indications for Blood Transfusion. Nurs. Mir., *124*:17, 1967.

Sylvester, B.: Factors Associated with Infiltration During Continuous Intravenous Therapy. Nurs. Res., *15*:255, 1966.

Tovey, G. H.: Nursing Care During Blood Transfusion. Nurs. Mir., *124*:35, 1967.

Controlling the
Spread of Disease

In order to practice efficiently the various techniques in controlling the spread of disease, the nurse must: (1) have a sufficient knowledge of the environmental factors which permit, inhibit, and destroy the growth of disease-producing organisms; (2) understand the degrees of seriousness of infectious diseases (the common cold is highly contagious but is not considered a critical disease); (3) be aware of the predisposing factors influencing the susceptibility to contagious diseases; (4) acquaint herself with the bodily portals of entry and exit of pathogenic organisms; and (5) familiarize herself with the terminology used in controlling the spread of disease.

HANDWASHING TECHNIQUES

Since the advent of pHisoHex, the time spent on handwashing can be reduced to about one half the time of that spent using soaps and other solutions. pHisoHex is a liquid, nonalkaline detergent containing hexachlorophene 3 per cent. It has a penetrating, lasting bacteriostatic effect and is not irritating to the skin. pHisoHex is being used for both the surgical scrub and for general handwashing purposes. Nearly all hospitals now have pHisoHex dispensers located at all sinks frequently used by nursing personnel for handwashing. A brush and orangewood stick need not be used with pHisoHex unless the nails need special attention; however, a number of authorities still prefer the use of a brush for the surgical scrub.

SURGICAL SCRUB

The surgical scrub using pHisoHex is done like this:

Wet the hands and forearms; then spread a few drops of pHisoHex (about the size of a dime) over the hands and forearms. After the hands and arms have been rubbed a few times, they will become rather sticky and dry. To get more suds, add more water, NOT more pHisoHex.

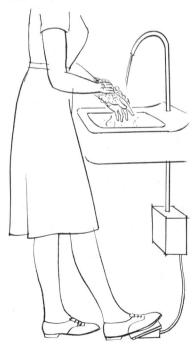

Rinse well under running water, holding the hands like this:

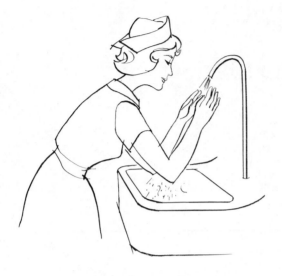

so that contaminated soil is not rinsed down over the clean area. This preliminary cleaning removes most of the infectious material that would act to reduce the detergent quality of pHisoHex if used over a more prolonged period of washing.

Next clean under the nails with an orangewood stick; then wet the hands and forearms again. Spread about one teaspoonful of pHisoHex over the hands and forearms. If a brush is to be used for the surgical scrub, the brush is used at this point. In this event, pHisoHex is put on the brush (first wetted) instead of on the hands. Again work the cream into suds by adding small amounts of water from time to time.

Wash for 2 to 4 minutes, rinse thoroughly holding the hands higher than the elbows, and dry with a sterile towel. Dry the hands first, then the forearm, working up toward the elbow. Never use the towel on the hands after drying the area next to the elbow, as the towel may have become contaminated by touching the upper arm.

GENERAL HANDWASHING

When using pHisoHex for general handwashing purposes, do it like this:

Wet the hands and spread an amount of pHisoHex about the size of a dime over the hands, adding water as necessary. If a hand-operated water faucet is used, leave the water running for this entire procedure. Never add extra pHisoHex to the suds but rinse and repeat the lathering if necessary.

When rinsing, hold the hands like this:

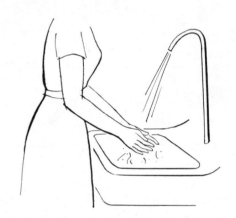

Remember, in medical asepsis the nurse is considered free of contamination; thus the hands are held in this position to keep contamination away from the forearms.

Dry with a paper towel. If hand-operated faucets are used, use the towel to turn off the water. This handwashing procedure should last about 20 seconds.

USE OF GLOVES

The nurse wears gloves to protect the patient from pathogenic organisms on the nurse's hands and to protect herself from disease-producing organisms which may be acquired from the patient. Clean but unsterile gloves are worn when the nurse wishes to protect herself from contamination as in the insertion of vaginal or rectal suppositories and rectal tubes and for handling dressings that are extremely soiled. Sterile gloves are worn to prevent contamination of the patient as in the postoperative care of surgical wounds and in carrying out procedures requiring surgical asepsis.

Gloves are usually packaged in a billfold-type muslin wrapper. The glove is folded to form a cuff several inches wide around the top. A small package of sterile powder is usually packed in one side of the folded muslin.

PUTTING ON STERILE GLOVES

Before putting on sterile gloves, the hands should be washed and dried. Then proceed like this:

Open the glove wrapper and locate the powder by gently shaking one side of the wrapper (both sides if necessary) until the packet of powder falls to the center as shown:

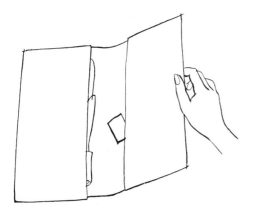

Powder both hands and remove the first glove by grasping the folded edge of the cuff like this:

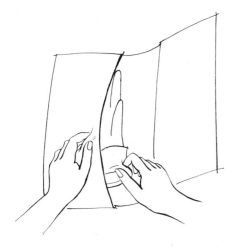

Pull it from the wrapper. It makes no difference which hand is gloved first. The first glove is placed on the hand by pulling on the folded

edge of the cuff like this:

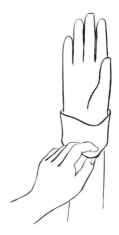

In doing this, be careful not to touch the exterior surface of the glove with the fingers of the ungloved hand. If there is difficulty in getting the fingers fully fitted into the glove fingers, disregard it momentarily, and make this adjustment after both gloves are placed on the hands.

Remove the second glove from the wrapper by placing the fingers of the gloved hand under the cuff like this:

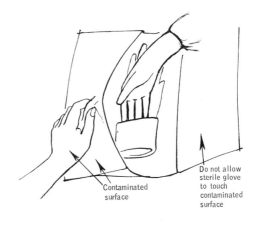

Contaminated surface

Do not allow sterile glove to touch contaminated surface

Place this glove with the fingers under the cuff, being careful not to touch the gloved fingers to the ungloved hand and wrist.

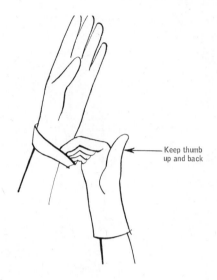

Keep thumb
up and back

Any adjustment in fitting the fingers on both hands is now made.

When wearing sterile gloves for a lengthy or major surgical procedure, you should first cleanse the hands as recommended in the surgical scrub (p. 101), and an assistant should open and hold the glove wrapper so that the operator need only touch the powder wrapper and the gloves (see p. 103). If an assistant is not available, open the glove wrapper and locate the powder before performing the surgical hand scrub.

USE OF GOWNS

In caring for a patient with a cummunicable disease, the nurse must wear a gown to protect her clothing. The gown should be large enough to cover the clothing entirely. It should have tightly cuffed sleeves, a belt, and open down the back with a fastener at the back of the neck. The surgical gowns worn by operating room personnel are usually the type used. The standard hospital gown worn by patients should never be worn for this purpose by nurses.

It is imperative that a gown be worn each time the service required by the patient is such that the nurse's clothing may become contaminated. For instance, a gown need not be worn when merely entering the patient's room to talk to the patient or to hand articles to the patient.

The only safe gown technique is the discard method. In this method a clean gown is worn each time. When removing the gown, place it in the "contaminated" laundry bag (see Isolation Techniques, p. 107). Actually, however, the ideal method is not always the method used in a given hospital situation, and the gown is sometimes worn several times before it is discarded.

PUTTING ON A PREVIOUSLY WORN GOWN

When the same gown is worn repeatedly, everyone must use exactly the same technique in putting it on and taking it off. This in itself is next to impossible. The gown is hung just inside the entrance to the patient's room. To help simplify the steps in gown technique, keep in mind that the inside of the gown and the area surrounding the fasteners of the gown are to be kept free of contamination. You should keep the back away from the patient as much as possible while wearing the gown to prevent unnecessary contamination of this area.

Before putting on the gown, you must make sure that your hands are free of contamination. *To put on the gown*, proceed as follows:

Lift the gown from the hook, touching only the inside surface like this:

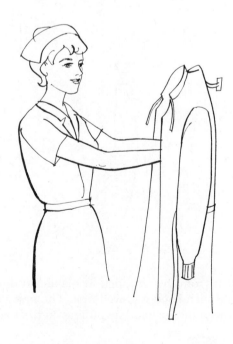

(The gown should always be hung with the contaminated surface on the outside.)

Slide the gown over the hands and arms by holding the arms forward and slightly above the head like this:

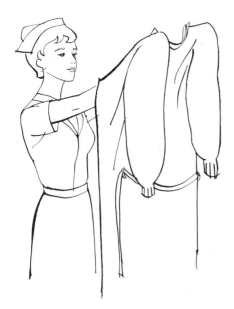

If it is difficult to get the hands through the tight sleeve cuffs, the first sleeve may be pulled on with the opposite hand still inside the sleeve as shown:

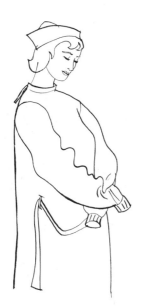

When one sleeve is completely pulled on, it is usually easier to manipulate the fingers of the other hand through the cuff. Remember, at this point the hands are still to be kept free from contamination; therefore, do not touch the outside of the gown with the hands. If perchance the hands accidentally touch the outside surface of the gown, they must be recleansed and dried before proceeding with the closure of the gown. (The fasteners are to be kept free from contamination.)

Fasten the gown at the back of the neck, then grasp the gown at the waistline in the back, and try to overlap the edges as much as possible.

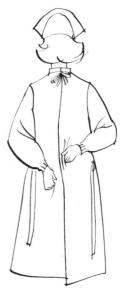

While holding the overlapping edge with one hand, grasp one end of the belt with the other hand, and pull it around the back.

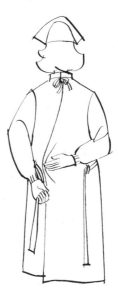

Draw the other belt end into place and fasten.

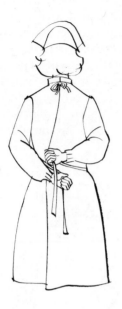

REMOVING THE GOWN TO BE WORN AGAIN

First untie the belt in the back; then wash and dry the hands. Unfasten the neck of the gown, and pull off the first sleeve by slipping the fingers under the cuff like this:

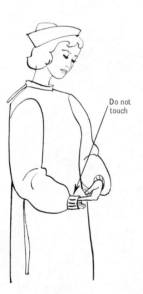

Do not touch the outside surface of the cuff because the outside is contaminated and the hands are now clean.

Remove the second sleeve by grasping it through the first sleeve like this:

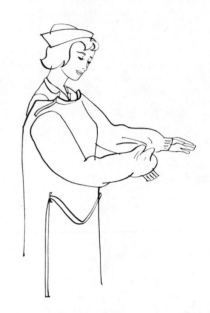

Without touching the outer surface of the gown, fold the gown lengthwise by bringing the shoulder seams together. Hold the gown away from the uniform like this:

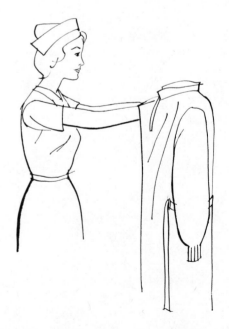

With one hand remaining on the inside of the gown and one hand grasping the neckband, place the gown on the hook. You should wash your hands thoroughly again before leaving the unit.

USE OF MASKS

A mask is worn to reduce the danger of transmitting disease-producing organisms. It acts as a filter to the air. In surgical asepsis the mask is worn to protect the patient from contamination by droplet infection. In medical asepsis the mask is worn to protect the nurse from a patient with a communicable disease that may be transmitted through the respiratory passages. In some cases the patient who is properly instructed may wear the mask. The mask should consist of six layers of gauze (42 × 42 threads per square inch). Materials which offer resistance are not suitable for a mask because it causes the wearer to rebreathe expired air. A mask should fit the face closely to prevent the escape of air around the sides. It should cover the mouth and nose like this:

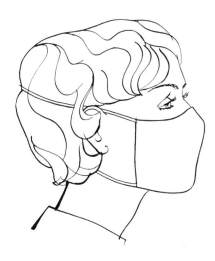

The mask should be worn only once and then only for a short period of time. A large number of masks is needed with separate containers for the clean and contaminated masks.

Using a Mask in Medical Asepsis
1. A container of clean masks should be kept in a clean area near the handwashing facilities.

2. Put on the mask with clean hands before going into the contaminated area. If the discard technique in using gowns is NOT used (see p. 104), the mask must be put on before the gown. In the discard technique for gowns, whether the gown or the mask is put on first is unimportant, since both are clean and both are kept in a clean area.
3. To remove the mask in the discard gown technique, remove the gown, wash hands, remove mask by touching the strings only, then wash the hands again. When the gown is not to be discarded, wash hands, remove the gown, remove the mask, then wash hands again.
4. A mask should be worn no longer than one hour.

Putting on a Clean Mask while Working in a Contaminated Area
Wash the hands, remove the soiled mask, wash the hands again, then put on the clean mask.

Using the Mask in Surgical Asepsis
When putting on the mask, adjust the hair covering, place the mask, perform the surgical scrub, then put on the sterile gown.

The Disposable Mask
Paper and cellulose film masks have been designed to be discarded after use. These masks are used in promoting medical asepsis.

ISOLATION TECHNIQUES

A patient is isolated when there is danger that his infection may be communicable. The extent of isolation precautions used depends upon the disease. The equipment needed to set up an isolation unit depends upon the physical facilities of the hospital as well as the type of disease the patient has. Because there are many varieties of situations involved in carrying out isolation techniques, only general factors in the care of the isolated patient on the general hospital unit will be discussed here. The following points are suggested for the care of the isolated patient. It should be understood that the list is not all-inclusive and that the efficient nurse usually discovers additional ways to apply the principles of medical asepsis.

1. The patient must be segregated for the protection of others.
2. All unnecessary equipment and furniture should be removed from the patient's unit.
3. All equipment needed for the care of the patient should be kept in the unit.
4. The nurse must wear a gown over her uniform when attending the patient (see p. 104).
5. Hands must be washed each time the patient receives care (see p. 102).
6. If there is no sink in the patient's unit, a basin with a disinfectant solution is kept in the unit. This solution should be changed several times daily.
7. All food is transferred from the clean tray to the dishes kept on a tray in the patient's unit. The clean tray may be placed on a table covered with clean newspapers while the food is being transferred. The individual who performs this procedure need not wear a protective gown over her uniform.
8. Linen used by the isolated patient is kept separate from all other soiled linen by placing it in a laundry bag labeled "contaminated." The bag containing the contaminated linen should be kept clean on the outside.
9. Feces and other body excretions can usually be poured directly into the hopper. When a hopper is not conveniently located, the excreta must be placed in a container of chlorinated lime. The excreta should be mixed thoroughly with the chlorinated lime solution and be left standing for 4 hours before discarding.
10. Solid waste materials such as food or soiled tissues should be collected in paper bags or newspapers and burned.
11. Dishes, basins, and similar articles should be disinfected before storage or use for other patients. Boiling for fifteen minutes is considered adequate. Articles contaminated by spore-forming bacteria must be autoclaved.
12. Books, magazines, and papers must be burned following contamination. Single sheets of paper may be read or signed without becoming contaminated by placing them between a newspaper and a paper towel like this:

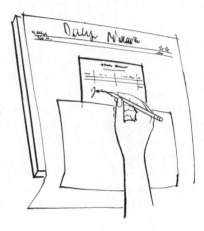

13. Articles that are too large for sterilization or are destroyed by heat should be washed with a detergent and aired for 12 hours.
14. Items such as a nurse's watch may be kept free from contamination by being placed in a small plastic bag. After use, slide the item from the bag onto an uncontaminated surface.
15. The patient, his relatives, and, if necessary, other patients on the ward should be instructed in the procedures in medical asepsis in order to promote a thorough safeguard against the spread of infection.

REVERSE ISOLATION

In the treatment of certain disease conditions which render the patient extremely susceptible to infection, a reverse isolation technique is used. Currently, this technique is being used mainly in the care of patients with extensive burns and for patients who are receiving extensive chemotherapy (cytotoxic drugs) which cause bone-marrow depletion, thus lowering the body's resistance to infection.

In reverse isolation the main objective is to keep the patient's environment as free of disease-producing organisms as possible (as is done in the operating room). Some institutions now have a special reverse isolation unit which can accommodate a number of patients. In other hospitals the patient may be confined to a private room and placed on "reverse isolation."

Regardless of whether the patient is in a reverse isolation unit or in his own private room, the techniques of reverse isolation are the same, as follows:

1. All doors leading to the unit are kept closed.
2. All persons must scrub as for a surgical scrub (p. 101) before entering the patient unit.
3. Sterile gown, mask, and gloves are put on before entering the unit.
4. All clothes, linens, plastic ware, and metalware are sterilized before going into the unit.
5. The patient's hair is initially shampooed with pHisoHex, and a pHisoHex bath is given. PHisoHex baths are then given once or twice daily.
6. Books, magazines, and newspapers are sterilized in hot air for 1 hour at 150° centigrade (300° F.).
7. Cutlery and china are autoclaved.
8. Cooked food is considered germ free and can be served on sterile paper plates, then wrapped in plastic by kitchen personnel trained in the procedure; or it can be served directly from the serving cart onto sterile china at the patient unit door.
9. Beverages such as milk, canned juices, and so forth are poured directly into sterile drinking containers at the door of the patient's unit. All drinking water is sterilized. Containers of distilled water from central supply can be kept in the refrigerator for this purpose.
10. Dry food articles such as instant coffee, tea, and so forth can be stored in sterile containers in the patient area.
11. When the patient must be transferred from the unit to x-ray, for example, the stretcher is first scrubbed with a disinfectant solution. The stretcher and the patient are then covered with sterile sheets. All those attending to the patient must then wear sterile gowns, masks, and gloves. When the patient returns to his unit, he is given a pHisoHex bath, and the room is cleaned with a disinfectant solution.
12. All sterile containers that are stored in the patient's room are resterilized and replaced periodically, and the room is thoroughly cleaned with a disinfectant solution daily.
13. Some foresight is required in preparing sterilized items to be passed into the unit. A single wrapper can be used on items that require no further special handling, such as a comb, a blood pressure cuff, or a drinking glass. Double wrappers are used on all items requiring surgical asepsis such as sterile procedure trays.

As with any type of isolation, only those items absolutely necessary in the care of the patient are kept in the room. When the physician prescribes reverse isolation, it may take several days to prepare the patient and his room. Culture swabs of all bodily orifices such as the eyes, nose, mouth, ears, vagina, urethra, and so forth are usually taken, and the patient may be placed on a bowel-cleansing and antibiotic therapy regimen. pHisoHex baths or showers may be given several days prior to entry. Sterile linen is also used for bathing during the pre-entry regimen. After the pre-entry cleansing, the patient is given sterile bed clothes, a robe, slippers, and bed linen.

Preparation of the reverse isolation unit includes daily disinfecting and culturing until it is felt that the room is safe.

When the precise time has arrived to transfer the patient from his room to the isolation room, he is given a pHisoHex bath and redressed in fresh sterile clothes. He is placed on a disinfected stretcher and covered with sterile sheets. The nurses aiding in the transfer also wear sterile gowns, masks, gloves, and caps. After the patient is placed in the isolation unit, the floor is mopped and the furniture is cleaned with a disinfectant solution.

Before transferring the patient to the isolation unit, the procedure should be explained to him as well as to his family. At the same time the nurse will learn which personal belongings as well as occupational-therapy items must be sterilized for transfer. It should also be explained that telephone, television, music, and visiting privileges are available if the proper techniques are used.

THE ISOLATOR

Most recently developed and not yet widely used is a device called the "isolator." The isolator was designed as a single unit in which to isolate a patient. The isolator looks similar to the tank type of respirator illustrated in Chapter 5, except that the entire tank is made of see-through plastic. Two types of isolators have been designed, one used for the patient in isolation for a communicable disease and the other for the patient on reverse isolation. The isolator used for communicable diseases has an air circulator attached to one end. It circulates and cools the air inside the isolator, then filters the air before returning it to the outside. On the isolator used for reverse isolation, just the opposite occurs; the air-circulation cooler filters the room air before blowing it into the canopy. One model isolator is constructed of rigid plastic. Another model is flexible plastic. Both types have entry portholes as shown below.

The isolation principle and technique in caring for the patient in an isolator are the same as when placing the patient in isolation or reverse isolation in his room.

Special situations peculiar to each type of isolator are as follows:

Isolator Used for Communicable Diseases

1. All articles used inside the isolator are disinfected before removal through specially designed portholes. Trays containing disinfecting solutions are built into the isolator for this purpose. Articles that cannot be immersed in solution are wrapped in plastic bags, then placed in the solution before removal.

Isolator Used for Reverse Isolation

1. All items passed through the equipment portholes are sterile and are handled with an aseptic technique using sterile forceps. The pass-through portholes on this isolator are surrounded by ultraviolet lights. Items must be passed through quickly to prevent contamination of the interior. The nurse wears a mask during the pass-through procedure.
2. When placing the patient in the isolator, sterile sheets are draped around the outside of the opening on the canopy to prevent contamination of the patient. (The patient and the isolator will have been prepared as previously discussed in this chapter under "Reverse Isolation.")

While the patient is in the isolator, the nurse is responsible for housekeeping of the isolator. The inside and outside are scrubbed daily with a disinfectant solution. Periodic cultures are made from the inside of the isolator canopy.

Occupational therapy is of extreme importance while the patient is in an isolator because he cannot ambulate. There is, however,

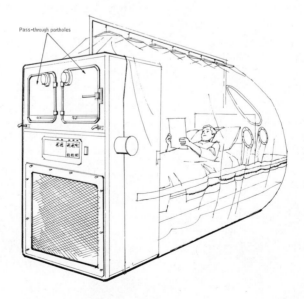

Pass-through portholes

a new type of isolator currently under design which permits ambulation.

An electrical outlet located on the inside part of the headboard permits the use of such items as an electrical heating pad or a shaver.

After the patient is removed from the isolator, the mattress and feather pillow are encased in a double plastic cover and are sterilized by gas. The inside of the isolator can be thoroughly cleaned with a spray of 500 cc. 2 per cent peracetic acid solution. All port-holes are closed after spraying the interior, and the circulating fan is turned off for 30 minutes. The fumes can then be removed by turning the isolator ventilator on and connecting a hose between it and an air vent in the room.

In reverse isolation, daily cultures are made from the isolator to decide when it is safe for the next patient to enter.

Additional Procedures that may be required when the patient is in isolation are as follows:

Lumbar puncture

Bone marrow aspiration (p. 236)

Administration of I.V. solution (p. 85)

Administration of oxygen (p. 30)

Tracheotomy care (p. 353)

Use of Bird or Bennett respirator (p. 56)

BIBLIOGRAPHY

Adams, R.: Preventions of Infections in Hospitals. Am. J. Nurs. *58*:344, 1958.

Benson, M. E.: Handwashing—An Important Part of Medical Asepsis. Am. J. Nurs., *57*:1136, 1957.

Bonney, V.: Handwashing in the Home. Am. J. Nurs., *55*:557, 1955.

Bower, A., Pilant, E., and Crafton, N.: Communicable Diseases. 8th ed. Philadelphia, W. B. Saunders Co., 1958.

Brown, A. F.: Medical Nursing. 3rd ed. Philadelphia, W. B. Saunders Co., 1957. (Chapter 27.)

Deschambear, E. R.: Chart Helps Nurse Select Correct Isolation Procedure. Mod. Hosp., *109*:66, 1967.

Donovan, C.: Reverse Barrier Nursing. Nurs. Times, *63*:791, 1967.

Gallivan, G. J., et al.: Isolation for Possible and Proved Staph. Am. J. Nurs., *67*:1048, 1967.

Griffith, R.: Isolation Cart Wins Award in Achievement Contest. Hosp. Top., *45*:125, 1967.

Johnson, A.: Aseptic Techniques. Nurs. Times, *63*:252, 1967.

Juzwiak, B.: Newest Infection Control: The Plastic Isolator. RN, *28*:58, 1965.

Seidler, F.: Nurs. Clin. North America, *1*:587, 1966.

Smendek, P., and Kurtagh, C.: Isolation in the Home. Am. J. Nurs., *56*:575, 1956.

Streeter, S., et al.: Hospital Infection a Necessary Risk? Am. J. Nurs., *67*:526, 1967.

The Proper Use of Surgical Supplies

Although the use of surgical supplies is one of the basic procedures demonstrated to student nurses, it is a technique that requires constant practice in order for the nurse to maintain an assured degree of dexterity. Nurses who have not worked in a surgical department for some time usually feel insecure when confronted with procedures that require the art of handling sterile articles and applying dressings. This chapter affords an opportunity for the nurse to review the most commonly encountered procedures in the application of surgical asepsis.

HANDLING STERILE SUPPLIES

Sterile equipment should never be touched with the bare fingers. Some sterile equipment is handled with sterile gloves. Most sterile equipment used in a hospital surgical department is handled with the handling forceps kept in a jar of antiseptic solution.

Removing the Handling Forceps from the Container of Antiseptic Solution

Grasp the forceps by the handle, and withdraw in a vertical line, being careful not to touch the tip of the forceps to the side of the jar. Always hold the forceps in the vertical position with the tip down. This must be done to prevent the solution from running back and forth over both sterile and unsterile portions of the forceps. *See illustration at the top of the following page.*

Removing a Lid from a Container of Sterile Supplies

If the lid is held, it should be held with the

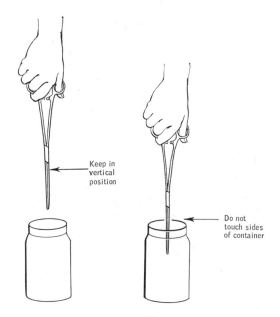

inner surface downward to prevent contamination.

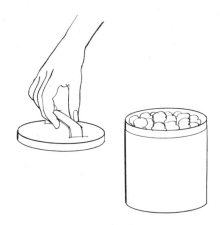

If the lid is placed on a table, the outer surface is placed downward to prevent contamination to the inner surface.

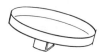

Handing a Sterile Instrument to Someone

Remove the instrument from the container of antiseptic solution by grasping the tip end

with the handling forceps like this:

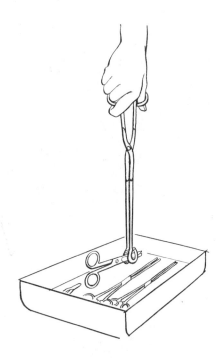

Hand the instrument like this:

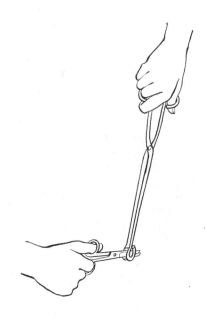

Removing Sterile Gauze or Cotton Balls from a Container

Remove the cotton ball with the handling forceps, being careful not to touch the inside of the can with the unsterile portion of the forceps.

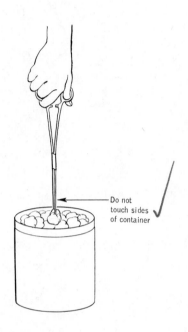

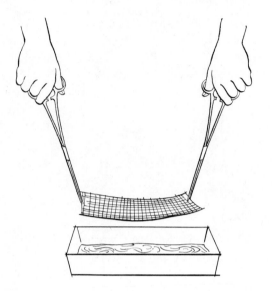

The forceps may not be used to remove another piece of petrolatum gauze from the container if they are used on the patient or have become contaminated in any other way.

Using a Tongue Blade in Removing Sterile Ointments from a Jar

Remove the tongue blade from its container with a handling forceps, and place the sterile tongue blade in the jar of sterile ointment like this:

Handing a Sterile Piece of Gauze or Cotton Ball to Someone

Remove the cotton ball as shown previously, and hand it like this:

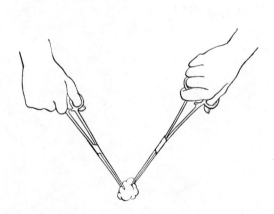

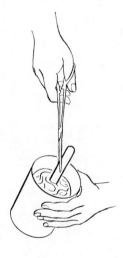

If the blade is handed to someone, the forceps must be used to dip the tongue blade into the ointment and to hand the tongue blade.

If the blade is not handed to anyone, you

Removing Sterile Petrolatum Gauze from Its Container

Two forceps must be used like this:

may grasp the top of the blade with the bare fingers, being careful not to touch the inside of the jar.

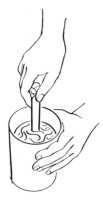

Opening Sterile Packs

Sterile dressings, drapes, towels, small basins, treatment and diagnostic trays and some instruments are first wrapped in muslin and sterilized in the autoclave. When these supplies are needed, they must be opened in such a way that the fingers do not touch the inside of the wrapper or the sterile article.

If the pack is large, it must be placed on a table to open. Loosen the wrapper fastener (fasteners are usually straight pins, string, or gummed tape); then fold back one flap at a time like this:

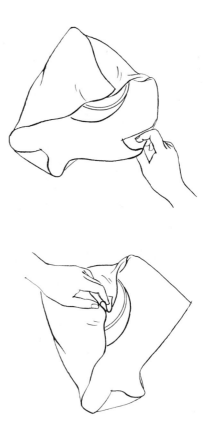

Note the method of grasping the wrapper so that the fingers never touch the inside.

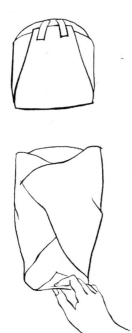

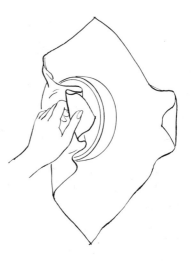

Commercially presterilized packages are opened by either tearing or peeling the package at one end. The two types are shown here:

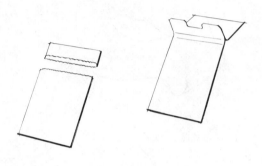

The opening of the packet must then be held apart so that the contents can be removed with sterile forceps without touching the outside of the packet.

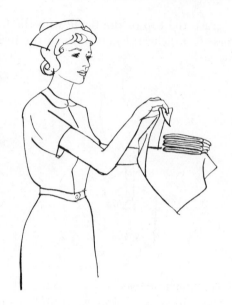

Continue to hold the opened pack away from the body while the other individual picks up the sterile article.

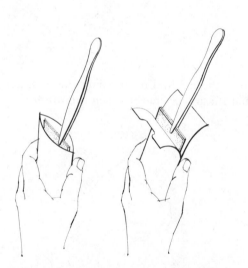

Handing an Opened Sterile Pack to Someone Wearing Sterile Gloves. After loosening the fastener of the wrapping, hold the pack in one hand, and open it with the other. A right-handed individual should hold the pack in the left hand and open it with the right hand. Hold the pack up and away from the body so that the inside does not become contaminated. The pack should be held so that the last flap is opened toward yourself like this:

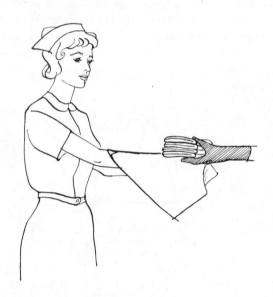

Placing Sterile Articles on a Previously Opened Sterile Tray. Occasionally after a sterile tray has been opened for the physician's use, additional sterile articles may be needed. If the tray remains sterile, the nurse removes the desired sterile article from an opened pack or container with the handling forceps <u>and drops</u> the article on the opened tray.

If an article stored in a disinfecting solution is transferred to an open sterile tray, it must be dropped in a sterile basin. If the linens on a sterile tray accidentally become wet, the tray is considered contaminated.

Pouring Sterilized Solutions into a Sterile Basin or onto Sterile Dressings and Wounds. If the bottle containing the solution has a screw top or paper cap, do not touch the outer part of the bottle rim, or the inside of the cap as these are considered sterile.

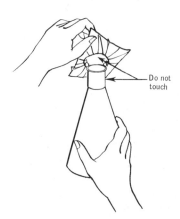

Do not touch

Open the outer wrapper of the tray as shown on page 115; then fold the sterile towel covering back with a handling forceps. Grasp only a very small part of the towel with the forceps, and stand away from the opened outer wrapper to prevent contamination as shown:

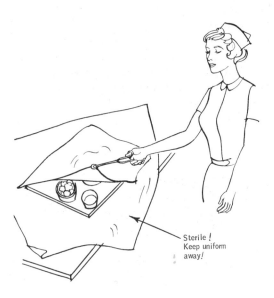

Sterile *!* Keep uniform away*!*

If a Sterile Tray Must Be Opened and Closed Before Taking It to the Patient's Room for Use. This is not considered good practice; however, an occasion may arise that makes it necessary. For example, the nurse may need to pour sterile cleansing solutions in the basins on a sterile catheterization tray before taking the tray to the patient's bedside. It is done like this:

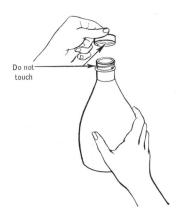

Do not touch

Pour the sterile solution into the basin. With the handling forceps place the towel covering back over the tray. Make certain that the disinfectant solution from the tip of the handling forceps does not drip on the tray or any part of the tray covering.

Replace the wrapper by touching only the outside layer. This is done by sliding the hand under the wrapper like this:

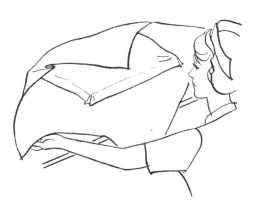

Setting Up a Tray Containing Sterile Articles in an Emergency Situation

Occasionally the nurse will be called upon to assemble several articles for a sterile procedure for which there is no routine sterile tray available. This practice should be avoided except for emergency situations.

Select a tray (unsterile) suitable in size. With handling forceps remove a sterile towel from an opened wrapper or can. (Sterile towels are kept on hand for this purpose.) Using two forceps, grasp two corners of the towel, and unfold until the towel remains folded in half. Place the towel, folded in half, on the unsterile tray like this:

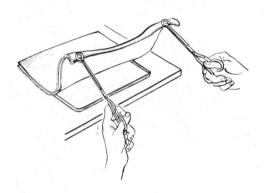

Do not allow the forceps to touch the tray. The towel should extend slightly over the edges of the tray. A double thickness of towel is necessary to filter out the particles of dust. If the tray is too large to be completely covered by a towel folded in half, two unfolded towels must be used.

Then with the forceps place the desired sterile articles on the towel, well in from the edges of the tray like this:

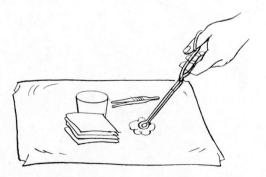

With two handling forceps unfold another towel, and place it, double thickness, over the sterile articles, making certain that the articles are completely covered. The tray may then be carried to the patient's bedside.

Assisting the Physician in Putting on Sterile Gloves

Touching only the outside surface, unfold the glove wrapper like this:

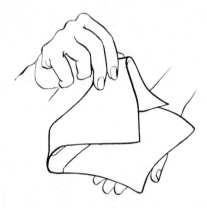

Shake the powder packet toward the center of the glove folder like this:

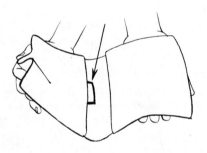

Hold the glove folder like this so that the physician can pick up the powder without touching the inside of the folder:

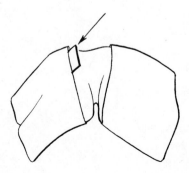

Hold open the pocket for one glove as shown:

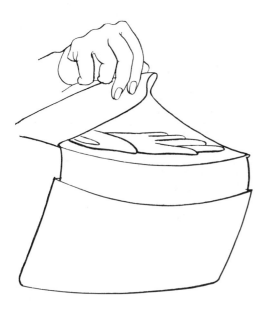

Then hold open the other pocket the same way.

Putting on Sterile Gloves. See page 103.

Warming Sterile Solutions

Place the bottle of solution in a basin of hot water like this:

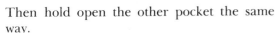

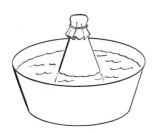

Make certain there is <u>not too much</u> water in the basin, as this will cause the bottle to tip over.

Using a Sterile Applicator to Apply Medication

Remove the applicator from its container with a handling forceps.

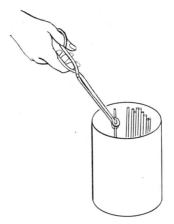

Insert the tip into the medication jar, being careful <u>not to touch</u> the applicator to the sides or the top of the jar.

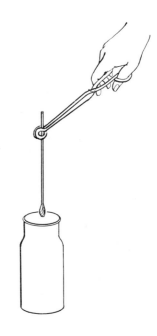

Hand the applicator, still grasping it with the handling forceps.

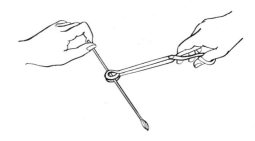

If you yourself are applying the medication with an applicator, you may touch the top of the applicator stick with the bare fingers after using the handling forceps to remove it from the sterile container.

Using Caustic Sticks

Caustic sticks are *not* sterile. Shake the caustic stick from the bottle like this so that the physician can grasp the wooden end:

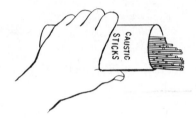

Caustic sticks are used only by the physician.

USE OF THE SURGICAL DRESSING CART

The surgical dressing cart is no longer recommended and has been abolished in most hospitals because of the danger of cross infection. The recommended procedures that have replaced the use of the dressing cart include the use of individually wrapped sterile packs such as suture-removal packs and dressing packs. Additional sterile supplies that are needed are wrapped individually, i.e., tongue blades, cotton applicators, drains, syringes, towels, gauze packing, safety pins, and instruments. Many of these items, including suture-removal packs, are commercially available, are prepackaged and sterilized, and are ready for use. The recommended procedure for changing a dressing, using a dressing pack, is discussed later in this chapter under "Changing Dressings."

It has been noted, however, that a few institutions still use the dressing cart. Since cross infections are almost always directly related to improper use of a surgical dressing cart, we feel obligated to include a discussion on the proper technique.

The instruments commonly found on a dressing cart are these:

The curved and straight hemostat

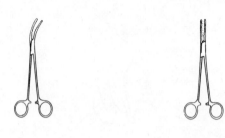

Handling forceps   Plain thumb forceps

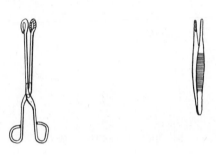

Rattooth thumb forceps   A probe

A groove director   A scalpel

Curved and straight surgical scissors

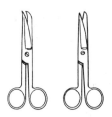

Supplies used frequently in changing dressings are kept on a dressing cart. The cart enables the nurse to locate quickly supplies needed by the physician and to transport them conveniently to the patient's bedside. The articles contained on the dressing cart vary with each institution; however, similar articles would serve the same purpose. Most dressing carts are supplied and arranged somewhat like the one shown below.

In order to use the dressing cart properly, the nurse should remember these points:

1. The dressing cart should be kept aseptically clean at all times.
2. The only parts of the cart which should be touched with contaminated hands or articles are the basin used as a receptacle for contaminated instruments and the bucket used as a receptacle for contaminated dressings.
3. When a number of dressings are changed, two carts should be used, one for sterile supplies and one for contaminated articles.
4. When possible, two individuals should use the dressing cart, one person to change the dressings on the patient and the other person to hand the supplies from the dressing cart.
5. The dressing cart should be cleaned and reset with clean sterile supplies every 24 hours.
6. The dressing cart should be used only for the purpose for which it is intended. It should not be used as a storage area for odds and ends.
7. Soiled equipment should be taken to the workroom after each dressing. Instruments are washed and sterilized. Soiled dressings are placed in covered disposal cans.
8. When using the dressing cart, always keep it at such a distance from the patient's bed as will prevent its becoming contaminated by bed linen. When a nurse changes dressings and has no one available to assist her

Surgical Dressing Cart

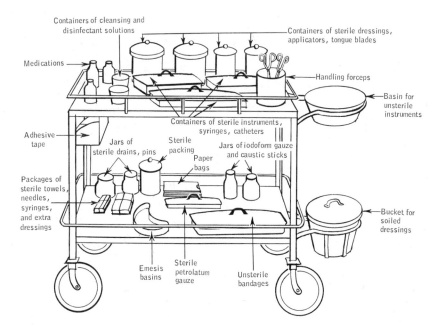

with the use of the dressing cart, she does it like this:

Remove the soiled dressings, and place them on several thicknesses of newspaper at the foot of the patient's bed as shown:

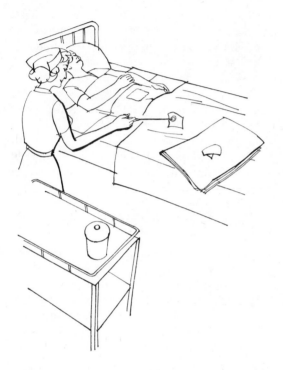

Soiled dressings should never be handled with bare fingers. Dressings, soiled or not, that touch a surgical wound should never be touched with the bare fingers.

Place the contaminated handling forceps used in removing dressings in the basin; then wash the hands thoroughly before touching containers or any other article on the dressing cart. Cleansing the surgical area and reapplying the sterile dressings can usually be accomplished without touching the patient or the patient's bedclothes with the bare hands. If it becomes necessary to touch the patient or the bedclothes with the fingers, this can usually be done with one hand. For instance, if the nurse is right-handed, she could allow her left hand to become contaminated and keep the right hand free of contamination. This would permit the use of the right hand for opening and closing containers and lifting sterile supplies with the handling forceps.

Make certain the lids are replaced on the containers on the dressing cart; then proceed to fasten the patient's dressings in place with whatever device is to be used. (If adhesive tape is used, this should be cut and placed on the side of the cart before beginning the procedure.) Both hands are now considered contaminated; therefore, do not touch a clean area on the dressing cart until after the hands are washed.

DRESSINGS

Some nurses have never acquired the knack of applying a neat-looking dressing that will remain in place. Because of this, dressings are dealt with in great detail in this book. Suggestions are given here on the general application of dressings. Additional details on the uses of dressings for specific disease conditions are given in Part Two. Dry sterile dressings are used to protect wounds from contamination and to absorb drainage.

Dressing Materials

Dressings may be made from a variety of materials, the selection depending on the preferences of the physician and/or the institution.

Dressings for Dry Surgical Wounds. These dressings may include gauze 3 × 3's, 3 × 6's, 4 × 4's, and 4 × 8's.

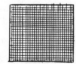

Steripak* is a nonadhering dressing available in 4 × 4's or 4 × 8's. It looks like this:

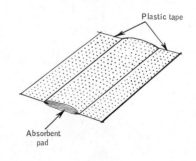

Plastic tape

Absorbent pad

*Trade name.

A spray-on dressing is available that is used by some surgeons. The dressing is sprayed over the incision in the operating room. When the spray comes in contact with the skin, it forms a transparent, waterproof protective film over the area. The incision is clearly visible through this film, and at first glance there appears to be no covering over the area. This dressing enables close observation of the incision. To remove the dressing, grasp it with a forceps and peel it from the skin like this:

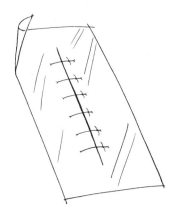

Dressings for Moderately Draining Wounds. This type of wound usually requires changing once daily. Dressings may include petrolatum gauze:

4 × 8 gauze:

or Adaptic.* Adaptic is a nonadhesive rayon fabric available in 3 × 8 and 3 × 16-inch sizes. The rayon strips are packaged in a sterile envelope like this:

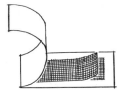

---

*Trade name.

Dressings for Profusely Draining Wounds. These require changing every few hours. For this type of dressing, several layers of gauze 4 × 8's or gauze fluffs as shown

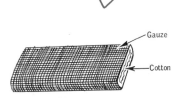

are placed over the wound and covered with absorbent pads, also called ABD pads, which look like this:

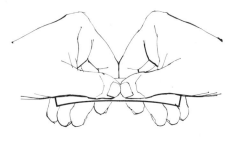

Gauze
Cotton

Materials Used to Hold Dressings in Place

Dressings are held in place with Scotch tape, plastic tape, adhesive tape, liquid adhesive, binders, or bandages.

How to Tear Adhesive. How many nurses know how to tear adhesive tape? It's easy when you know how. Grasp the adhesive as shown:

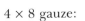

Note that the two index fingers are touching. Now, keeping the top of the adhesive in a straight line, pull it apart in opposite directions like this:

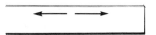

NOT like this:

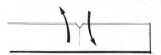

Montgomery Tapes. Adhesive straps, commonly referred to as Montgomery tapes, are used to secure dressings that must be changed frequently. Montgomery tapes are made by folding a strip of 1-inch adhesive like this:

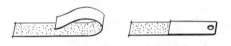

The tapes are either tied over the dressing like this:

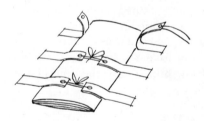

or they are secured by using broken applicator sticks and rubber bands like this:

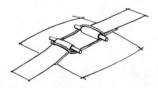

Montgomery tapes should be removed as soon as they are soiled.

Adhesive tape should not be placed on skin that is not shaved. Adhesive tape that is difficult to remove may be soaked with benzine or ether applied with a cotton ball like this:

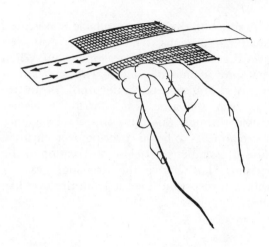

Never apply benzine or ether to irritated areas of the skin, as this will cause a severe burning sensation.

Elastic Tape. An elastic adhesive tape is available that offers advantages over the regular type adhesive tape from the standpoint of patient comfort and a reduction in skin irritations. Elastic adhesive tape is made of a cotton elastic cloth with an adhesive surface on one side. The elastic adhesive tape is recommended for applying dressings over areas of the body where motion in involved, such as joints.

Scotch tape and plastic tape may be used to secure small dressings anywhere on the body but are used mostly on the face for purposes of appearance. Scotch tape is transparent, and plastic tape is flesh-colored.

Liquid Adhesive. Liquid adhesive is a fairly recent development. It is a creamy white substance supplied in tubes. It is applied directly to the skin and is convenient for use in dressing small wounds located at areas difficult to bandage. Liquid adhesive is removed by gentle rubbing, which causes it to form small balls and fall off the skin. This shows a suitable method of applying a small dressing with liquid adhesive:

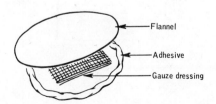

Bandages and Binders. Bandages and binders are used to hold dressings in place on areas where support is needed and where adhesive cannot be used. Bandages are made of gauze, muslin, flannel, woven elastic, and knitted cotton. Binders most commonly used are the straight, scultetus, and T binder, female and male, shown here:

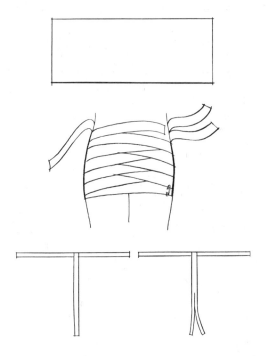

The straight binder and the scultetus binder are very seldom used as the sole means of holding a dressing in place. The T binder is used to hold dressings in place over the perineal area.

Some of the common errors made in securing dressings in place, with suggestions for correction are as follows:

1. Use of too narrow adhesive tape on large areas of the body.

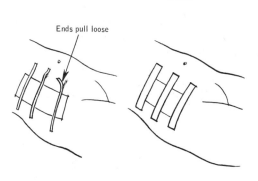

2. Length of adhesive either too short or too long.

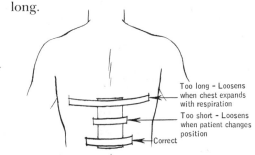

3. Improper spacing of adhesive tape.

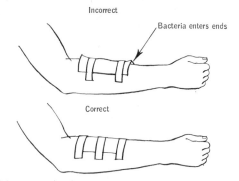

4. Adhesive tape running in wrong direction on motion areas of the body.

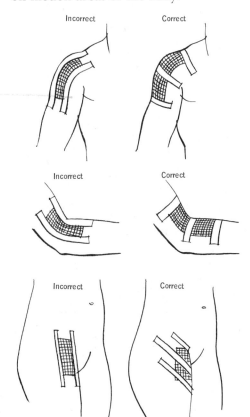

5. Insufficient amount of bandage applied loosely and improperly secured.

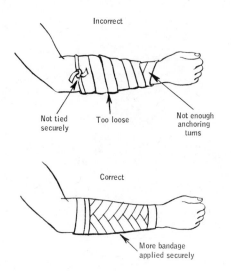

Incorrect

Not tied securely   Too loose   Not enough anchoring turns

Correct

More bandage applied securely

6. Binders improperly secured.

Changing Dressings

Most hospitals now use dressing trays or dressing packs to change dressings. The items found on the dressing tray vary with the institution and the type of wound. An aseptic technique is used for the procedure, and all items used are sterile with the exception of adhesive tape.

Before changing dressings on any type of wound, make certain there is a doctor's order to do so. Often dressings are not to be disturbed unless there is hemorrhage or excessive drainage. Sometimes, even with excessive drainage, the nurse may be asked to reinforce rather than change dressings. In other cases the physician makes the initial dressing change, then delegates the remaining changes to the nurse.

Changing Dressings on Nondraining Wounds.

To do this one needs the following basic items:
1. Sterile towel
2. Sterile cup to hold disinfectant solution
3. One or two sterile handling forceps
4. Four to six 1" × 1" sterile gauze squares or cotton balls to cleanse wound
5. Sterile dressing materials 3 × 3 or 3 × 6 gauze
6. Disinfectant solution such as 70 per cent alcohol
7. Adhesive tape

8. Paper bags
9. Paper towels

A dressing tray may include items 1 through 4 or items 1 through 5. Some institutions use commercially packaged dressings. In this case these would be carried separately.

Collect all the items required and proceed to the patient's room. If the nurse is assisting the doctor in suture removal and dressing changes on several patients, she would collect a dressing tray and a suture-removal tray for each patient and carry all the equipment on a cart. In the patient's room, remove all the items needed for the patient from the cart, and place them on the bedside table.

Open the dressing tray and fill the cup with disinfectant.

Place the jar of disinfectant solution on the bedside table; open a paper bag, folding the top down slightly so that it will remain upright on the bedside table.

Remove the soiled dressings. Adhesive tape is removed with short quick pulls; always pull toward the wound to prevent strain and pain on sutures:

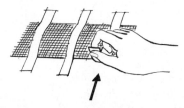

Remove the soiled dressings from the tray with a forceps (or with a disposable glove); place the soiled dressings (or disposable glove) in the paper bag. The forceps are not used for further handling of sterile dressings. Place the forceps on a paper towel on the bedside table.

Remove the second sterile forceps from the dressing tray; place the sterile towel (if used) across the patient as shown:

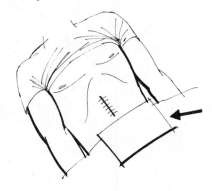

Be careful not to contaminate the forceps by touching the bed clothes. Next use the same forceps and cleanse the wound with small gauze squares saturated in disinfectant solution. Use each gauze square only once, then discard it in the soiled dressing bag. If sutures are to be removed, it is done at this point. Place the forceps on the sterile towel and proceed, opening the pack to assist the physician in suture removal. If no sutures are to be removed, use the forceps to remove sterile dressings from the tray and place them on the wounds. If individual packs of dressings are used, place the forceps on the sterile towel, and open the dressing pack with both hands; then use the forceps to remove the dressings from the pack and place them on the wound.

Secure the dressings in place. Place the soiled instrument and the cotton towel on the dressing tray. Twist shut the top of the paper bag containing soiled dressings, and discard it in the wastepaper can. Make the patient comfortable; then wash your hands and remove the flask of disinfectant and the used tray from the bedside.

Changing Dressings on Draining Wounds. The procedure and steps in handling the equipment are the same as for nondraining wounds. Draining wounds are cleansed with larger sponges, first with sterile water and then with a disinfecting solution that is nonirritating. Allow the skin to dry; then apply the clean sterile dressing. When the patient has a draining wound that requires frequent changes of dressings, all the necessary equipment is usually kept at the bedside.

BIBLIOGRAPHY

Suddarth, D. S.: Individual Dressing Packs. Am. J. Nurs., *60*:991, 1960.

9

Preoperative Procedures

The preparatory care of the operative patient includes psychological and physical preparation.

PSYCHOLOGICAL PREPARATION

The patient who is admitted to the hospital for elective surgery usually has been told by his physician several days or weeks prior to admission that surgery is necessary. During the waiting period before admission there is much time for the development of apprehension and fear. The nurse can do a great deal to alleviate the patient's fears by first evaluating what the patient already knows about his operation and whether his knowledge is correct, and by explaining in detail what series of events will take place during the preoperative, operative, and postoperative periods.

The psychological preparation for each patient varies somewhat because the needs of individuals vary, according to age, sex, family-group position, occupation, diagnosis, and so forth. However, there are specific points which may be applied to all patients. A patient usually wants to know:

1. Which procedure will be done and why?
2. What will be expected of him before, during, and after surgery?

3. Will he have pain after surgery, and what can be done about it if he does?
4. May he have visitors?
5. When and what can he eat? If intravenous fluids are to be given postoperatively, he should be told prior to surgery.
6. How long will he be in the operating room?
7. How long will he be incapacitated postoperatively? Will the operation be a success?
8. What type of anesthesia will be given, how will it be given, and what effect will it have on him? In most hospitals this is explained by the anesthesiologist, who visits the patient prior to surgery.

If the patient is to be transferred to another room after surgery, he should be told before going to surgery. If the postoperative regimen includes the use of special equipment such as that used with oxygen administration, a respirator, suction and drainage equipment, blow bottles, and so forth, the use and purpose of these should be explained and demonstrated, if necessary, preoperatively.

PHYSICAL PREPARATION

Preoperative procedures used in the physical preparation of the patient may be categorized according to the time during which they

128

are performed before surgery. Patients are usually admitted to the hospital one day prior to surgery. In certain types of major surgery and when the patient's physical condition must be improved for surgery, the patient may be admitted several days or weeks prior to surgery.

PREPARATIONS ON THE DAY OF ADMISSION

1. The physician conducts the physical examination with special attention to the heart, lungs, and kidneys.
2. Laboratory studies are made. The routine studies include a urinalysis, red and white blood cell count, hemoglobin determination, blood typing, test for syphilis, and chest x-ray.
3. A permit for surgery is signed by the patient on admission.
4. Physical symptoms and mental reactions are observed closely.
5. The intake of fluids is increased, and a nourishing diet is given.
6. Instructions are given to the patient regarding postoperative activities.
7. Attention is given to good personal hygiene.
8. The assurance of rest is important.

PREPARATIONS ON THE EVENING BEFORE

1. The skin is prepped.
2. A cleansing enema is given.
3. A sedative is administered.
4. The patient receives a light evening meal.
5. All food and oral fluids are omitted after midnight.

PREPARATIONS ON THE DAY OF SURGERY

1. Temperature, pulse, respiration and blood pressure are taken and recorded. Any deviation from normal must be reported.
2. The patient's valuables such as wrist watch and rings are put in a safe place. If the patient does not wish to remove her wedding band, it may be secured to the hand as shown later.
3. False teeth and prosthetic eyes are removed.
4. Cosmetics such as rouge, lipstick, and nail polish are removed so that cyanosis, if it occurs, may be recognized.

5. The bladder must be emptied just before the patient goes to the operating room. If the patient is unable to void, he must be catheterized.
6. The patient wears loose stockings and a hospital gown to the operating room. Patients with medium-long hair should wear a covering over their hair to keep it in place. Long hair on female patients should be braided.
7. The preoperative medication is administered. This should never be given until all other steps of the prep have been completed.

The schedule for preoperative preparation varies somewhat with surgery on different parts of the body and in emergency situations when the entire preparation must take place in a short time. These variations are discussed in Part II.

Few of the nursing techniques involved in preparing the patient for surgery are new. Details of the following procedures may be of concern to the nurse who is not familiar with the care of the surgical patient.

SKIN PREP

In many hospitals a team of nurses from the operating room is responsible for performing all the skin preps on the day before the scheduled surgery, in which case the nurse who works in the surgical department would be relieved from this responsibility except in emergency situations.

The tray setup for the surgical prep looks like this:

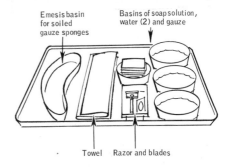

Emesis basin for soiled gauze sponges

Basins of soap solution, water (2) and gauze

Towel   Razor and blades

A disposable prep tray is also available from several companies. Each is similar in design and contains these items:

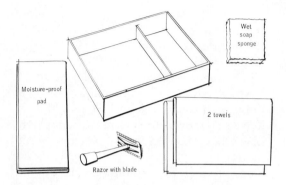

The tray is made of plastic and is used as a receptacle for the water used in cleansing the skin. In addition to the tray, a good light is an absolute necessity.

A soap solution is first applied to the area of skin to be shaved. If the area to be prepared is large, only a small portion should be moistened at a time.

Using a sharp razor, remove the hair by shaving with one hand while stretching the skin with the other. The razor is held at about a 30° angle to the skin as shown:

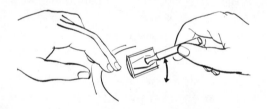

Using long, gentle strokes, pull the razor in the direction in which the hair grows. Repeatedly remove the excess hair from the razor.

The skin must be repeatedly inspected under direct light to make certain it is free of all hair. On areas where the hair is barely visible, inspect the skin by bending forward so that the eyes are on the same level as the skin as shown.

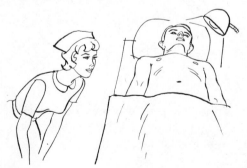

After the hair has been removed, the skin is cleansed with soap and/or an antiseptic solution. The use of pHisoHex (see p. 101) as a cleansing agent is becoming widely accepted. Vigorous rubbing should be avoided, since this may abrade the skin. Warm water is used to rinse the skin following the use of soap.

Applying Sterile Dressings to the Operative Site

Disinfection of the skin and the application of sterile dressings are usually not included in the preparation of the skin for general surgery. This procedure, however, is still widely used in the preparation for orthopedic surgery. When applying sterile dressings:

The skin is first shaved as described for the usual skin preparation; then the skin is cleansed using surgical aseptic precautions. Again the cleansing agent(s) vary with the institution. The gauze sponge used to apply the cleansing agent must be sterile. If water is used to rinse the area, it must be sterile. When applying the cleansing agent, start at the top and work downward using only three or four strokes with one gauze sponge. Each stroke should cover the entire width of the area being prepared, as shown here:

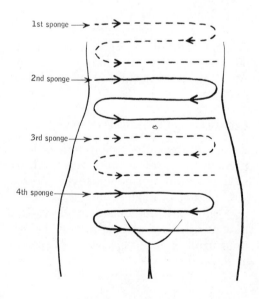

After the first three or four strokes, discard the gauze sponge and use a fresh sterile one for the next cleansing strokes. Cleanse the entire area in this manner. Never go back over the area just completed with the used sponge. If several cleansing agents are used, the entire area is cleansed with one agent before applying another.

A disinfecting agent is usually applied after the skin has been thoroughly cleansed. Alcohol 70 per cent, iodine, or Zephirin is commonly used as the disinfecting agent. The disinfecting agent is applied in the same manner previously described for applying the cleansing agent.

The area is then covered with sterile gauze.

Sterile towels are placed over the gauze and secured in place. The method used in securing the entire dressing in place requires some forethought and planning. In the first place, if one is not careful in applying the sterile towels, the sterile gauze will become displaced and contaminate part of the dressing. When applying the dressing, one should also keep in mind that the dressing is applied the day before surgery. Therefore, the dressing should not be too bulky, causing discomfort and preventing rest, and the dressing must be secured well enough that it does not become dislodged during the night. When several towels are needed, they should be overlapped a few inches. The overlapping edges may be held in place with small strips of adhesive or scotch tape as shown:

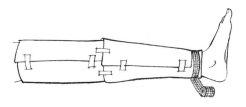

An expertly applied bandage seems to be the best method for securing the towels in place. When this type of preparation is done on the extremities, an assistant is needed to support the part. The assistant must support the limb at an area that will not interfere with the sterile technique.

Size of Skin Area to Be Prepared

The area of skin prepared is always much larger than the immediate area around the incision. Most physicians include specific instructions in the preoperative orders regarding the size of the area to be prepared. These are the sites usually prepared for specific types of surgery.

In abdominal surgery, the area includes the space between the nipple line and the upper thighs.

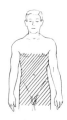

The area prepared for kidney operations is as shown:

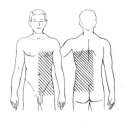

In thoracic surgery this area is prepared:

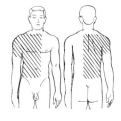

If a lateral incision is used in heart surgery, the same area is prepared. If a median sternotomy is used, the entire front of the chest must be prepared. Some heart surgeons prefer to have the entire trunk shaved, both front and back. If the heart machine is used for extracorporeal circulation during heart surgery, the cannula site must also be shaved (see p. 245).

For radical breast surgery, this area is shaved:

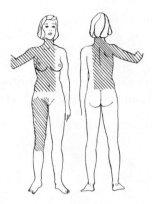

When a skin graft is contemplated in breast surgery, an area on the thigh is shaved as shown on the left.

The area for operations on the cervical spine is shown on the left and for operations on the thoracic spine (black) and lumbar spine (lined) on the right.

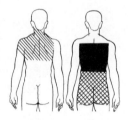

This shows the area prepped for an inguinal hernia,

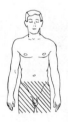

and this for rectal and perineal surgery.

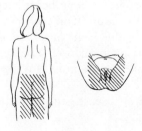

For an amputation of the foot, the area shaded in black is done, and for an amputation at the knee, the area in lines. The area on the arm shows that done for an amputation at the wrist.

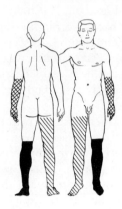

Cleansing the Umbilicus

In preparing the patient for surgery, special attention must usually be given the umbilicus. An ordinarily immaculate individual may have particles of dirt lodged within the umbilicus. Cotton swabs saturated in ether or hydrogen peroxide help to dislodge the dirt. Further cleaning may be done with cotton swabs saturated in soap solution.

Securing a Ring to the Hand

If the patient does not wish to remove the wedding band before going to surgery, it may be secured to the finger either with adhesive tape like this:

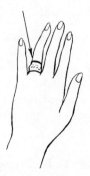

or with bandage like this:

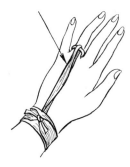

ADDITIONAL TECHNIQUES USED IN SPECIAL TYPES OF SURGERY

Gastrointestinal Surgery
1. Colonic irrigations (see Chap. 11)
2. Administration of systemic antibiotics
3. Gastric lavage (see Chap. 11)
4. Insertion of gastric tube (see Chap. 11)

Urological Surgery
1. Placement of indwelling catheter
2. Insertion of ureteral catheter (see Chap. 15)
3. Bladder irrigation (see Chap. 15)
4. Administration of systemic antibiotics

Gynecological Surgery
1. Antiseptic vaginal irrigations
2. Placement of indwelling catheter
3. Insertion of vaginal suppositories

Eye Surgery
1. Eye irrigations (see p. 336)
2. Instillation of eye drops (see p. 335)
3. Eyelashes trimmed short
4. Close observation for atropine toxicity when atropine dye instillations are used

5. Special adaptations of procedures for blindness
6. Use of eye shields (see p. 339)

Cardiac Surgery
1. Administration of diuretics and digitalis
2. Patient usually on complete bed rest
3. Application of elastic bandages to extremities (see p. 245)

PREANESTHETIC MEDICATIONS

1. Atropine—given subcutaneously about 20 minutes before the administration of anesthesia to inhibit secretions in the mouth and air passage.
2. Scopolamine—used to take the place of atropine. Produces a sense of well-being in addition to drying secretions.
3. Demerol—a synthetic drug with the same effects as the opiates. A depressant given to quiet the patient and allay fears.
4. Morphine—an opiate, also used to quiet the patient and allay fears.
5. Chlorpromazine, mepazine, and other synthetic tranquilizers—given to quiet the patient. These are given intramuscularly.

BIBLIOGRAPHY

Bird, B.: Psychological Aspects of Preoperative and Postoperative Care. Am. J. Nurs. 55:685, 1955.

Davis, L.: Christopher's Textbook of Surgery. 9th ed. Philadelphia, W. B. Saunders Co., 1968.

Harmer, B., and Henderson, V.: Textbook of the Principles and Practice of Nursing. 5th ed. New York, The Macmillan Co., 1958. (Chapter 38.)

Montag, M. L., and Swenson, R. P. S.: Fundamentals in Nursing Care. 3rd ed. Philadelphia, W. B. Saunders Co., 1959. (Chapter 24.)

Postoperative Procedures

After the patient has been taken to the operating room, the nurse prepares the patient's unit for his return. The equipment needed in preparing the unit depends upon the type of surgery and the hospital routines and facilities. Most hospitals now have a unit to which the patient is transferred immediately following surgery. The patient is kept in this unit and observed until fully recovered from anesthesia. This unit is commonly called the recovery room. The recovery room is usually located near the operating room suite and is equipped with all the necessary articles used in administering to the needs of the postoperative patient in all types of surgery and postanesthesia emergencies. Immediately at hand in the recovery room are oxygen equipment, suction apparatus, mouth gag, tongue forceps, artificial airway, blood pressure apparatus, sterile supplies, drugs and solutions, linen and utensils. Emergency equipment includes tracheotomy and phlebotomy sets, instruments for open-chest cardiac massage, an electric cardiac defibrillator, a heart pacemaker, and a respirator.

In institutions with no recovery room, the nurse should know where to locate articles that may be needed in postoperative emergencies. Equipment needed for the immediate postoperative care of the patient is placed on the patient's bedside table.

The patient's bed is prepared for his return as shown:

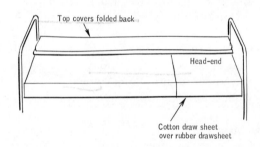

Top covers folded back

Head-end

Cotton draw sheet
over rubber drawsheet

In some institutions there is a standard doctor's postoperative order sheet for the surgeon's convenience in writing the postoperative orders. The sheet may look like this:

POSTOPERATIVE ORDER SHEET

1. Check vital signs q. 15 min. × 4 then
                q. ½ hr. until stable then
                q. 2 hrs. × 24 hrs.
2. Position of patient: _____ Trendelenburg; _____ flat; _____ semi-Fowler's.
3. Hemoglobin stat. and in A.M.
4. Turn, cough, hyperventilate q. 2 hrs. × 24 then q. 4 hr. until up.
5. Oral suction p.r.n.
6. Continuous gastric suction. Check p.r.n. at least q. 2 hr., and irrigate p.r.n. with _____ solution.

7. Connect drainage to catheter. Irrigate p.r.n. with
_____

8. Urine to laboratory daily for chlorides until gastric tube is removed.
9. Chart specific gravity of urine b.i.d. 8-6.
10. Weigh daily.
11. Sedation. Morphine sulfate gr. _____ q._____ h.
        p.r.n. for pain.
        Codeine sulfate gr._____ q._____ h.
        p.r.n. for pain.
        Demerol _____ mg. q. _____ h.
        p.r.n. for pain.
        Methadon _____ mg. q. _____ h.
        p.r.n. for pain.
        Other _____
12. Penicillin _____ U q. _____ h.
        Streptomycin _____ Gm. q._____ h.
        Aureomycin _____ mg. q._____ h.
        Other: _____
13. Fluid order: ADD:
    _____ cc. 5% glucose in distilled water
    _____ cc. 5% glucose in normal saline
    _____ cc. 10% glucose in distilled water
    _____ cc. 10% glucose in normal saline
    Transfuse _____ cc. whole blood
    _____ cc. plasma
14. Privileges: _____
15. Diet: _____
16. Chest x-ray stat.
17. Oxygen therapy: _____ tent _____ nasal:
    _____ Liters
18. A.M. Fluid order

Postoperative nursing care centers upon the prevention of postoperative discomforts and complications and the rehabilitation of the patient. The methods of accomplishing these objectives are begun when the patient is transferred from the operating room to the recovery room or other designated patient unit. Because most institutions have adopted the use of the recovery room, the nursing techniques employed in postoperative care will be classified according to (1) those applied while the patient is recovering from anesthesia and (2) those applied after the patient has fully recovered from anesthesia. In this chapter only those procedures which apply to general surgery are discussed. Procedures which apply to specific types of surgery are discussed in detail in Part II.

DURING RECOVERY FROM ANESTHESIA

The objectives of nursing care during this period and the methods used in accomplishing these objectives are as follows:

MAINTAINING AN OPEN AIRWAY

The airway is kept open by the use of artificial airways, proper positioning of the patient, suctioning secretions from the throat as necessary, changing the patient's position as necessary, and close observation for nausea and vomiting and supervision during vomiting.

Artificial Airways

An airway is inserted in the patient's mouth before or after going into the recovery room. The airway holds the patient's tongue forward and ensures unobstructed breathing through the hollow opening. Airways are made of plastic, hard or soft rubber, and metal. This shows an airway in place:

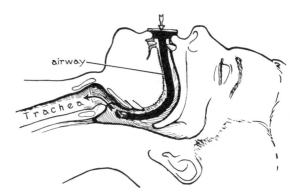

The airway is removed when the patient begins to gag or push the airway out with his tongue. This indicates the return of the swallowing reflex.

If an artificial airway is not in place and the air passage becomes obstructed from the tongue falling back into the pharynx, the nurse can open the patient's mouth. First locate the angle of the jawbone,

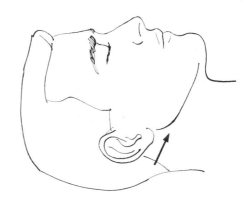

then press forward on the angle of the jaw-bone and down on the chin like this.

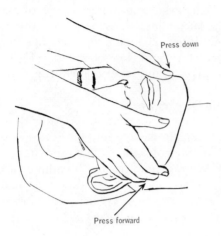

A mouth wedge may be needed to help force the patient's teeth apart and to hold the teeth apart temporarily for suctioning the throat. The mouth wedge may be made from tongue blades as shown:

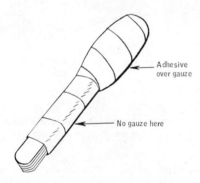

In some instances it may be necessary to pull the patient's tongue forward. To do this, grasp the tongue with gauze-covered fingers like this:

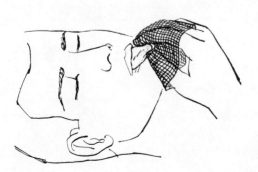

Proper Position of the Patient

Under ordinary circumstances the patient should be placed on his side, as shown, to prevent aspiration of secretions.

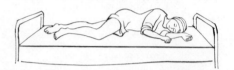

If the side-lying position is contraindicated, as in some types of surgery, the patient should be placed on his back with the head turned to one side as shown.

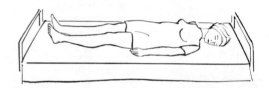

To Suction Secretions from the Throat

Until the patient's swallowing reflex has returned, secretions should be suctioned from the throat as necessary. A whistle-tip catheter connected to an electric or wall suction apparatus is inserted into the throat through the mouth. One type of wall suction apparatus looks like this:

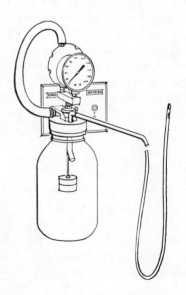

If the mouth cannot be opened, the catheter must be inserted through the nostril. When inserting the catheter through the nostril, pinch the catheter as shown during insertion and removal to prevent damage to the mucous lining.

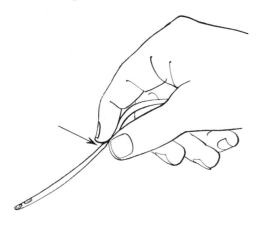

PREVENTING THE PATIENT FROM FALLING OUT OF BED

The patient is protected from falling out of bed by bedsides and close observation. The anesthetized patient should never be left alone.

Use of Bedsides. If the patient returns to his own room from the operating room, bedsides should be placed on his bed. The type of bed used in the recovery room is equipped with bedsides like the one shown here:

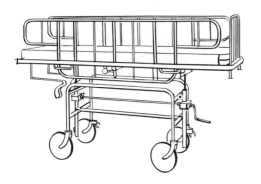

ADDITIONAL PROCEDURES

Additional aspects of the care given during the immediate postoperative period are outlined here:

Relief of Pain
1. Use of analgesics such as morphine, codeine, Demerol, and Methadon
2. Careful handling of patient
3. Avoid noise and confusion
4. Frequent change of position and proper positioning
5. Correct anchorage of drainage tubing

Observation for Shock and Hemorrhage
1. Observe and record vital signs every fifteen minutes until otherwise directed
2. Frequently observe dressings for hemorrhage
3. Observe vomitus and drainage for presence of blood

Attention to Fluid and Electrolyte Balance
1. Record intake and output
2. Administration of intravenous fluids as ordered (see Chap. 6)

Attention to Personal Hygiene
1. Change linen and gown as necessary
2. Wipe secretions and perspiration from face

Observance for Signs of Awakening
1. Involuntary motion, swallowing, blinking, and response to painful stimuli precede a return to consciousness.
2. A patient is not fully conscious until he responds to his name, answers questions correctly, and performs coordinated movements in response to definite requests.

Record Maintenance
Keep an adequate up-to-the-minute record of the observations made and the nursing care and treatments performed.

Recovery from anesthesia is considered complete when the patient is fully conscious. If there is no special problem demanding intensive care, the patient is discharged from the recovery room when he is fully conscious. The decision to return the patient to his room is made by the surgeon or his assistants or by the anesthesiologist.

AFTER RECOVERY FROM ANESTHESIA

Many of the aspects of nursing care during recovery from anesthesia are carried over into the period following recovery from anesthesia. The attentions of the nurse during this period are outlined here:

Relief of Pain
1. Use of analgesics as needed, usually for 48 hours postoperatively. Analgesics should be given only when the patient's discomfort cannot be relieved by other nursing methods.
2. Use of other nursing measures as mentioned in the previous topic.

Attention to Personal Hygiene
1. A cleansing bath is given shortly after the patient fully recovers from anesthesia. At this time a clean hospital gown is placed on the patient, and bed linens are changed as necessary.
2. Oral hygiene is important because the mouth feels dry and because nothing may be permitted orally for several hours. When mouth care is not given, the tongue and mucous membranes become irritated, and parotitis may occur. Teeth should be brushed several times daily, and the patient's mouth rinsed with mouthwash. If the patient is allowed nothing by mouth for an extended period of time, special mouth care (see p. 159) is given every hour.
3. Assistance with hygienic needs is usually required several days postoperatively.

Observation for Shock and Hemorrhage
Observation for symptoms, especially those of hemorrhage, should be made frequently during the first 24-hour period.

Aiding the Gastrointestinal Tract in Returning to Normal
1. Methods used to relieve nausea and vomiting are: (1) instruct the patient to breathe deeply; (2) instruct the patient to lie still for a short while; (3) when moving the patient, move him slowly. Nausea and vomiting persisting more than several hours after the patient has recovered from anesthesia should be reported to the physician. Sometimes medications such as Dramamine and chlorpromazine are administered.
2. Water may usually be given as soon as nausea and vomiting cease. Tea or bouillon may be allowed before water.
3. Milk, cocoa, and orange juice should be avoided for the first day because they cause gas.
4. The diet is prescribed by the physician in accordance with the type of surgery and the condition of the patient.
5. Some physicians prescribe a laxative or enema to promote defecation. A normal defecation indicates that the gastrointestinal tract has returned to normal.
6. For relief of gas pains, (a) instruct the patient not to swallow air, especially while drinking; (b) eliminate gas-forming foods from the diet; (c) instruct the patient to move about in bed and/or get the patient out of bed; and (d) with the doctor's permission, insert a rectal tube. A rectal tube is prepared for use as a flatus tube as shown here:

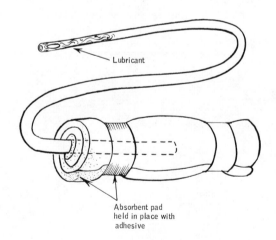

Lubricant

Absorbent pad held in place with adhesive

The surgeon may prescribe medications such as Pitressin, surgical Pituitrin, Urecholine, and

Prostigmine, which stimulate contraction of the intestines.

Prevention of Respiratory Complications

1. Change the patient's position at least every 2 hours.
2. Assist the patient with deep breathing exercises. One or more of the following methods to produce deep breathing may be used, depending upon the surgeon's preference:
   a. Instruct the patient to inhale deeply, then cough several times. It may be necessary for the nurse to hold the patient's incision during this procedure, since coughing causes pain in the incision. The patient should be informed as to the value of this exercise so that he will cooperate in coughing as deeply as possible.
   b. Instruct the patient to inhale and exhale 10 to 15 times into a paper bag held over his face as shown:

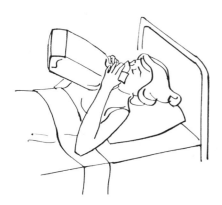

   The accumulation of carbon dioxide within the paper bag stimulates deep breathing. This exercise is usually done every 1 to 2 hours.
   c. Carbon dioxide inhalations may be used (see p. 53).
   d. The physician may order the blow bottle to be used every 1 to 2 hours. The patient is instructed to blow into the bottle with enough force to create bubbles in it. A blow bottle is made like this:

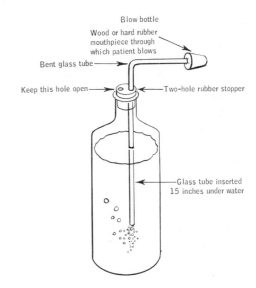

Blow bottle

Wood or hard rubber mouthpiece through which patient blows

Bent glass tube

Keep this hole open

Two-hole rubber stopper

Glass tube inserted 15 inches under water

Prevention of Circulatory Complications

1. Early ambulation.
2. Instruct the patient to flex and extend both arms and legs several times every hour while in bed.

Attention to Urinary Output

1. An accurate record of intake and output, at least for 24 hours postoperatively.
2. If the patient does not void 200 to 400 cc. within 6 to 8 hours postoperatively, this should be reported to the physician.
3. An order for catheterization may be written if the patient does not void within 6 to 8 hours postoperatively.
4. Drugs such as Doryl and Urecholine may be prescribed to help the patient void.
5. Observations should be made for symptoms of retention with overflow (voiding small amounts frequently).

VARIATIONS OF POSTOPERATIVE CARE WITH DIFFERENT TYPES OF ANESTHESIA

Spinal Anesthesia

1. Avoid unnecessary pressure on legs and toes.
2. Time of motor and sensory return is noted.

3. Keep patient flat in bed with a small pillow until directed otherwise.

Cyclopropane
1. Degrees of restlessness more pronounced.
2. Small amount of nausea and vomiting.

Vinyl Ether, Nitrous Oxide, and Ethylene
Used for short surgical procedures—recovery rapid.

Ether
Nausea and vomiting common.

Ethyl Chloride
Nausea and vomiting uncommon.

BIBLIOGRAPHY

Barker, H. G.: Supplementation of Protein and Caloric Needs in the Surgical Patient. Am. J. Clin. Nutrition, 3:466, 1955.

Bird, B.: Psychological Aspects of Preoperative and Post-operative Care. Am. J. Nurs. 55:685, 1955.

Bland, J. H.: Disturbances of Body Fluids. Philadelphia, W. B. Saunders Co., 1956.

Davis, L.: Christopher's Textbook of Surgery. 9th ed. Philadelphia, W. B. Saunders Co., 1968.

Harmer, B., and Henderson, V.: Textbook of the Principles and Practices of Nursing. 5th ed. New York, The Macmillan Co., 1958. (Chapter 39.)

Hosler, R. M.: Cardiac Resuscitation. Am. J. Nurs. 54:841, 1954.

Maddock, W. G.: Gastrointestinal Distention. Am. J. Nurs., 56:893, 1956.

Sadove, M. S., and Cross, J. H.: The Recovery Room. Philadelphia, W. B. Saunders Co., 1956.

PART TWO

Specific Nursing Techniques

11

Diseases of the Digestive System

DIAGNOSTIC PROCEDURES

X-RAY EXAMINATIONS

Gastrointestinal Series (G.I. Series)

Description. In the x-ray department the patient is given barium sulfate to drink. Fluoroscopic studies are made while the barium passes from the esophagus into the stomach. Several x-ray pictures are taken during this time. An x-ray picture is taken six hours after the administration of the barium. Sometimes an x-ray picture is also taken 24 hours after the administration of the barium. The barium, an opaque substance, outlines the gastrointestinal tract on the x-ray picture.

Preparation of Patient

1. Nothing by mouth after midnight. **NPO**
2. Allow nothing by mouth until after the 6-hour pictures have been taken.
3. An enema or cathartic may be ordered after the 6-hour picture has been taken.
4. If 24-hour pictures are ordered, do not

142

give a cathartic or laxative until after they have been taken.

Barium Enema or Colon Series

Description. The patient is given an enema of barium solution while under the fluoroscope. X-ray pictures are taken as indicated. The patient expels the enema before leaving the x-ray department.

Preparation of Patient

1. A cathartic, usually 2 fluid ounces of castor oil, is given between 2 and 6 P.M. the day before. Castor oil may be mixed with a glass of orange juice and a pinch of bicarbonate of soda.
2. A clear liquid diet may be ordered for the evening meal the day before and for breakfast the day of the studies.
3. Cleansing enemas until the return flow is clear are usually ordered to be given in the morning. "Until the return flow is clear" means that enemas should be given until there is no *solid* fecal matter expelled in the enema solution. For best results in giving enemas until the return flow is clear, the solution should be administered while the patient is in the position shown:

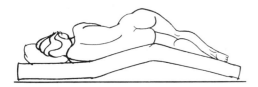

The temperature of the solution should not be less than 105° F., as the patient cannot retain water that is too cool. Around 500 cc. of solution should be administered and retained for at least ten minutes.
4. Some physicians order a cathartic to be given following the barium enema.

Cholecystogram or Gallbladder Series

Description. A drug that outlines the gallbladder is administered to the patient either orally or intravenously. An x-ray picture is taken; then a high-fat-content meal (i.e., buttered toast or cream) is given. Another picture is taken 15 minutes, 30 minutes, and 1 or 2 hours after the fatty meal until maximal emptying of the gallbladder is seen and until best visualization of the common duct is obtained.

Preparation of Patient

1. On the day before the examination, a light, fat-free meal is given at 6:00 P.M.
2. If an oral dye is used, it is administered following the meal. The drugs presently used are Telepaque, Teridax, Monophen, and Priodax. All these drugs depend upon their iodine content for visualization of the gallbladder. The tablets should be taken one at a time with several glasses of water. The oral dye must be taken 12 to 14 hours before the first x-ray examination of the gallbladder.
3. Nothing is allowed by mouth after the dye is administered until after the first x-ray examination the next morning.
4. A cleansing enema may be ordered in the morning before the examination.
5. If an intravenous dye is used, it is administered two to four hours prior to the first x-ray picture. Intravenous Cholografin is the drug most commonly used. This drug is usually administered in the x-ray department.
6. The patient may return to his room for the fatty meal with instructions stating the time he is to return to the x-ray department for the remaining pictures. In most institutions the patient remains in the x-ray department for the entire examination procedure, including the administration of the fatty meal.

Cholangiogram (Bile Duct Visualization)

Description. An opaque substance (Urokon) is injected into the bile ducts through a tube surgically placed in the bile duct. An x-ray picture is taken to outline the bile ducts. This procedure may be used either during or after surgery to aid the physician in further surgical procedures.

Preparation of Patient. None.

GASTROENTEROSCOPIC EXAMINATIONS

Gastroscopy

Description. The interior stomach is inspected by the physician through an instrument (gastroscope) inserted in the stomach through the esophagus.

Preparation of Patient

1. The patient is allowed nothing by mouth 8 hours prior to the examination.
2. Drugs such as atropine sulfate and sodium phenobarbital may be given ½ hour prior to the examination.
3. Depending upon the patient's probable diagnosis, a gastric lavage may be ordered before the gastroscopic examination. For techniques used in the gastric lavage, see page 168.
4. The patient is taken to a special examination room for the gastroscopy. In the examination room a rubber gastric tube is placed in the stomach, and the secretions are drained from the stomach with the patient in the position shown.

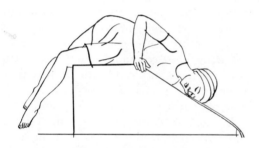

A local anesthetic is sprayed on the pharynx before insertion of the gastroscope.

5. When the patient returns to his room following the gastroscopic examination, he is allowed nothing by mouth for several hours because of the danger of aspirating food or fluid into the trachea before the anesthesia has worn off.

Sigmoidoscopy

Description. The sigmoid is inspected by the physician through a hollow lighted instrument inserted into the large intestine through the anus.

Preparation of Patient

1. A laxative is given the evening before the examination.
2. Liquids only are allowed for breakfast.
3. Enemas, until the return flow is clear, are given shortly before the patient is taken to the examination room.

4. For best results with enemas, see step 3 under the discussion of the preparation of the patient for a barium enema, page 143.

Proctoscopy

Description. The rectum is inspected by the physician through a hollow lighted instrument inserted through the anus.

Preparation of Patient. Same as for sigmoidoscopy.

Esophagoscopy

Description. The interior esophagus is inspected by the physician through a hollow lighted instrument.

Preparation of Patient

1. Nothing by mouth for 6 to 8 hours prior to the examination. Clear liquids are allowed for breakfast if the examination is done in the afternoon.
2. Drugs such as atropine sulfate and sodium phenobarbital may be given ½ hour prior to the examination.
3. Depending upon the probable diagnosis, a gastric lavage may be ordered before the examination. For technique used in the lavage, see page 168.
4. The patient is taken to a special examination room for the examination. A local anesthetic is sprayed on the pharynx before the insertion of the esophagoscope.
5. When the patient returns to his room following the examinations, he is allowed nothing by mouth for several hours because of the danger of aspirating food or fluid into the trachea before the anesthesia has worn off.

Peritoneoscopy

Description. The peritoneal cavity is inspected through a hollow lighted instrument (peritoneoscope) introduced into the cavity through a tiny incision in the skin.

Preparation of Patient

1. Nothing by mouth for 6 to 8 hours prior to the examination.
2. Drugs such as Demerol and Nembutal may be given one half hour prior to the examination.
3. An abdominal skin prep is done as for surgery.

4. Prothrombin time is taken.
5. The patient is taken to a special examination room for the procedure.
6. Following the peritoneoscopy, pulse and blood pressure are checked every two hours for 12 to 18 hours.

LIVER STUDIES

TESTS FOR ALTERATIONS IN SERUM PROTEINS

The following are tests used for the detection of alterations in the serum proteins as a manifestation of functional liver damage:

Determination of Serum Albumin and Globulins (A and G ratio)

Description. Ten cubic centimeters of blood is withdrawn from the patient. The serum is examined for albumin and globulin content. The normal is 1.5:1 (1.5 gm. of albumin to 1 gm. of globulin). In liver disease the globulin content is higher than the albumin content.

Preparation of Patient. Withhold breakfast.

Cephalin-Cholesterol Flocculation Test (Hanger's Test)

Description. Whole blood is withdrawn, and the serum is tested with a cephalin-cholesterol mixture for the amount of precipitation. Readings are made at 24- and 48-hour periods. Normally no precipitation should be present.

Preparation of Patient. Withhold breakfast.

Thymol Turbidity Test

Description. Whole blood is withdrawn, and the serum is tested with a thymol solution. The reaction is calibrated in degrees of cloudiness (turbidity). Patients with liver damage usually have turbidity readings above 4 units. Normal values vary from 0 to 4 units.

Preparation of Patient. Withhold breakfast.

Thymol Flocculation Test

Description. This is simply an extension of the thymol turbidity test. The specimen is allowed to stand overnight, and the degree of flocculation is noted in 0 to ++++ readings. Normal: negative or 1+.

Preparation of Patient. Withhold breakfast.

Zinc Turbidity Test

Description. Whole blood is withdrawn, and serum is tested for antibody formation. This test is used mainly in determining the course of infectious hepatitis. Normal values are 4 to 12 units.

Preparation of Patient. Withhold breakfast.

Transaminase Level in the Serum
GOT or SGOT

Description. The enzyme glutamic oxalacetic transaminase is present in large amounts in the heart, liver, muscles, and kidneys, and serum levels are increased whenever acute destruction of one of these organs occurs. The enzyme level increases in cardiac infarction and liver necrosis. Normal: 1 to 40 units; liver necrosis: 50 to 1000 units.

Preparation of Patient. Withhold breakfast.

GPT or SGPT

Description. The enzyme glutamic pyruvic transaminase is present in many tissues and, although the absolute amounts are less than those of GOT, there is a greater concentration of it in the liver than in the heart and muscles. SGPT elevations are more specific of liver cell damage than SGOT elevations. Normal: 5 to 35 units; liver disease: 20 to 500 times normal.

Preparation of Patient. Withhold breakfast.

TESTS FOR DISORDERS OF METABOLIC FUNCTION

Tests used for the detection of disorders of the metabolic functions of the liver are as follows:

Hippuric Acid Test

Description. The findings of this test are based on the fact that benzoic acid and aminoacetic acid are synthesized in the liver and excreted in the urine in the form of hippuric acid. A low output of hippuric acid occurs in some forms of hepatitis, carcinoma, and cirrhosis. Normal output of hippuric acid should be about 3 gm. in 4 hours.

Preparation of Patient

1. A light breakfast of toast and coffee is given.

2. One hour later the patient is requested to void. Discard this urine.
3. Sodium benzoate is administered either orally or intravenously. If administered orally, the drug is mixed with an ounce of water and flavored with a few drops of peppermint. One half a glass of water is given following the oral administration. If administered intravenously, the drug is dissolved in 20 cc. distilled water and must be given over a period of 8 minutes.
4. Request the patient to void immediately following the administration of the drug. Discard this specimen.
5. One hour later collect another urine specimen. In the intravenous method this is the only specimen collected and sent to the lab. If the patient cannot void, an order should be secured for catheterization.
6. In the oral method a urine specimen is collected every hour for 4 hours. Each specimen, including the fourth, is sent to the laboratory.

Urobilinogen Excretion in the Urine

Description. Urine is examined for the amount of urobilinogen present. In liver disease the amount is increased.

Preparation of Patient. None, other than to obtain a specimen of freshly voided urine.

Galactose Tolerance Test

Description. This test depends upon the ability of the liver to assimilate simple sugar and convert it into glycogen. Galactose is administered to the patient, and either the blood or urine is tested for the amount of sugar present. Abnormally high amounts of sugar present in the blood or urine indicate liver damage.

Preparation of Patient for Oral Method
1. Nothing by mouth after midnight.
2. Omit breakfast.
3. Collect a urine specimen.
4. Give the patient 40 gm. of pure galactose in 500 cc. of water flavored with lemon juice.
5. Collect a urine specimen every hour for 5 hours. Send all six urine specimens to the laboratory.
6. During the test the patient may drink water but should not take food.

Preparation of Patient for Intravenous Method
1. Nothing by mouth after midnight.

2. Omit breakfast.
3. The doctor withdraws blood from the patient and places it in an oxylated tube.
4. A prescribed amount of a 50 per cent solution of galactose is injected intravenously.
5. Seventy-five minutes later another sample of blood is withdrawn.

Cholesterol Esters in the Serum
(plasma cholesterol)

Description. In hepatic disease the cholesterol esters tend to disappear from the blood regardless of whether the total cholesterol is increased or decreased. Normally cholesterol esters should constitute 60 to 75 per cent of the total cholesterol count. The total cholesterol count is normally 160-270 mg., and the cholesterol ester count is 100-180 mg. per 100 ml. of blood.

Preparation of Patient. Withhold breakfast.

Prothrombin Content of the Blood
(prothrombin time)

Description. Blood is withdrawn, and the plasma is tested for prothrombin content. The prothrombin time is normally 14 to 18 seconds. In liver damage the prothrombin time is prolonged.

Preparation of Patient. None.

Blood Ammonia

Description. About 5 cc. of blood is withdrawn and tested for ammonia content. Blood normally contains 75 micrograms of ammonia per 100 ml. In liver damage the content is increased.

Preparation of Patient. Withhold breakfast.

TESTS FOR DEGREE OF IMPAIRMENT OF EXCRETORY FUNCTION

The following tests are used to determine the degree of impairment of the excretory function of the liver:

Serum Bilirubin (also called van den Bergh's test)

Description. Ten cubic centimeters of blood is withdrawn, and the serum is examined for the bilirubin content. Three readings are usually requested: the total, direct, and indirect reactions. Normally the total reaction is 0.1-0.8 mg. per 100 ml. liters of blood.

Preparation of Patient. Omit breakfast.

Bromsulphalein Excretion Test (BSP Test, Rosenthal's Test)

Description. There are several methods of doing this test, Rosenthal's method being one of them. In all methods the dye, Bromsulphalein, is injected intravenously; then blood is withdrawn to determine the amount of dye that has not been utilized by the liver and remains in the blood. When 5 mg. of dye for each kilogram of body weight is injected, not more than 5 per cent of the dye should remain in the blood one hour later.

Preparation of Patient

1. Weigh patient.
2. Doctor calculates amount of dye and administers it intravenously. In one method the dye is given diluted.
3. The physician withdraws 5 cc. of blood from the other arm. A *dry* syringe, needle, and test tube must be used. Blood is withdrawn one hour after the administration of the dye. Samples of blood may also be drawn at 15- and 30-minute intervals following the administration, depending upon the amount of dye given and the condition of the patient.

Alkaline Phosphatase in the Serum

Description. Ten cubic centimeters clotted blood is used to determine the alkaline phosphatase level in the serum. Alkaline phosphatase is increased in cases of biliary obstruction. Normal amounts of alkaline phosphatase per 100 ml. are: 1-4 units (Bodansky method), 8-14 units (King-Armstrong method).

Preparation of Patient. Withhold breakfast.

Total Serum Cholesterol

Description. Total cholesterol levels are sometimes increased when there are lesions involving the smaller bile ducts. For further explanation see description of cholesterol esters on page 146.

Preparation of Patient. Withhold breakfast.

Liver Biopsy

Most diseases of the liver cause uniform changes throughout the organ. Because of this a needle liver biopsy may be helpful in diagnosing liver disease.

Description. A special liver biopsy needle is inserted through the skin, either in the subcostal or intercostal area, and a small sample of liver tissue is obtained. A liver biopsy may be obtained during the peritoneoscopic examination (see p. 144).

Preparation of Patient

1. Bleeding and clotting time and prothrombin time are determined before the biopsy because patients with liver disease frequently have a bleeding tendency.
2. Food and fluids are withheld if general anesthesia is used.
3. A mild sedative is administered about ½ hour prior to the time of the biopsy.
4. If the peritoneoscope is used, the patient will be taken to a special examination room for the biopsy. If local anesthesia is to be used, the biopsy may be done at the patient's bedside. In this event the nurse is responsible for setting up the necessary equipment as shown:

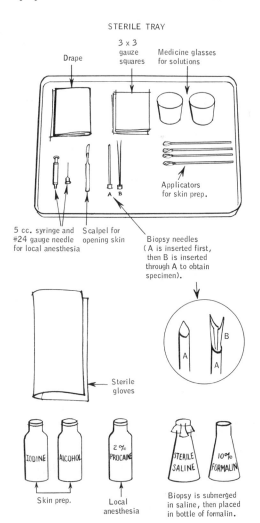

STERILE TRAY

Drape

3 x 3 gauze squares

Medicine glasses for solutions

Applicators for skin prep.

5 cc. syringe and #24 gauge needle for local anesthesia

Scalpel for opening skin

Biopsy needles (A is inserted first, then B is inserted through A to obtain specimen).

Sterile gloves

IODINE · ALCOHOL · 2% PROCAINE · STERILE SALINE · 10% FORMALIN

Skin prep.

Local anesthesia

Biopsy is submerged in saline, then placed in bottle of formalin.

5. Following the procedure to obtain the biopsy, the patient must be observed closely for signs of internal hemorrhage. Blood pressure and pulse must be checked frequently for 24 hours as ordered. In some institutions it is customary to place the patient on his right side with pressure applied to the operative site by means of a pillow or rolled sheet to prevent hemorrhage. The patient is usually instructed to remain in bed for 24 hours.

GALLBLADDER STUDIES

Biliary Drainage (Gallbladder Drainage)

Description. A tube is inserted into the duodenum through the mouth. Duodenal contents are withdrawn and sent to the laboratory for chemical and/or microscopic examination.

Preparation of Patient

1. Nothing by mouth for 12 hours prior to test except for occasional sips of water.
2. The tube is inserted into the patient's stomach. Either the Rehfuss or Jutte tube are usually used (see p. 152). For instructions in passing the tube, see page 153.
3. Withdraw stomach contents (usually discarded).
4. Place on right side with hips elevated as shown.

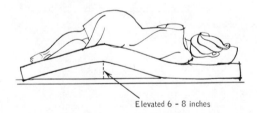

Elevated 6 - 8 inches

5. Patient is instructed to swallow 1 to 2 inches of tube every 5 minutes until second mark on tube is reached.
6. Golden yellow bile from the common bile duct begins to flow through the tube. Collect this in a sterile specimen bottle and label "A."
7. Fifteen cubic centimeters of magnesium sulfate solution is injected directly into the tube, and the tube is clamped for 5 minutes.

8. The next portion of bile that appears is a darker color and is supposed to come from the gallbladder. Collect this color bile in a sterile bottle labeled "B." Bile of this color usually amounts to from 30 to 75 cc.
9. After this, the bile is clear light yellow, assumed to be freshly secreted from the liver. This should be collected in a sterile bottle labeled "C." If there is difficulty in obtaining any specimen, several cubic centimeters of warm water can be injected into the tube. This usually stimulates the flow of bile.
10. The tube is removed. If the nurse is removing the tube and the tube offers resistance, the removal must be completed by the doctor.

If a microscopic examination of the bile is desired, the fluid must be examined within a few minutes after it is secured.

Direct Serum Bilirubin (see p. 146)

Serum Alkaline Phosphatase (see p. 147)

Urine and/or Feces for Urobilinogen (see p. 146)

Description. When bilirubin of the bile reaches the intestine, it is reduced to the substance urobilinogen. In biliary obstruction bilirubin does not enter the intestine; thus urobilinogen would not be contained in the feces or be excreted by the kidneys.

Cholecystogram and Cholangiogram (see p. 143)

Examination of Stools for Presence of Amebas (see p. 149)

MICROSCOPIC EXAMINATIONS

Leukocytes and pus cells appear if there are ulcers of the intestinal tract. A gram-positive stool is suggestive of intestinal ulceration and is sometimes striking in cases of carcinoma of the stomach. Bacteria of the typhoid-dysentery group indicate intestinal disorders or a carrier. Presence of ova and parasites also indicate intestinal disorders.

COLLECTION OF STOOL SPECIMEN

In tests for protozoa and amebas, the stool must be warm and cannot be mixed with water or urine.

When an enema is ordered to collect the specimen, the bedpan should be left standing for at least 5 minutes; then the top fluid can be discarded, and the sediment can be placed in the specimen jar.

EXAMINATION OF GASTRIC CONTENTS

The examination of the fasting contents of the stomach is used in the diagnosis of gastric disease. The examination of gastric secretions is called gastric analysis. Gastric secretions are examined for food content (presence of food content ingested the night before indicates pyloric obstruction) as well as for a number of other substances discussed on p. 150.

METHODS TO STIMULATE STOMACH SECRETIONS

Methods used to stimulate stomach secretions include test meals and certain drugs.

Test Meals

All test meals are given on an empty stomach. Here are three test meals commonly used.

Ewald's Test Breakfast
1. Contents:
   One roll or two slices of bread without butter
   300 to 400 cc. of water or tea without cream or sugar
2. Remove gastric contents 1 hour after the time of the *beginning of the ingestion* of the meal.

Riegel's Test Meal
1. Contents:
   400 cc. bouillon
   150 to 200 gm. broiled beefsteak
   150 gm. mashed potatoes
2. Make certain meal is thoroughly masticated.
3. Remove 1 hour after the time of the beginning of the ingestion of the meal.

Motor Test Meal
1. Include spinach or raisins or both in Riegel's test meal.
2. Remove gastric contents 8 hours later.

Drugs

Alcohol, histamine, and insulin are some-times used to stimulate stomach secretions. The procedure for each is given here.

Alcohol. Fifty cubic centimeters of a 7 per cent alcohol solution is instilled into the stomach through a stomach tube.
1. Give nothing by mouth after midnight prior to the test.
2. Aspirate the empty stomach every 5 minutes three times before instilling the alcohol.
3. Aspirate the stomach (approximately 10 cc.) at 10-minute intervals for 1 hour following the instillation of alcohol.

Histamine Hydrochloride or Histamine Phosphate (administered subcutaneously)
1. The stomach is aspirated before and after the administration of the drug.
2. Toxic reactions to the drug include flushed face and tachycardia.

Insulin (Insulin Tolerance Test)

A specific amount of insulin is given intravenously. The insulin causes a drop in blood sugar which in turn stimulates the vagus nerve, thus causing an increase in the flow of gastric secretion.
1. The stomach is aspirated before and after the administration of the drug.
2. Orange juice (if permitted) and glucose should be available in the event that symptoms of insulin shock appear.

REMOVING GASTRIC CONTENTS

The tubes most commonly used to remove gastric secretions for diagnostic studies are the Rehfuss, Jutte, and Sawyer (see p. 152). Most institutions have a gastric analysis tray which contains all the necessary equipment as shown here:

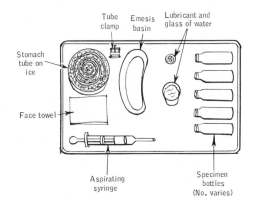

The responsibility of inserting the gastric tube and withdrawing the stomach contents may be assigned to the doctor, nurse, or laboratory technician, depending upon hospital policy. When the doctor performs the procedure, the nurse collects the necessary equipment and assists with the test. See page 153 for techniques of inserting the gastric tube.

The number of gastric specimens needed and the time for withdrawing each specimen varies somewhat with the laboratory's preference in each institution and with the method of stimulating stomach secretions. When the entire gastric analysis procedure is the responsibility of the nurse, she should consult the hospital procedure manual for details concerning the number of specimens needed and the times they are to be withdrawn. A minimum of 10 cc. is needed for each specimen. The specimens should be sent to the laboratory for examination immediately after withdrawal.

Tubeless Gastric Analysis (Diagnex Blue Test)

In this test the stomach contents are not removed for examination. This procedure can indicate whether free hydrochloric acid is present in the stomach, but it cannot be used to determine how much of this acid is present. Azure A (azuresin, Diagnex Blue), a blue dye, is given to the patient. If free hydrochloric acid is present, the dye is released and excreted in the urine.

1. Breakfast is withheld until the test is completed. Water may be taken as desired.
2. Discard the first morning's urine.
3. Caffein sodium benzoate 500 mg. is taken orally with a glass of water to stimulate gastric secretion.
4. One hour later collect a urine specimen for control, and administer to the patient 2 gm. of Diagnex Blue or azuresin mixed in one-half glass of water.
5. Two hours later collect the urine, and save the entire voided specimen.
6. Send both specimens of urine to the laboratory.

The presence of blue color in the 2-hour urine specimen indicates a secretion of free gastric hydrochloric acid.

This test cannot be performed within 48 hours after the ingestion of barium, iron, calcium, magnesium, aluminum, quinine (as in some soft drinks), and steroids. The test is used primarily in the diagnosis of gastric achlorhydria.

THERAPEUTIC AND REHABILITATIVE PROCEDURES

GASTROINTESTINAL INTUBATION

Gastrointestinal intubation is one of the commonest procedures used in the surgical department. Tubes are inserted into the stomach and intestine to remove gas and fluids. They are especially useful postoperatively in preventing vomiting. Gastrointestinal tubes are also used prophylactically to prevent obstruction following abdominal surgery. In this event the tube is inserted the night before surgery. Gastrointestinal tubes are usually left in place after surgery until peristalsis has resumed, as shown by the expulsion of gas through the rectum.

Most tubes are made of rubber; some are plastic. They come in sizes 12 to 16 French.

Size 14 French is used most frequently for the adult patient.

TYPES OF GASTROINTESTINAL TUBES

The tubes most commonly encountered are described here:

Levin Tube

This is the simplest tube and the one used most generally. It is made of rubber or plastic and may be inserted through the nostril. It is used diagnostically and therapeutically. The Levin tube looks like this:

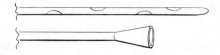

Gastric Lavage Tube (Ewald)

This is a large-lumen tube passed through the mouth and into the stomach for the purpose of washing poisons or other substances from the stomach and in aspirating large amounts of substances from the stomach (i.e., to empty barium from an obstructed stomach following x-ray).

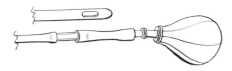

Harris Tube

This is a long tube used for passage into the intestine. On the distal end is a small rubber bag that is filled with 4 cc. of mercury, then tied in place with black silk.

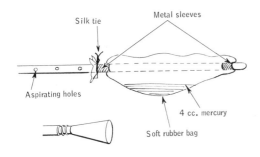

All air is removed from the bag before securing it in place.

Points on the passage of the Harris tube include these: If well lubricated, the tube may be passed through nostril. With the patient in a sitting position, the mercury makes passage into the stomach easy. The patient is then placed in a right Sims's position so that peristaltic motion will carry the tube into the small intestine. During this time the tube is not secured to the nose but is allowed to pass at will. It should be kept in mind that any tube long enough to travel the entire length of the intestinal tract should not be removed if there is suspicion that it has passed the ileocecal valve. Tubes of this type are removed several inches every 4 or 5 minutes.

Miller-Abbott Tube

This is a long double-lumen tube used for intubation of the small intestine. One lumen has an outlet at the distal end, and the other lumen has an outlet into a small rubber bag near the distal end like this:

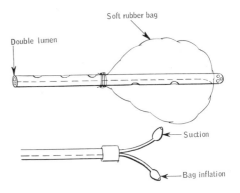

Passage of tube: This tube, well lubricated, is passed through the nostril into the stomach. After the tube is passed into the stomach, mercury or air is used to inflate the balloon. The balloon then helps the passage of the tube through the remainder of the gastrointestinal tract.

Abbott-Rawson Tube

This is also a double-lumen tube with one lumen extending about 8 inches beyond the other. It is used in gastric surgery so that feeding and suction can both be done through the same tube; the more distal lumen is attached to a metal bulb. The Abbott-Rawson tube is shown here:

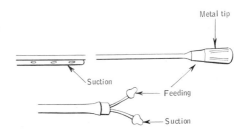

Passage of Abbott-Rawson tube: The tip of the tube without the metal bulb is inserted into the nostril; then the tip of the tube is pulled out through the mouth with a hemostatic forcep, and the bulb is attached. The patient then swallows the bulb with small sips of water.

Rehfuss Tube

This is a rubber tube with a metal bulb attached to the distal end. It is used to withdraw gastric and duodenal secretions for diagnostic purposes. This tube is passed through the mouth.

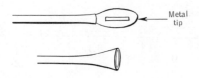

Metal tip

Jutte Tube

This is a rubber tube with a small wire mesh bulb tip at the distal end. It is passed through the mouth and is used to withdraw gastric and duodenal secretions for diagnostic purposes.

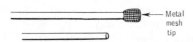

Metal mesh tip

Sawyer Tube

This is a rubber tube which looks like the Levin tube. The walls are thicker and harder than other rubber tubes, allowing less flexibility and promoting an easy passage. The Sawyer tube is passed through the nose or mouth and is used diagnostically and therapeutically.

Colon Tube

All nurses are familiar with the colon or rectal tube, a short rubber tube used for insertion into the colon through the anus. Size 26 French is usually used.

Cantor Tube

The Cantor tube is a long tube used for intubation of the small intestine. A small rubber bag is fastened to the distal end like this:

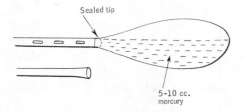

Sealed tip

5-10 cc. mercury

With sterile technique, 5-10 cc. of mercury is injected into the bag with a syringe and needle like this:

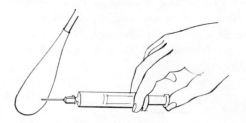

(the needle hole will not allow mercury to escape). The Cantor tube, well lubricated, is inserted through the nose with the aid of forceps like this:

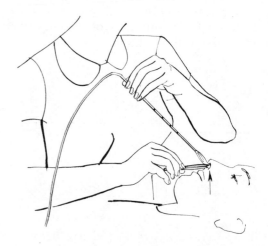

Blakemore-Sengstaken Tube

This tube, commonly called the Blakemore tube, is made of rubber and has a dual purpose: to stop hemorrhage from esophageal and gastric varices and to suction contents from the stomach. The Blakemore-Sengstaken tube looks like this:

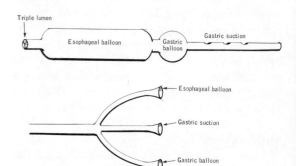

Triple lumen

Esophageal balloon

Gastric balloon

Gastric suction

Esophageal balloon

Gastric suction

Gastric balloon

The physician passes the tube through the nose.

The details of insertion of this tube and care of the patient after its insertion are discussed on p. 154.

Linton Tube

This tube is used for the same purpose as the Blakemore-Sengstaken tube. It is also a triple-lumen tube as shown:

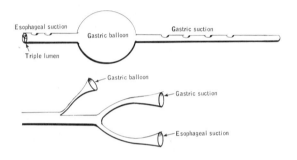

Details of insertion are shown on p. 154.

Passing the Tube

In most instances the gastrointestinal tube is passed by the physician. The nurse may be called upon to pass a tube through the mouth into the stomach for diagnostic studies and gastric tube feedings. Regardless of the reason for passing the tube, it is done like this:

To make the tube easier to pass, a rubber tube is made firmer by chilling it in a bowl of chipped ice for several minutes; a plastic tube is made softer by placing it in warm water. Next lubricate the tube well with surgical jelly. If the nurse is right-handed, she stands to the right of the patient and holds the tip of the tube in the right hand and the remainder of the tube in the left. Instruct the patient to open his mouth; then pass the tube over the top and middle of the tongue. When the tip of the tube reaches the posterior pharynx, tell the patient to close his mouth lightly on the tube and swallow. When swallowing, the patient should be instructed to hold his head in this position, as this is the natural position for swallowing:

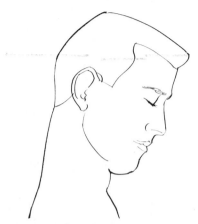

As the patient swallows, push gently and firmly on the tube. Don't try to pass the tube faster than it is normally carried by the swallowing process because gagging will result. If there is any question about the tube entering the trachea, ask the patient to hum. It is impossible to hum when the tip of the tube is located between the vocal cords.

Wait until the patient resumes deep breathing through the mouth; then have him swallow again, and gently push the tube downward. This procedure should be repeated until the tube has been inserted as far as desired. Gastrointestinal tubes are marked, usually with small black rings like this

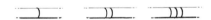

indicating the length of tube to be inserted into the stomach, pylorus, and duodenum. If the tube is not marked, the length of the tube to be inserted into the stomach may be measured before insertion as the distance between the bridge of the nose to the tip of the xyphoid processes as shown:

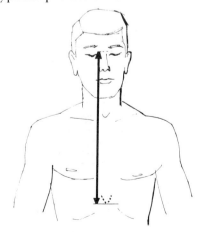

It is not necessary to hurry the patient in swallowing the tube. It is also important to keep the patient relaxed. Mouth breathing is encouraged during the entire process until the desired length of the tube is passed. After the tube has been passed to the desired length, it may be placed between the patient's teeth and cheek.

CONTROLLING HEMORRHAGE FROM ESOPHAGEAL VARICES

When hemorrhage from esophageal varices occurs in cirrhosis of the liver, a Blakemore-Sengstaken or Linton tube is passed by the physician to stop the bleeding as shown on p. 153. These tubes are also used sometimes to differentiate between bleeding from esophageal varices and other causes of upper gastrointestinal hemorrhage. If bleeding stops after the passage of the tube, it is certain that esophageal varices are the source of hemorrhage.

Before insertion of the tube the physician inspects the tube and tests the balloons by inflating them with air. The tube is then passed through the nose as is done with the Cantor tube shown on p. 152. After the tube is passed, the gastric balloon is inflated with air (150 to 200 cc. for the Blakemore-Sengstaken tube and 400 to 500 cc. for the Linton tube). Next, some form of traction is applied on the external portion of the tube. This pulling force on the tube pushes the gastric balloon tightly against the gastric mucosa, thus stopping the bleeding. A number of devices are used to create traction on the tube. One readily available and satisfactory device is an ordinary football helmet used as shown:

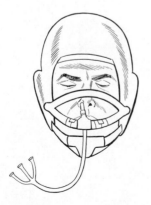

A traction helmet, manufactured for the purpose, looks like this:

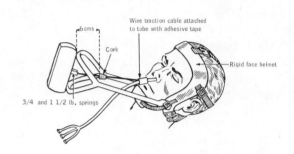

If neither of these devices is available, a pulley, rope, and weight or a baseball catcher's mask can be used to create traction. Traction can also be attained by simply pulling on the tube, then taping the tube to the nose and face. This latter method, however, is not recommended by most authorities because it exerts too much pressure on the tip of the nose, thus causing skin necrosis.

After traction has been applied, the esophageal balloon on the Blakemore tube is inflated to a pressure of 20 to 25 mm. as shown:

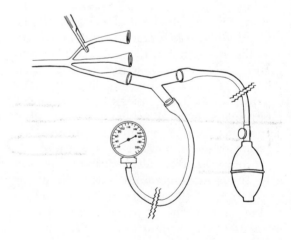

This balloon also serves to stop hemorrhage.

Continuation of Care

The patient with bleeding esophageal varices is usually critically ill and requires a great deal of nursing supervision. Nursing care may include the following:

1. Checking vital signs every 15 minutes until hemorrhage stops.
2. The patient is on nothing by mouth while the tube is in place; thus he requires frequent mouth care and removal of blood from the mouth.
3. Gentle suctioning of the throat and mouth may be needed. This should be done only on doctor's orders.
4. Nostrils must be checked for tissue injury because of irritation from the tube. Keep the nostrils clean and lubricated. Cotton or a small piece of sponge rubber can be placed in the nostril around the tube.
5. Oxygen by tent or catheter may be administered (see Chapter 4).
6. Blood transfusions are given to replace loss of blood (see p. 93). Fresh whole blood is used rather than stored blood because refrigerated blood does not contain prothrombin, and cirrhosis of the liver also depletes the patient's prothrombin level.
7. Check the manometer attached to the esophageal balloon of the Blakemore-Sengstaken tube to make sure the pressure reading remains constant. If the pressure changes, the physician makes the necessary adjustment.
8. An extra tube must be kept on hand in the patient's room in the event there is damage to the one being used. All tubes have the date of manufacture stamped on them. Tubes more than 1 year old should not be used because of possible deterioration of rubber.
9. Nasogastric suction, mild cathartics, and enemas are used to rid the gastrointestinal tract of blood. (The intestinal bacterial action on blood produces ammonia which, in turn, overtaxes the liver.)
10. The patient is on complete bed rest.

Complications resulting from the use of the Blakemore and Linton tubes and their preventive care include the following:

1. *Esophageal and gastric mucosal erosions.* To prevent this, the tube is seldom kept in place longer than 48 hours. Traction is released every 15 to 20 minutes for a few minutes as prescribed by the doctor. The nurse should receive instruction from the doctor as to how this is done if it is to be her responsibility.
2. *Pharyngeal obstruction.* This occurs when the inflated tube accidentally pulls out and it happens more frequently with the Blakemore tube than with the Linton tube because the gastric balloon on the Blakemore tube is smaller. The nurse must check to make sure the tube is not pulling out. Both tubes have centimeter markings along the entire length of the tube. Count the number of markings between the tip of the nose and the adhesive used to fasten the traction to the tube; record this number so that a continual check on the position of the tube can be made.
3. *Esophageal perforation.* Observe the patient for symptoms of this, which are rapid development of back pain, pain in the upper part of the abdomen, shock, and fluid in the chest.
4. *Pneumonia.* This occurs sometimes from aspiration of secretions into the tracheobronchial tree. If secretions in the mouth and throat are a constant problem, notify the physician. A tracheotomy may be performed in this event (see p. 353).

Removal of Tube. The balloon or balloons are deflated gradually by the physician before he removes the tube. Observe the patient for indications of renewed bleeding. After removal of the tube, surgery is usually performed to reduce hypertension in the portal venous system (the cause of esophageal varices). Surgical procedures may include ligation of esophageal varices and an anastomosis in the portal venous system. These two surgical procedures may be done in separate stages or both at once. Two types of anastomoses currently being used are an anastomosis of the splenic vein to the left renal vein (splenorenal shunt) and an anastomosis of the portal vein to the inferior vena cava (portacaval shunt).

METHODS OF DRAINAGE

A number of methods of drainage are used in the medical and surgical treatment of diseases of the digestive tract. The techniques used in draining two specific areas are discussed here: drainage through the gastrointestinal tract and drainage from a surgical incision. In order to classify all types of drainage under specific headings we have categorized the drainage technique under drainage without suction and suction drainage. Those methods of drainage most commonly encountered are discussed here.

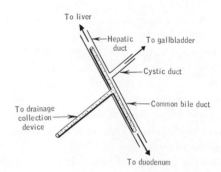

DRAINAGE WITHOUT SUCTION

Drainage without suction is usually the method employed in draining secretions from an abdominal incision. Tubes used for this type of drainage include the Penrose and cigarette drain, the T tube, and ordinary urethral catheters.

The Penrose drain is a flat soft rubber drain available in several widths:

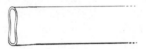

It is used to drain secretions through an incision in the skin. For example, in a case of peritonitis resulting from a ruptured appendix, the Penrose drain may be used to drain the purulent material from the peritoneal cavity following the removal of the appendix. Nurses do not insert or remove Penrose drains. The physician usually removes the drain an inch or two each day until the drain is completely removed. Surgical asepsis is used in removing the drain.

Cigarette drains are used for the same purposes as the Penrose drain. A cigarette drain is a soft rubber tube with a small diameter. The Penrose and cigarette drains are actually secured to the skin by the surgeon. They are then covered with dressings.

The *T tube* is frequently used in operations on the common bile duct to assure passage of the bile from the liver to the intestine as shown here:

There is usually several hundred cubic centimeters drainage of bile from the T tube in a 24-hour period. Because of this a drainage collection device must be attached to the T tube. If the T tube is clamped at the time the patient returns from surgery, it must be released immediately. The most suitable collection receptacle is one that is lightweight and can be secured to the patient when he is ambulatory. Such a setup can be made with a plastic blood storage unit as shown here:

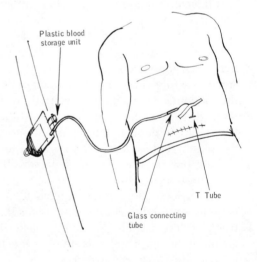

The drainage should be checked for color and amount every 2 hours on the day of operation. The tube may drain some blood-stained fluid during the first few hours postoperatively, but drainage containing large amounts of blood must be reported to the physician. Within 10 days postoperatively, the bile should be draining into the duodenum; the tube is then removed. If excessive drainage has continued for a prolonged time, the bile collected in the drainage bottle is administered to the patient to improve digestion (see p. 165).

Before removal of the T tube, tests may be performed to determine the patency of the biliary system. A cholangiogram (see p. 143) may be done by injecting radiopaque dye through the T tube. A *burette test* is frequently done by the doctor to decide whether to remove the T tube. A sterile burette tube is attached to the T tube as shown:

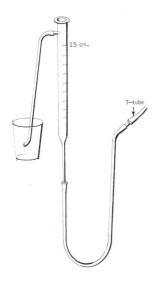

The center of the burette is hung at the level of the common bile duct. The burette is filled with sterile normal saline solution, usually to a level of 15 cm. The nurse checks and records the level of bile every hour for 4 to 24 hours. If the system is still obstructed, the level of bile will continuously rise in the burette tube, causing the normal saline solution to overflow. If this happens, notify the physician. The patient must remain flat in bed during this test. Moving, talking, coughing, and laughing by the patient will also cause the pressure to increase.

When the patient's condition is satisfactory, the physician removes the T tube by pulling it through the small incision in the skin. The T tube is small in diameter and is flexible; thus it can be removed with little discomfort to the patient. Reactions to observe and report after removal of the tube include fever, chills, and abdominal pain. As a rule, the skin incision

heals promptly without further drainage. In some instances the patient may be discharged from the hospital with the T tube in place. In this event the physician may cut the tube so that only a few inches show above the skin. The tube is clamped with a rubber band, and a dressing is placed over the area. Instruction of the patient is important to prevent the tube from becoming dislodged.

Biliary Flush

The biliary flush is a method of dislodging common duct stones which remain after cholecystectomy and choledochostomy by increasing the intraductal pressure and bile flow. The biliary flush is usually done over a 3-day period as follows:

1. The T tube is kept clamped during the 3 days to permit building up of intraductal pressure.
2. The patient is given 3 tablets of Decholin (to increase the flow of bile) with belladonna after each meal and at bedtime for 3 days.
3. One-half bottle (6 oz.) of magnesium citrate is given each morning before breakfast for 3 days.
4. Give 3 tablespoonful of pure cream or olive oil before the noon and evening meals for 3 days.
5. Place a nitroglycerine tablet (1/100 gr.) under the tongue before the evening meal for 3 days.

If this procedure is not successful, the chloroform and ether technique may be incorporated in the biliary flush regimen as follows:

1. On the first day of the flush regimen, the physician first attempts to aspirate bile from the T tube, then slowly instills 5 cc. of chloroform heated to 60° C. (140° F.). The T tube is then clamped.
2. This is repeated again on the second day of the regimen.
3. On the third day a nitroglycerine tablet is given under the tongue, and 5 cc. of ethyl ether is instilled through the T tube. The T tube is reclamped.

After the biliary flush, x-rays are taken. If the stones have not been dislodged, the biliary flush is repeated about a week later.

While the patient is on the biliary flush

regimen, the increased intraductal pressure may cause a great deal of pain. For relief of pain the physician will leave specific orders for the administration of morphine or for momentary release of the T tube.

Regular urethral catheters are generally used to drain secretions from surgical openings into the gastrointestinal tract such as the gastrostomy and ileostomy. The catheter is inserted and removed by the physician. It is the nurse's responsibility to make certain that the catheter remains in place. Shown here is a catheter draining fluid from an ileostomy.

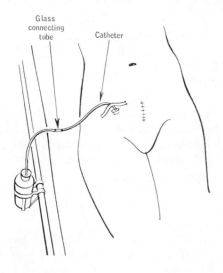

Glass connecting tube

Catheter

SUCTION DRAINAGE

Wangensteen Drainage

Drainage promoted by suction is used in removing gas and fluids from the digestive tract through the gastrointestinal tubes described on page 150. Some of the more common uses for gastrointestinal suction include: the prevention and treatment of postoperative distention in many types of surgery but particularly after surgery on the digestive tract, the treatment of an obstruction in the gastrointestinal tract, and emptying the stomach prior to surgery. Gastrointestinal drainage is commonly referred to as Wangensteen drainage or Wangensteen suction. Technically speaking, the water displacement suction

apparatus is really the Wangensteen suction apparatus; however, hospital personnel usually refer to all gastric suction as Wangensteen suction regardless of the type of suction machine used.

The original Wangensteen suction setup is now seldom used. An adaptation of this original setup is shown here:

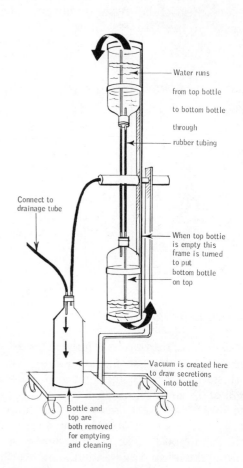

Water runs from top bottle to bottom bottle through rubber tubing

Connect to drainage tube

When top bottle is empty this frame is turned to put bottom bottle on top

Vacuum is created here to draw secretions into bottle

Bottle and top are both removed for emptying and cleaning

With this setup suction is promoted by water displacement. The force of the water flowing from the high bottle into the low bottle produces suction. To function properly, the bottles must all be airtight.

Another suction device used is the Gomco thermatic pump. This is an electrically operated pump, nonmechanical, which operates on the principle that air expands and contracts when subjected to heat variations. The Gomco pump looks like this:

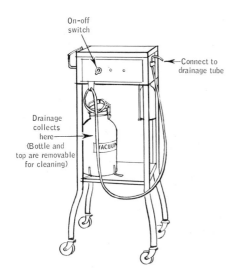

On-off switch

Connect to drainage tube

Drainage collects here (Bottle and top are removable for cleaning)

VACUUM

Many hospitals now have piped suction with wall-station outlets. The suction outlet is usually located next to the oxygen wall-station outlet (see Chap. 4). The apparatus used with wall suction in gastrointestinal drainage looks like this:

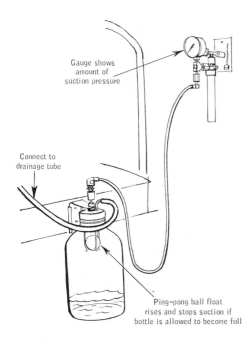

Gauge shows amount of suction pressure

Connect to drainage tube

Ping-pong ball float rises and stops suction if bottle is allowed to become full

Nursing procedures important to the patient on Wangensteen suction are:
1. Keep an exact record of intake and output.
2. The suction tube should be secured carefully to the patient and also to the bed by

means of a safety pin so that the patient has freedom of action without danger of pulling out the tube. A large safety pin should be used so that the pin does not compress the tube and block drainage. Better still, put tape around the tube and pin the tape to the bedding.

3. Special mouth care is given to prevent dryness and irritation of the mouth. Special mouth care must be given at least every 1 or 2 hours. When the patient is allowed nothing by mouth, the tongue and gums should be swabbed with a mixture of glycerin and lemon juice. The glycerin should not be too concentrated, as this in itself causes dehydration and irritation (one part glycerin to one part lemon juice is satisfactory). A thin coat of mineral oil or vegetable oil is applied to the nostrils. Cold cream, petroleum jelly, or lanolin may be applied to the lips. The patient should be instructed to rinse his mouth with mouthwash or some other prescribed solution before the application of the lubricant. When the patient is permitted, sips of water, hard candy, and chewing gum also help to prevent dryness of the mouth.

4. The tube is irrigated every hour or two, as ordered, to prevent it from becoming clogged. Always make certain that there is a doctor's order to irrigate the tube. This is not a routine procedure. To irrigate the tube, clamp the tube leading to the drainage apparatus, then disconnect it as shown:

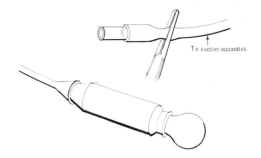

To suction apparatus

flush it with 30-60 cc. of normal saline. The saline is instilled slowly with a medication or Asepto syringe. If there is evidence that the tube is clogged, the water must be forced into the tube to clear it. When the irrigation is completed, connect the tube to the suction apparatus, and remove the clamp.

5. If at any time the suction does not seem to be functioning properly, notify the doctor.

6. An accurate record of the color, amount, and consistency of the drainage must be kept. Unless otherwise indicated, the solution used to irrigate the tube is withdrawn immediately after instillation. If the irrigating solution is not to be withdrawn or cannot be withdrawn during irrigation, the amount instilled into the tube must be recorded, as this will be suctioned through the suction apparatus.

Drainage from the Peritoneal Cavity

When the peritoneal cavity becomes infected following the perforation of any of the abdominal organs or from some other cause, it may be necessary to drain off the toxic fluid with a suction apparatus. Two methods of fixing the drainage tubing for this purpose are shown here. This is one drain used, the sump drain:

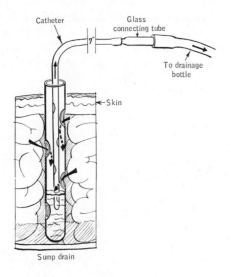

Sump drain

Another drain, the Chaffin tube, is shown here:

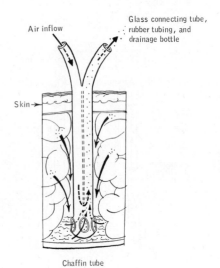

Chaffin tube

These drains are connected to a small drainage bottle, about one quart size, fastened to the side of the bed like this:

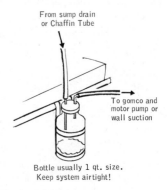

Bottle usually 1 qt. size.
Keep system airtight!

The system must be airtight.

A motor-driven pump like this may be used for this type suction drainage.

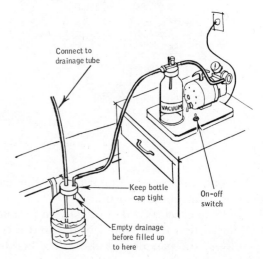

Important aspects of the nursing care of the patient with this type of drainage are:

1. Make certain that the tube is secured to the patient and to the bed in such a way that the tube will not be pulled from the skin wound. The drainage tube is usually sutured in place. If not, it must be taped in place (see p. 38).

2. Great care must be taken to prevent the skin around the tube from becoming irritated by seepage from the skin wound. Secretions from the upper digestive tract, as in stomach and duodenal perforation, may cause excoriation of the skin within a few hours following the first exposure. The area should be cleansed with tap water and soap and/or aqueous benzalkonium chloride solution every 1 or 2 hours. Special preparations such as aluminum hydroxide gel and Kaolin may be prescribed for application to the skin when the seepage consists of digestive secretions. Ointments seem to be of little value because the secretions burrow through or seep under them.

3. A record of the amount and character of the drainage must be kept.

4. A bed cradle may be used to hold the bedclothes off the area.

5. Dressings must be changed frequently, depending upon the amount of seepage around the tube.

SPECIAL FEEDING METHODS

GASTRIC GAVAGE

When the patient is unable to take feedings orally, a Levin tube may be inserted into the stomach, and the patient is fed through the tube. Feeding the patient through a tube inserted into the stomach is called gastric gavage. Depending upon the condition for which the gavage is used, the gastric tube may either be inserted through the nose and left in place for several days, or it may be inserted by the nurse prior to each feeding. For the technique of inserting the tube, see p. 153.

The type of feeding administered through the tube depends upon the physician's preference. The feeding is calculated so that the patient receives a diet consisting of the basic food nutrients. No more than 500 cc. are administered at one feeding. The usual amount prescribed is 150 to 200 cc. given every 3 to 4 hours.

After the tube is inserted, proceed with the feeding. First, make certain that the tube is inserted in the stomach by inserting the tip into a glass of water or asking the patient to hum. If the tube is inserted in the trachea, bubbles will appear in the water as the patient exhales and humming is impossible. The equipment used in giving the feeding is shown here:

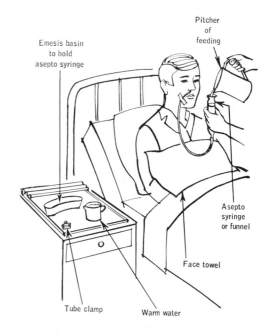

Note that the patient should be in a sitting or semi-Fowler's position while receiving the feeding.

One ounce of warm water (about 105°F.) is given first to make certain that the tube is open. (This step is not necessary if the tube is inserted prior to each feeding.) Then pour the feeding, also warmed to 105°F., to run slowly into the stomach. Feedings should always be given slowly. The rate of flow may be regulated by raising or lowering the syringe like this:

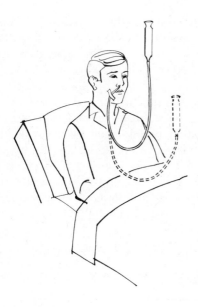

About 10 minutes should be allowed for the entire feeding. As soon as the solution empties to about this point, add more feeding. If the

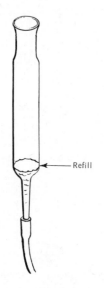

Refill

syringe is allowed to empty, an air pocket will form in the tube, causing air to enter the stomach.

After administering the entire feeding, an additional 1 to 2 ounces of warm water is given to prevent stoppage of the tube. Again the water should be poured into the syringe before it is completely emptied from the feeding. Unless otherwise prescribed, this water need not be given if the tube is to be removed following the feeding.

If the tubing is to be removed, clamp it or pinch it during the removal to prevent spillage and loss of part of the feeding. If the tube is to be retained, clamp the end with a Hoffman clamp or medicine dropper shown here:

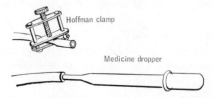

Hoffman clamp

Medicine dropper

When the tube is retained for a period of days, the tape used to anchor the tube to the face must be checked periodically to make sure that it is secure and that the skin is not becoming irritated. When the tube is retained, care is given to the mouth and nostril as described for the patient receiving continuous Wangensteen suction (p. 159). An accurate record is kept of the time and amount of feedings, including water.

GASTROSTOMY FEEDING

When gastric tube feedings are indicated and the tube cannot be inserted into the stomach through the esophagus because of disease conditions and/or surgery of the esophagus and upper portion of the stomach, feedings are given through a gastrostomy tube. As the term implies, the gastrostomy tube is a tube inserted directly into the stomach through a surgical opening in the abdominal wall. A small incision is made in the upper left abdomen, and a small opening is made into the stomach. A catheter is inserted into the opening. The area of the stomach around the catheter is sutured securely to the abdominal wall, and the incision is sutured tightly around the catheter to prevent leakage. The catheter is usually secured in place with the end of an elongated skin suture as can be noted in this diagram:

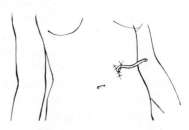

Approximately 10 days after this gastrostomy procedure, the incision surrounding the catheter is healed. This enables the physician to remove and replace the gastrostomy tube when necessary for cleaning purposes. Sterile dressings are always kept in place over the skin around the catheter. A dressing like this:

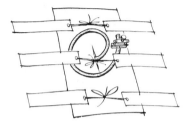

is most satsifactory because the tube feeding can be given without removing the dressing each time. Coiling the tube under the Montgomery ties also prevents the tube from pulling out.

The consistency, frequency, and amount of the feeding given through the gastrostomy tube is the same as that described for the gastric gavage. With one or two exceptions, the procedure for giving a feeding through the gastrostomy tube is also the same as for the gavage. For the gastrostomy feeding the patient remains flat in bed. After the feeding has been given, the gastrostomy tube must be clamped off before removing the funnel, because there is a backflow.

When the gastrostomy tube is no longer needed, the gastrostomy opening is closed by surgery.

ENTEROSTOMY FEEDINGS

When feedings cannot be administered through the stomach because of extensive disease as in advanced carcinoma of the stomach or because of extensive gastric surgery and gastric surgical complications, a tube may be inserted into the small intestine for the purpose of feeding. When the tube is inserted through a surgical opening into the duodenum, the term "duodenostomy tube" may be used. When the tube is inserted through a surgical opening into the upper portion of the jejunum, the term "jejunostomy tube" is generally used. The techniques for giving enterostomy feedings are the same as those for gastrostomy feedings.

MURPHY DRIP

The Murphy drip is a method of administering fluid into the gastrointestinal tract, drop by drop. This is accomplished with a specially designed tube, the Murphy drip tube, named after the surgeon who first used and described it. Most nurses are familiar with the drip tube, a glass tube like this:

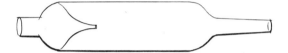

The Murphy drip method is used in administering fluids or nourishment into the colon (proctoclysis) and in administering fluids into the gastrostomy and enterostomy tubes when the patient cannot tolerate the usual amount of tube feedings at one time.

The equipment used in administering the fluid may vary somewhat with the institution. Some institutions have a proctoclysis tray that is reassembled and sterilized after each use. The equipment on this tray can be used for administering fluid into the gastrostomy and enterostomy tubes. One setup is shown here:

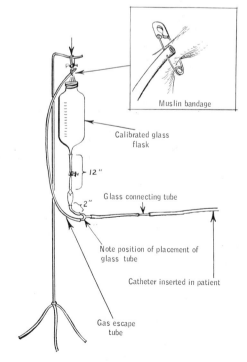

For the proctoclysis an enema can may be used instead of the glass flask.

For gastrostomy and enterostomy feedings, the gas escape tube is sometimes omitted, and the setup looks like this:

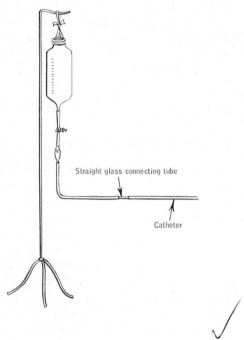

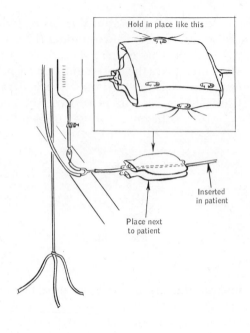

For the proctoclysis an enema is given 1 to 2 hours prior to the treatment. A size 18 to 22 French catheter, well lubricated, is inserted 4 to 5 inches into the colon and secured to the buttocks with adhesive or cellophane tape.

For gastrostomy and enterostomy feedings, the setup is connected to the tube already in place on the patient. The flask of solution is hung at a height of 12 inches above the area through which the solution is administered. The solution must be administered at a temperature of 100° and 104°F. This temperature must be maintained in order for proper absorption to take place. To do this, first heat the solution, then place hot water bottles around the flask or the tubing.

If hot water bottles are placed around the flask, they must be filled with water at about 130°F. and must be refilled every half-hour. The disadvantage of this method is that the solution cools as it runs through the tube.

The best method of keeping the fluid warm is to place the hot water bottles around the tubing like this:

Hold them in place with a face towel wrapped and pinned as shown. Hot water bottles filled at 110° to 112° F. will maintain the temperature of the solution in the tube at 100° to 104° F. The hot water bottles must be replaced every half-hour.

The flow of solution is regulated at a rate most suitable for absorption by the patient. This may vary from 10 to 60 drops per minute, as prescribed by the physician. The patient should receive 1000 to 2000 cc. in 24 hours. An accurate record of the amount of solution administered and the rate of flow is kept, and observations are made periodically to make certain the solution is flowing. Stoppage results from a clogged tube and inability of the patient to absorb the solution. If the tube becomes clogged, pinch it several times. If the solution is not being absorbed, notify the physician.

The position of the patient should be changed during the treatment. This usually lasts for a period of several days.

HARRIS DRIP

The Harris drip is sometimes used in giving the proctoclysis. With this method the flow of solution into the colon is regulated by placing the irrigating can on the level of the rectum. With the Harris drip the solution flows back and forth between the rectum and the irrigating can. The setup is like this:

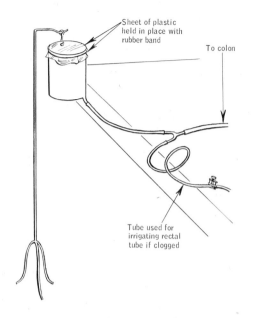

Note the following:
1. A large rectal tube (Number 28 French) is used so that flatus and fecal matter may pass through the tube when pressure increases within the rectum.
2. An irrigating can should always be used to hold the solution, as there will be a back flow of fecal matter that would be unsightly if visible.
3. A cover should be placed over the irrigating can in such a way as to retain the odor within the can.
4. The solution is warmed by the same method as is the Murphy drip.
5. The second tubing attached to the Y connecting tube is used to drain the rectum if necessary, to irrigate the rectal tube if it becomes clogged, and to empty the can for cleaning purposes.
6. If the solution in the irrigating can becomes too offensive, the can is drained and cleaned, and fresh solution is used.
7. Never allow the can to become empty, as this causes air to be drawn into the rectum.

This treatment may also be continued for several days. Records of observations, as with the Murphy drip, are kept during this time.

BILE FEEDINGS

After biliary tract surgery, the bile collected from T tube drainage is sometimes administered to the patient to aid in digestion.

The bile is stored in a refrigerator and is usually given in amounts of 120 cc. per feeding either via a nasogastric tube or orally. It is better not to tell the patient he is receiving bile. Instead, tell him he is receiving a special solution to aid in digestion. When the bile is to be given through a nasogastric tube, the procedure for administration is the same as described on p. 162 except that the Asepto syringe or funnel should be covered with a paper towel so that the patient cannot see the bile.

SPECIAL TYPES OF IRRIGATIONS

COLOSTOMY IRRIGATION

A colostomy irrigation is given for several reasons: to cleanse the intestinal tract and prevent obstruction and to establish a regularity of evacuation. In order to understand better some of the techniques used in irrigating the colostomy, a few comments about the types of colostomy encountered will be given here.

The three common sites for the colostomy are shown here:

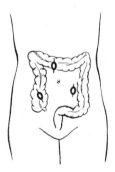

Colostomies are either temporary or permanent. They are made temporarily to rest a portion of the colon as in severe diverticulitis and extensive reconstructive surgery. A permanent colostomy is made when the lower bowel is removed as for cancer.

There are several methods used in creating the colostomy. One method the surgeon uses is to bring a loop of the colon through the abdominal wall and hold it in place like this:

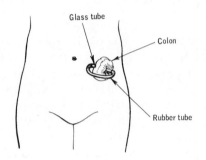

After the incision around the loop has adhered (usually 48 hours), an opening is made into the colon with a scissors or cautery while the patient is in his own room. No anesthesia is necessary for this procedure. After this the patient will have two open segments of bowel protruding on the abdomen. When two segments are protruding, it is called a double-barrel colostomy. One loop is the distal loop, and one is the proximal loop. Consequently, the proximal loop, or the one farthest from the anus, is the functioning loop. The location of the proximal and distal loops is shown here:

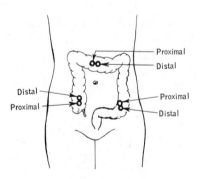

The double-barrel method is used for the temporary colostomy and for the first stage of a two-stage permanent colostomy. The permanent colostomy is usually performed in two stages, the first stage being the formation of the double-barrel colostomy and the second being the removal of the diseased portion of the colon.

Colostomy irrigations are usually prescribed once daily. When the irrigation is given to establish a regularity in bowel movements, it is given at the same time every day. The solutions usually prescribed are tap water, normal saline or soap solution. To be most effective, the solution should be given at a temperature of 105° F. Heat the solution to a temperature of 108° F., allowing for the cooling that occurs as it flows through the tube. The amount needed varies with each patient. The irrigation is given until the return flow is clear. This means until the return flow contains no fecal matter. This could require from 300 to 3000 cc.

The equipment used to give the irrigation varies from a simple enema type setup to the more elaborate commercial sets. There are several commercial irrigating sets on the market. These are purchased either after the patient is discharged or shortly before. The commercial sets are no more effective in cleansing the colon than the simple enema type setup, and they are much more expensive.

The setup the nurse begins with is shown here:

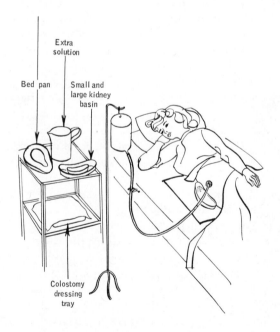

Note that the patient is placed on the side of the colostomy for the irrigation and that a sizable protective pad is needed. The irrigating can is hung about 18 inches above the colostomy. The large kidney basin is placed under the colostomy opening and as close to the patient as possible. The patient can be requested to hold the kidney basin in place.

The lubricated catheter (16 or 18 French) is injected 6 to 8 inches after the flow of solution is started. This makes it much easier to insert the tube. Allow at least 250 cc. and no more than 500 cc. of solution to enter the colon, then clamp the irrigating tube. Remove the catheter from the colostomy, and allow the solution and feces to drain into the kidney basin. One word of warning is necessary at this point. Forceful spurts of water may be emitted from the colostomy. The nurse can protect herself from these sudden spurts by making a shield with a small emesis basin held in front of the colostomy opening like this:

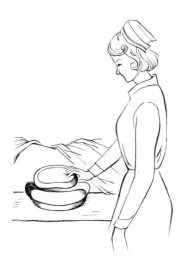

It may also be necessary to use this protection during the instillation of the irrigating solution.

When the kidney basin under the colostomy is almost filled, remove it, and replace it immediately with another kidney basin. Empty the fecal matter into a covered bedpan. The interchange of the two large kidney basins is continued throughout the treatment.

When all of the solution has drained from the colostomy, reinsert the catheter as before, and allow more solution to enter the colon. This process is repeated until the return flow is free of fecal matter. It usually takes about 10 to 15 minutes for the solution to drain from the colostomy each time and about an hour to perform the entire procedure. The entire object of the treatment is lost if the colon is not cleansed properly and completely; therefore there is no short-cut method.

After the irrigation has been completed, make certain all of the solution is drained from the colostomy; then cleanse the patient, and apply the colostomy dressing (see p. 170). Again there is no point to haste. If the dressing is put on before the solution has completely drained, you will only discover that in a short time the patient's dressings, gown, and bedcovers are saturated.

As the nurse and the patient progress, the following variations in the technique may be helpful:

1. Depending upon the size of the remaining colon and the ease of inserting the catheter, the catheter may be inserted as much as 12 inches. With the catheter inserted this distance, there is usually no leakage of solution from the colostomy while the solution is being instilled.

2. After the patient's condition permits, it is easier to have him sit on a chair or preferably on the toilet. Make a plastic apron and tie it around the patient to direct the flow of evacuation like this:

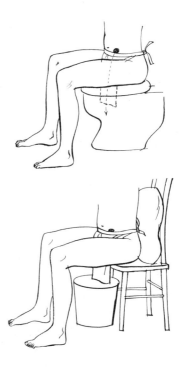

An ordinary plastic housewife's apron may be purchased by the patient for use at home.

3. A week or more after the patient receives daily colostomy irrigations, he may be able to retain more than 500 cc. of solution at one time.

The patient who has a permanent colostomy will in time develop his own routine for the colostomy irrigation. Many patients also design their own equipment. Here is a setup for the irrigation that can be suggested to the patient. It is made of inexpensive materials: a flexible plastic glass and a plastic tube sewn from a sheet of plastic material. Cut the end out of the glass, and cut a small hole in the side of the glass for the insertion of the catheter, and assemble it like this:

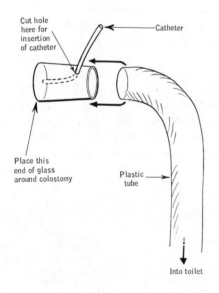

Irrigating Both Colostomy Loops. When a temporary colostomy is to be closed, preoperative care usually includes an irrigation of both loops. The distal loop is irrigated the same way. If there is no obstruction in the distal portion of the colon, the irrigating solution may be expelled through the rectum.

PERINEAL IRRIGATION

Following some types of rectal surgery such as a perineal resection, the physician may order perineal irrigations to keep the area around the rectum clean and prevent infection. The solution most frequently used is normal saline solution heated to 105° F. The sterile solution is heated as shown on page 119. The irrigation is done with an Asepto syringe with the patient in the position shown:

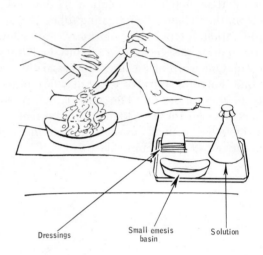

Dressings   Small emesis   Solution
                       basin

GASTRIC LAVAGE

The term "gastric lavage" means to wash out the stomach. The lavage is used most frequently as an emergency treatment in gastric dilatation and poisoning. It is also sometimes done to rid the stomach of toxic substances in preparation for an emergency surgery and to cleanse the stomach for gastric surgery.

A Levin tube or special lavage tube (see p. 150) is used for the lavage. When the contents of the stomach consist of undigested food particles, the gastric lavage tube must be used because it has a large lumen. The lavage tube is always passed through the mouth.

In emergency situations for poisoning, the stomach is lavaged until the return flow is clear. This requires several gallons of solution (usually soda bicarbonate).

When the lavage is ordered as part of the preoperative preparation for gastric surgery, the order usually includes the amount and type of solution to be used.

The equipment used for the lavage is shown here:

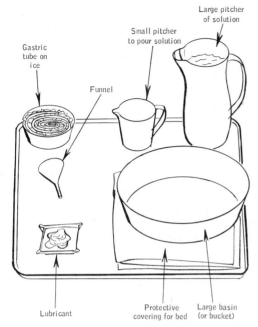

Large pitcher of solution

Small pitcher to pour solution

Gastric tube on ice

Funnel

Lubricant

Protective covering for bed

Large basin (or bucket)

The stomach tube is inserted as described on page 153. Five hundred cubic centimeters of solution is given at a time, then siphoned from the stomach. To start the siphonage action, allow the last funnel-full of solution to enter the stomach; then pinch the tube immediately so that the tube does not empty itself of solution, and quickly invert the funnel over the drainage receptacle. As the solution allowed to remain in the tube drains off, a siphonage effect is produced, and the entire stomach is emptied. Very seldom is any suction needed to empty the stomach.

Continue the introduction and drainage of solution until the prescribed results are obtained; then pinch the tube and withdraw it quickly. In cases of poisoning the tube is sometimes left in place and used to administer a dose of antidote.

DRESSINGS

The types of dressings most commonly encountered in caring for patients with diseases of the digestive system include those for specific draining wounds, colostomy dressings, ileostomy dressings, and rectal dressings.

DRAINING WOUNDS

The various draining wounds one may encounter include these:

1. Bile drainage from the opening through which a T tube has been removed after biliary duct surgery.
2. Seepage of duodenal secretions through an abdominal incision when a duodenal fistula occurs as a complication following a gastrectomy and as a complication following biliary duct surgery when the common bile duct is implanted in the duodenum.
3. Drainage from the peritoneal cavity when peritonitis occurs as a complication before or after surgery and when surgical drainage is used in treating an abscess formation on an organ in the peritoneal cavity.
4. Drainage from the paracentesis wound in ascites.

When dealing with dressings on draining wounds, there are a number of factors to be considered. Special care should always be used when removing the dressings from these wounds because there may be a cigarette or Penrose drain in place that could become dislodged.

Dressings on all draining wounds must be changed frequently, and the skin must be thoroughly cleansed and dried each time to prevent excoriation of the skin. The amount of drainage of course determines the frequency required. Prevention of skin irritation is the most difficult when the drainage consists of digestive juices. Dressings on wounds of this type should be changed every hour.

One or more of a variety of medications may be prescribed either to prevent or to treat excoriated skin. Substances used to protect the skin from digestive juices include powdered aluminum rubbed into the intact skin, brewer's yeast, tannic acid in lanolin, Kaolin, aluminum hydroxide gel, and egg white. Sterile soap solution and water seem to be the best cleansing solutions. Ointments and powders should be removed with each cleansing, then freshly reapplied.

One point frequently overlooked when placing a dressing is that the drainage on a wound located on the side of the abdomen flows to the side. When dressing a wound at this location, the thickest portion of the dressing should be placed on the lower side of the wound at about this position:

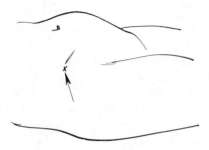

rather than directly on top of the wound, especially when the patient is obese.

When a suction drainage tube is in place in the wound, the gauze is placed around the tube and covered with absorbent pads overlapped like this:

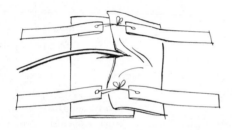

Montgomery tapes are used to hold the dressings in place unless the skin becomes irritated from the adhesive. If this occurs, a binder must be used.

A record should be kept of the time dressings are changed, the amount and character of the drainage, and the appearance of the skin surrounding the wound.

COLOSTOMY DRESSINGS

When the patient returns from the operating room following the colostomy operation, the colostomy dressings usually consist of sterile petrolatum gauze wrapped around the stoma and covered with a thin layer of dry gauze. Some surgeons paint the skin around the stoma with collodion to protect against infection. For the first day or two, the surgeon usually changes the dressings. The first dressing may be difficult to remove because of dried secretions on the stump. The nurse should have sterile water or saline on hand to soak the dressings loose.

The first bowel evacuation usually occurs on the second or third day. The feces are liquid or semi-liquid in consistency at first and continue to be so until the patient's diet is regulated and his anxieties have diminished. Until the bowel evacuation is regulated, the colostomy dressing must be changed usually every 1 to 4 hours. A colostomy is considered well regulated when a formed stool is eliminated once or twice daily with no drainage from the opening between eliminations. The elimination should occur with regularity at the same time daily. This perfection in colostomy behavior is rarely attained during the usual hospital stay following surgery.

A colostomy dressing tray is used to change the dressings. The tray should include all the materials needed to cleanse and dry the skin and redress the area. A supply of newspapers is needed as a receptacle for the soiled dressings.

Protective coverings which may be used for the skin include Kerodex, petrolatum gauze, and ointments such as aluminum paste, Desitin ointment, and zinc oxide. Ointments must be gently removed each time the skin is cleansed and freshly reapplied. Soap and water (unsterile, because this is not a sterile procedure) are the best cleansing agents.

We would like to suggest two methods for dressing a colostomy. One method is this: Take a 2-inch strip of absorbent pad or several layers of gauze and fold it, forming a doughnut. Hold this together with a long, narrow rubber band like this:

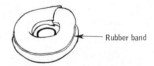

Place this around the stoma; then cover it with several thicknesses of 4 × 8 gauze and an absorbent pad held in place like this:

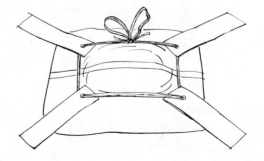

Another method is this: Cut a small hole in the center of a sheet of plastic, and cement it with rubber cement to the skin here:

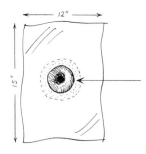

Wrap petrolatum gauze around the stoma like this:

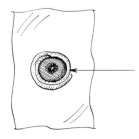

Then place gauze and an absorbent pad over the stoma, and fold the plastic over the dressings like this:

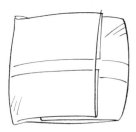

Hold the dressing in place with Montgomery straps.

When the colostomy becomes regulated, the dressing is kept simple. A small piece of gauze or disposable tissue covered with Saran Wrap and held in place with an elastic belt or panties is sufficient.

There are several types of colostomy bags available. Most patients with a permanent colostomy find that these are not necessary.

ILEOSTOMY DRESSINGS

The care of an ileostomy is much more difficult and exasperating than the care of a colostomy. Prevention of skin excoriation is extremely difficult with the ileostomy. The discharge from the ileostomy is green and watery and contains digestive juices that, as mentioned before, are irritating to the skin. The watery discharge from the ileostomy also tends to be constant. Some patients with a permanent ileostomy state that after 6 months to 1 year the drainage becomes more formed because the ilium takes over water absorption. The most recent and most effective management of the ileostomy includes the use of bags cemented to the skin around the ileostomy stump. At the operation a disposable plastic bag that looks like this

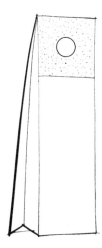

is cemented to the skin around the ileostomy. This bag is used only temporarily until the ileostomy stump completes shrinkage. (An ileostomy stump usually continues to shrink for 6 weeks after surgery.) The secretions are thus kept from coming in contact with the skin. The bag is emptied and the contents measured when it becomes full. After the stump is healed and shrinkage is complete, the patient is fitted with a permanent rubber bag cemented to the skin with rubber cement.

The permanent bag is removed only if leakage occurs or if ordered by the physician. The patient is advised to have two permanent bags. Most permanent bags look similar to this. The back of the bag or the part cemented to the skin is shown here:

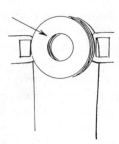

The bag held in place looks like this:

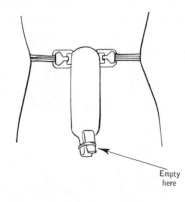

Empty
here

To clean the ileostomy bag while it is cemented in place on the patient:
1. Open the bottom and empty into a bedpan.
2. With an Asepto syringe instill warm soapy water in the open end.
3. Hold the end shut, and manipulate to cleanse the bag thoroughly.
4. Drain and instill plain warm water for rinsing. (A few drops of vinegar may be added to the rinse water to control the odor.) Drain off rinse water; then close the end.

The bag should be emptied frequently to prevent its pulling off because of excessive weight.

To remove the bag, empty it, and follow these steps:
1. With a medicine dropper apply a small amount of solvent (benzine) around the edge of the disc and very gently and carefully pull the disc away from the skin. Continue to apply small amounts of solvent around the disc until the entire disc is free. Do not force the disc from the skin; this causes skin trauma.
2. Place the bag in a basin; then proceed to cleanse gently and dry the skin.
3. If prescribed, apply medication to skin.

To apply a clean bag:
1. Apply a thin coat of rubber cement to skin around ileostomy stump. The area covered by cement should extend about one inch beyond the area the disc will cover.
2. Apply a thin coat to the disc. Allow both to dry completely.
3. Apply another thin coat of cement to skin and disc; then place the disc on the skin, and hold firmly until adhesion takes place. Ask the patient to remain in one position until the bag has firmly adhered to the skin.
4. Talcum powder may be applied to the cement-covered area of skin around the disc.
5. Adjust straps comfortably around waist.

Cement is removed from the disc with solvent. The extra permanent bag is washed, rinsed, soaked in water to which a teaspoon of vinegar has been added, then dried and stored in the patient's unit.

When surgical dressings are used over the ileostomy, the same methods are used as when dressing the colostomy.

RECTAL DRESSINGS

Following rectal surgery either moist or dry dressings may be prescribed. Rectal dressings are held in place with the T binder. Continuous warm moist dressings are placed on the patient in this arrangement:

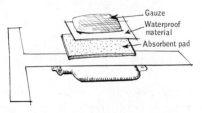

Gauze
Waterproof material
Absorbent pad

Moist dressings are changed every 3 or 4 hours. The hot water bottle is changed more often as needed.

THERAPEUTIC EXERCISE

Specific exercises are seldom prescribed for patients recovering from diseases of the digestive tract. Exercise, however, is an important aspect in the recovery from any type of abdominal surgery. The nurse should review the postoperative exercises discussed in Chapter 10.

A program of early ambulation is now considered desirable following surgery. The patient should be taught how to get in and out of bed and how to walk with the least effort.

To help the patient get out of bed, first tell him to turn on his right side like this:

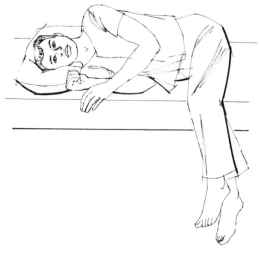

Then tell him to push himself to a sitting position as shown:

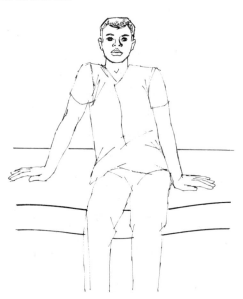

He can then ease forward to a standing position. The nurse stands in front of the patient to prevent any possible fall.

Most patients with abdominal surgery stand like this:

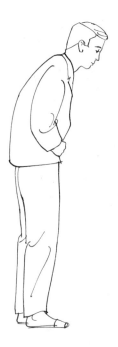

Most patients are not aware of the way they are standing and must be reminded by the nurse to stand up straight.

ADDITIONAL PROCEDURES TO REVIEW

Paracentesis
Colloid baths
Sitz baths
Retention and nonretention enemas
Hot and cold moist compresses
Parenteral therapy (Chap. 6)
Intramuscular injections (Chap. 6)
Oxygen therapy (Chap. 4)
Assisting with rectal examination
Isolation techniques (Chap. 7)
Occupational therapies

DIETS TO REVIEW

Bland	High protein
Low residue	High carbohydrate
High residue	Low salt
Low fat	Ulcer diets

EXAMINATION OF FECES

MACROSCOPIC EXAMINATIONS
(Those made by naked eye)

EXAMINATION	NORMAL	ABNORMAL INDICATIONS
Color	Light or dark brown	Golden yellow due to unchanged bilirubin Putty colored due to absence of bile Tarry black due to digested blood Red due to fresh blood
Odor	Offensive	Sour due to diarrhea in older children Strong foul stench suggests malignant or syphilitic ulceration of rectum
Mucus	Occasional small amounts	Excessive amounts indicate inflammation or irritation

CHEMICAL EXAMINATIONS

EXAMINATION	NORMAL	ABNORMAL INDICATIONS
Reaction	Slightly acid or slightly alkaline	Acidity due to excess of carbohydrates Alkalinity due to excess of proteins
Fermentation	None	Presence indicates thrush
Blood	None	Indicates hemorrhage Traces of blood (occult blood) always present in carcinoma of the stomach and intermittently present in gastric ulcer
Bile	None	Presence indicates catarrhal conditions of small intestine
Urobilin	100-250 mg. in 24 hours	Absent in catarrhal jaundice and biliary obstruction Increase indicative of excessive destruction of erythrocytes

STUDIES OF GASTRIC CONTENTS

Tests conducted on the gastric contents are listed here:

TEST	NORMAL	ABNORMAL INDICATIONS
Reaction	Acid	Neutral or slightly alkaline in some cases of gastric carcinoma or severe chronic gastritis or when containing a large amount of saliva
Mucus	Small amount	Large amount in chronic gastritis
Bile	Trace	Large amount rare, points to duodenal obstruction
Blood	None	Indicates gastric hemorrhage or injury from tube
Particles of food		Those eaten hours or days previously indicate deficient motor power or pyloric obstruction
Free acids (hydrochloric)	Positive	Negative suggests gastric carcinoma, gastric ulcer, and neurosis Excessive amount suggests duodenal ulcer
Lactic acid		Present when hydrochloric acid is abnormally decreased
Yeast cells	Few	Excess suggests retention and fermentation
Lactobacillus of Boas-Oppler	None	Rare in any disease except carcinoma of stomach; occurs in majority of cases of carcinoma

MEDICATIONS TO REVIEW

Antacids. Bismuth magma (Cremo-Bismuth, Lac-Bismo); bismuth subcarbonate (Cremo-Carbonates); bismuth subgallate; sodium acetate; aluminum hydroxide (Aludrox SA, Aludrox Suspension, Aludrox Tablets, Amphojel Suspension and Tablets, Co-Gel, Donnalate, Estomul, Gelusil, Kolantyl, Kudrox, Maalox, Magnatril Suspension and Tablets, Marblen Suspension and Tablets, Modutrol, Mylanta, Polymagma Suspension and Tablets, Robalate, Sigmagen, Silain-Gel, Spasmasorb, Trisogel, WinGel).

Antiemetics. Bucladin, Torecan.

Smooth Muscle Relaxants and Tranquilizers. Isovex-60, Spasodil, Trocinate; Compazine, Librium, Meprospan, Meprotabs, Miltown, Softran, Tybatran, Vistaril.

Digestants. Arco-Lase, Bilogest, Butibel-Zyme, Canz Tablets, Combichole, Convertin, Convertin-H, Converzyme, Dactilase, Digestant, Digolase, Donnazyme, Entozyme, Enzypan, Festal, Gastroenterase, Geramine, Gustase, Kanulase, Kanumodic, Kutrase, Ku-Zyme, Lipan, Pentazyme, Phazyme, Pro-Gestive, Therabile.

Anticholinergics and Combination. Akalon, Belbarb, Butibel, Combid Spansule capsules, Cyclo-Bell, Darbid, Daricon, Donnalate, Donnatal, Enarax, Murel, Nembu-donna, Pamine, Pathibamate, Pathilon, Piptal, Pro-Banthine, Prydon Spansule capsules, Prydonnal, Robinul, Tral Gradumet and Filmtab, Tral with phenobarbital, Transentine hydrochloride, Trest, Valpin.

Antidiarrhetics. Gel-Kote, Kaopectate.

Anti-infectives. Coly-Mycin, Furoxone, Kaomycin, Kectil Suspension, Mycifradin, Paremycin Elixir, Polymagma Suspension and Tablets.

Laxatives. Agoral, Bilron, Fleet Enema, Metamucil, Kondremul, Peri-Colace, Neoloid, Phospho-Soda, Senokot.

BIBLIOGRAPHY

Adson, M. A.: Emergency Portal-Systemic Shunts. Surg. Clin. North America, 47:4, 1967.

Barton, K. M.: Gastric Ulcer: Individualization in Diagnosis and Therapy. Med. Clin. North America, 64: 103, 1964.

Beeson, P. B., and McDermott, W.: Cecil-Loeb Textbook of Medicine. 12th ed. Philadelphia, W. B. Saunders Co., 1967.

Bielski, M. T., and Molander, D. W.: Laennec's Cirrhosis. Am. J. Nurs., 65:82, 1965.

Borosini, A. V.: Bowel Conditions and Your Posture. Life & Hlth., 80:33, 1965.

Boxall, T. A.: Current Trends in Rectal Surgery. Nurs. Mir., 122:583, 1966.

Brown, A.: Medical Nursing. 3rd ed. Philadelphia, W. B. Saunders Co., 1957.

Cunningham, L.: The Patient with Ruptured Esophageal Varices. Am. J. Nurs. 62:69, 1962.

Davidsohn, I., and Henry, J. B.: Todd-Sanford Clinical Diagnosis by Laboratory Methods. 14th ed. Philadelphia, W. B. Saunders Co., 1969.

Davis, L.: Christopher's Textbook of Surgery. 9th ed. Philadelphia, W. B. Saunders Co., 1968.

Dericks, V. C.: Rehabilitation of Patients with Ileostomy. Am. J. Nurs., 61:48, 1961.

Drummond, E. E.: Gastrointestinal Suction. Am. J. Nurs., 63:109, 1963.

Eisenberg, S.: Proctosigmoidoscopy. Am. J. Nurs., 65: 113, 1965.

Eisenmenger, W. J.: Viral Hepatitis. Am. J. Nurs., 61: 56, 1961.

Fason, M. F.: Controlling Bacterial Growth in Tube Feedings. Am. J. Nurs., 67:1246, 1967.

Glenn, F.: Surgical Treatment of Biliary Tract Disease. Am. J. Nurs., 64:88, 1964.

Goldsteen, F.: New Approaches to the Management of Peptic Ulcer. Med. Clin. North America, 49:1253, 1965.

Harmer, B., and Henderson, V.: Textbook of Principles and Practice of Nursing. 5th ed. New York, The Macmillan Co., 1958.

Henderson, L. M.: Nursing Care in Acute Cholecystitis. Am. J. Nurs., 64:93, 1964.

Katona, E.: Learning Colostomy Control. Am. J. Nurs., 67:534, 1967.

Klug, T. J.: Gastric Resection and Nursing Care. Am. J. Nurs., 61:73, 1961.

Kurihara, M.: The Patient with an Intestinal Prosthesis. Am. J. Nurs., 60:852, 1960.

Linton, R.: The Treatment of Esophageal Varices. Surg. Clin. North America, 46:485, 1966.

McKittrick, J. B.: Ulcerative Colitis. Am. J. Nurs., 62: 60. 1962.

Meschan, I.: Roentgen Signs in Clinical Practice. Vols. I and II. Philadelphia, W. B. Saunders Co., 1966.

Molander, D. W.: Liver Surgery and Care of the Patient with Liver Surgery. Am. J. Nurs., 61:72, 1961.

Montag, M., and Swenson, R.: Fundamentals in Nursing Care. 3rd ed. Philadelphia, W. B. Saunders Co., 1959.

Remine, W. H. and Ferris, D. O.: Surgery for Biliary Structures. Surg. Clin. North America, 47:4, 1967.

nursing techniques in the care of

Diseases of the Musculoskeletal System

DIAGNOSTIC PROCEDURES

BLOOD TESTS

Blood Chemistry Tests

In the tests as shown on the top of page 177, 3 to 5 cc. of whole blood is withdrawn, and either the serum (oxalated specimen tubes are not needed) or plasma is examined. In all these tests the blood should be withdrawn before breakfast.

Blood Hematology Tests

No preparation of the patient is necessary for these tests.

Serological Tests

Serological tests are performed for the detection of antibodies in the serum. No preparation of the patient is necessary. The serological tests shown on the bottom of page 177 are used in the diagnosis of rheumatoid arthritis:

TEST	DESCRIPTION OF APPLICATION	NORMAL PER 100 ML.	ABNORMAL IMPLICATIONS
Aldolase	An enzyme normally present in the serum	7-14 units per cc.	Increased in muscular dystrophy
Alkaline phosphatase	Phosphatase is an enzyme that liberates organic phosphates	1.5-4 units	Increased in cystic osteofibrosis, osteogenic sarcoma, and other diseases which cause bone changes
Calcium	Calcium is stored in bones, from which it is metabolized for physiological needs	9-11 mg.	Increased in bone tumors
Fibrinogen	Aids in coagulation	0.15-0.3 gm.	Increased in malignant tumors, rheumatoid arthritis, and closed fractures
Formol gel test	Means of testing increased amounts of globulins	Negative	Positive in atrophic arthritis
Mucoprotein	Little known concerning formation	8-14 mg.	Increased in rheumatic arthritis, gout, cancer, myeloma
Phosphorus (serum-phosphate)	Absorbed in ratio to amount of calcium	3-4.5 mg.	Increased in myeloma and healing fractures
Protein (total) Gamma globulin Alpha 2 globulin	Globulin is thought to form in bone marrow	15-25% of total protein 8-13% of total protein	Both are increased in rheumatoid arthritis, osteomyelitis, and myeloma

The Antistreptolysin Test. Antistreptolysin is formed in the serum by certain strains of hemolytic streptococcus.

The RA Test. Latex coated by gamma globulin is mixed with serum. If rheumatoid arthritis is present, the serum agglutinates. Other substances that may cause agglutination in the rheumatoid serum are sheep cells and bentonite. These tests are called the sheep-cell test for rheumatoid factor and the bentonite flocculation test for rheumatoid factor.

Blood Culture

To obtain a culture, 5 cc. whole blood is placed in a culture medium, and the bacterial growth is examined microscopically. Blood culture may be used in the diagnosis of osteomyelitis and arthritis. No preparation of the patient is necessary.

URINE TESTS

Certain urine tests are sometimes useful in diagnosing orthopedic diseases. These are

TEST	ABNORMAL IMPLICATIONS
Hemoglobin	Decreased in anemia associated with arthritis
W.B.C.	Increased in joint and bone inflammations and in sarcoma
W.B.C. differential	Eosinophils increased in bone neoplasm, Basophils increased in chronic infections of bony sinuses
Sedimentation rate	Increased in chronic and localized infections

listed in the table below.

URINE TEST	NORMAL VALUE	SPECIMEN NEEDED	ABNORMAL IMPLICATIONS
Albumin	None	Fresh, voided	Present in myeloma
Bence-Jones protein	None	Fresh, voided	Present in myeloma, sarcoma, and bone metastases of carcinoma
Creatine	Less than 100 mg. in 24 hours	24-hour specimen	Increased in muscular dystrophy (Creatine is used in muscle metabolism. The wasted muscle therefore cannot retain creatine.)
Urine culture	No bacteria	Sterile, catheterized	Bacteria may indicate systemic infection

OTHER TESTS

Aspiration and Study of Synovial Fluid

Occasionally the physician will wish to remove synovial fluid (joint fluid) for laboratory examination. This is a simple procedure and can be done in the patient's room. The skin at the withdrawal site is anesthetized with an injection of 1 per cent procaine; then the same needle is pushed further into the joint, and the fluid is aspirated. The withdrawn fluid is placed in a sterile test tube or small sterile flask.

In various forms of arthritis, the leukocyte count is increased (normal: 200 or less per cu. m.), and the fluid is cloudy (normal: clear).

Bone Marrow Examination

A bone puncture may be made to examine the marrow. The technique for bone puncture is described in Chapter 14. L. E. (lupus erythematosus) cells may be present in the bone marrow in arthritis.

Cultures from Lesions on the Skin

These may be taken from lesions when present in osteomyelitis. A sterile culture tube containing a sterile applicator is used. With aseptic technique the applicator is removed from the tube and the tip rubbed on the lesion; then the applicator is replaced in the tube. The bacteria growth is examined microscopically to determine the disease-causing organism.

Biopsies

Small pieces of tumors or cysts may be removed for microscopic examination. This procedure is carried out in the operating room.

Metabolic Tests

Metabolic tests are prescribed when bone disease is caused by metabolic disorders (see Chap. 20).

X-rays

X-ray examination is one of the most frequently used diagnostic acids in diseases of the bone and joints. No preparation of the patient is necessary.

THERAPEUTIC AND REHABILITATIVE PROCEDURES

ORTHOPEDIC DEVICES

A number of devices are used in orthopedic therapy to immobilize parts of the body and to assist the patient with certain functions. Devices included in this chapter are casts, splints, braces, sandbags, crutches, walkers, traction, internal fixation methods, artificial limbs, and orthopedic beds and frames.

PLASTER OF PARIS CASTS

Plaster of paris casts are used to immobilize a part of the body in the treatment of certain types of fractures, dislocations, joint disorders, and skeletal deformities. The common areas of the placement of casts and the conditions for which they are used are shown here:

The Body Spica. Used for fracture and dislocation of the dorsal and lumbar spine. Worn about 3 months.

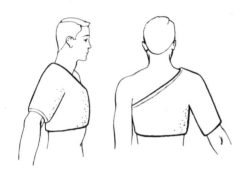

Shoulder Spica. Used for fracture of clavicle. Worn about 4 weeks.

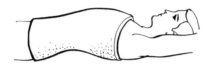

Hanging Cast. Used for a fracture of the lower shaft of the humerus and some fractures of the ulna. Worn 6 to 12 weeks.

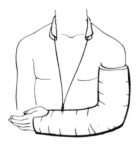

Forearm Cast. Used for fracture of wrist. Worn for about 6 weeks.

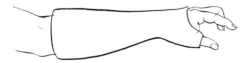

Hip Spica—Front and Side View. Used for fracture of femoral shaft. Worn about 12 weeks.

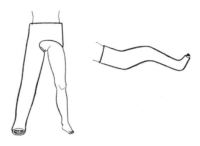

Hip Spica. For fractures of the upper femoral shaft and hip joint. Worn about 12 weeks.

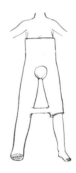

Full Leg Cast. Used for fractures of the femoral condyle, knee, shaft of tibia, and fibula. Worn 8 to 10 weeks.

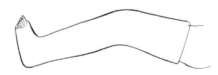

Short Leg Cast. Used in ankle and foot fractures. Worn 6 weeks.

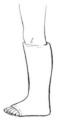

Application of Plaster of Paris Cast

The cast is applied by the physician, usually in the operating room or in a room designed for that purpose. Anesthesia or an analgesic drug is administered to the patient prior to the application of the cast in order to minimize pain and promote muscle relaxation during the procedure.

The equipment needed for the application of the cast varies with the physician's preference. The usual equipment includes a sterile

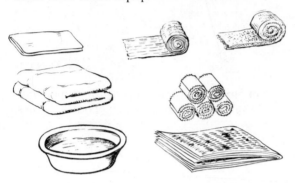

gown and gloves, stockinette and/or sheet wadding, plaster of paris bandage, a bucket or basin of water, and newspaper or other protective covering for the floor.

There is a plastic bandage available that may be used instead of plaster of paris. This bandage is immersed in acetone instead of water, and a special waterproof felt and cottonoid are used to protect the skin. This newer type of cast material is harder when dry than plaster of paris. (Additional information concerning the plastic casts is given under "Care of the Patient with a Cast.")

Sometimes small wooden splints, wire netting, or other strengthening materials are incorporated into the cast as reinforcements over areas likely to be subject to excess strain. One teaspoon of salt added to every 1000 cc. of water hastens the drying of plaster of paris.

The part to be covered by the cast is prepared by shaving, washing, and drying. The plaster of paris bandage is prepared for use like this: Remove the paper wrapping from the bandage, and place it on end in lukewarm water as shown:

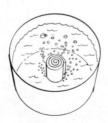

The bandage is ready to use when the bubbling stops. Allow the excess water to drain from the bandage while removing it from the water. If the physician prefers to have excess water squeezed from the bandage, hold the bandage in both hands, and gently squeeze with the fingers like this:

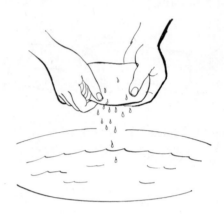

The squeezing removes plaster as well as water. If the bandage is too wet, it will telescope like this when being used:

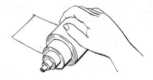

About 10 to 12 layers of bandage are applied with a circular motion. If the surgeon needs help in supporting the limb during the process, the nurse should hold the cast on the palm of the hand like this,

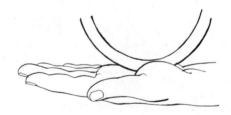

keeping the fingers away from the cast. After a sufficient number of layers have been applied, the cast is rubbed and molded for a few minutes. Some surgeons rub dry plaster on the cast.

Care of the Patient with a Cast

It may take from several hours to several days for a cast to dry, depending on the temperature of the air, the humidity, the amount of air circulation, the thickness of the cast, and the type of bandage used in the cast. Plaster of paris is available in slow, medium, and fast-setting types. Plaster of paris to which water-soluble plastic has been added dries in the same time as plain plaster of paris. The plastic bandage soluble in acetone is very slow in drying. A dry cast looks white and shiny; a wet cast is gray and dull.

During the drying process bedcovers should be held away from the wet cast with bed cradles, and if the cast is an extensive one, a bed board should be placed under the mattress to prevent sagging, which may cause the wet cast to break.

Sometimes a cast dryer is used to speed the drying process in slow-drying casts. One type of cast dryer looks like this:

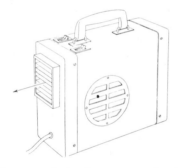

A heat lamp or hair dryer may also be used. These devices should be placed about 18 inches away from the cast.

The doctor leaves instructions as to how high the part should be elevated when the patient can be turned. Here are some methods used in elevating limbs.

This shows the use of a pillow and the Chandler leg elevator:

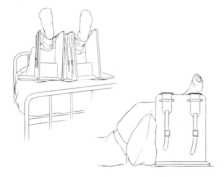

Here the entire mattress is elevated:

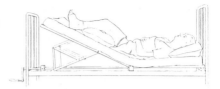

The arm can be elevated either with pillows alone or with the use of a pole:

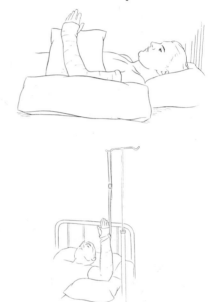

Under a wet cast it is better to use pillows that are firm and hard rather than soft and fluffy. The pillows must also have a waterproof covering, or they will become quite moist.

While the cast is drying and for about the first 24 hours, the fingers and toes must be checked frequently for symptoms of impairment of circulation: burning pain, cyanosis, swelling, coldness, and loss of sensation. These symptoms occur not only from a tight cast (the cast tends to shrink as it dries) but also from the swelling that sometimes occurs around the fracture.

Any seepage of blood through the cast should be encircled and dated like this:

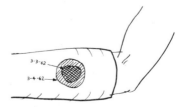

After the cast is dry, the cast edges should be finished. If the stockinette padding is long enough, bring it up around the edges and fasten it with adhesive tape like this:

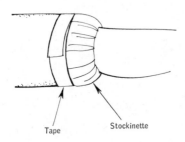

Tape   Stockinette

If the stockinette is too short, fix the edges with adhesive tape cut in short strips. To fix these, cut 2-inch lengths of 1- or 2-inch adhesive tape, and place them on wax paper like this:

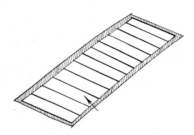

Then fold the paper in half, and trim the edges like this:

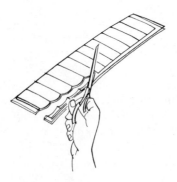

Now pull the strips from the wax paper,

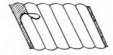

and place them around the edge of the cast like this:

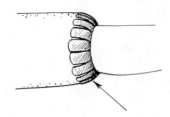

Any unused tape on the wax paper can be stored for future use.

Proper body alignment and positioning is extremely important to the patient in a cast for several reasons: One must prevent pinching of the skin and formation of pressure areas on the bony protrusions around the edges of the cast. With a body cast, positioning is also important to allow for maximum chest expansion in respiration. A number of well selected and properly placed supports are used to position the patient. These supports can be made from small and large pillows, folded or rolled bath blankets, folded sheets, and an assortment of sizes and shapes of sandbags. It is impossible to describe here the best kind of support for each type of cast-patient situation.

Here are several examples of the results desired. A support like this keeps pressure off the heel and keeps the cast from pressing into the top of the leg:

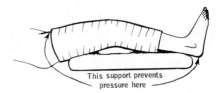

This support prevents pressure here

Here the supports under the head and back keep pressure off the abdomen, chest, and back, and the support under the leg keeps the cast edge from cutting into the skin:

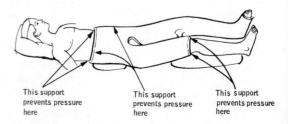

This support prevents pressure here

This support prevents pressure here

This support prevents pressure here

From these examples you can see that the amount of support required to promote body alignment varies with the size and weight of the patient, the thickness of the cast, and the extent of the area covered by the cast. Remember, the patient can usually tell whether or not he is comfortable!

While the patient is confined to bed, his position must be changed frequently. The patient with the hip spica cast is turned on his abdomen three or four times daily. Three or four persons are needed to do this.

With an extensive cast, explanations of turning procedures should be given to the patient to prevent added fear of falling out of bed. Some patients prefer to have bedsides until the fear of helplessness and of falling out of bed is overcome.

When one or both arms are free, a trapeze should be attached to the bed like this

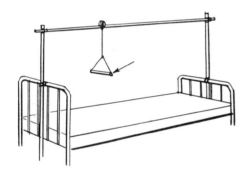

so that the patient can help in changing his position.

The patient with a hip spica can turn himself with a rope and pulley fastened overhead and on the side toward which he wishes to turn:

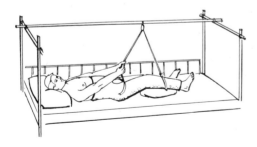

Patients with arm and leg casts in most instances can get out of bed. The patient with a leg cast gets into a wheelchair like this:

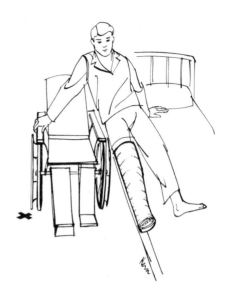

Note that the wheelchair is placed on the side of the affected leg. Also note the X on the floor. Stand on this spot, and steady the wheelchair with one leg, grasping the cast with both hands. Most patients with a walking cast must be reminded to walk with the foot forward. The usual tendency is to slant the foot outward as shown by the dotted lines here:

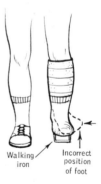

Walking iron

Incorrect position of foot

Note how the walking cast is protected by a sock with a hole cut in the sole.

Elimination usually presents problems to the patient in a hip spica. It is difficult to use a bedpan, and the edges of the case around the perineal area become soiled from excreta. It is better to take steps right at the start to prevent soiling of the cast, because once the cast becomes soiled and odorous, not too much can be done about it. To protect the cast, push sheets of plastic under the entire edge of the opening, both front and back, and tape the plastic to the outside of the cast like this:

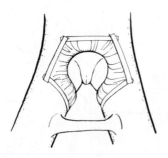

When placing the patient on a bedpan, keep the upper trunk and cast elevated so that excretions do not run up under the cast. Support the patient like this:

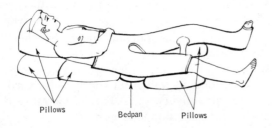

Pillows Bedpan Pillows

Voiding is especially difficult for the female patient in a hip spica. We have tried all sorts of methods and devices to reduce wetting accidents and have found the emesis basin to be the most satisfactory. Use a large emesis basin, and simply push it up under the patient like this:

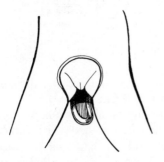

The skin along the edges of the cast should be washed, dried, rubbed, and inspected daily for irritation. Reach up under the cast like this to massage the skin and remove broken pieces of plaster:

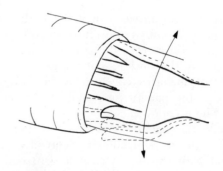

Meanwhile, note whether musty odors are coming from under the cast. An odor may indicate pus formation.

Devices for scratching under the cast include a scratcher made from tongue blades taped together like this:

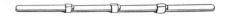

and a piece of muslin bandage pushed under the cast with a yardstick and tied like this:

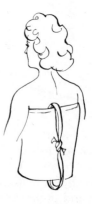

To clean a soiled cast, rub it with a small amount of scouring agent (Comet, Babo, etc.) on a damp cloth; then dry is promptly. Indelible stains may be covered with patches of adhesive tape and plaster of paris bandage or with white shoe polish. Plastic casts are waterproof and may be washed with soap and water. Plastic spray applied to a dry plaster cast protects it from soil.

Removal of the Cast

The cast is removed when it is no longer necessary for immobilization or when an x-ray must be taken as an aid in further treatment. The plastic cast need not be removed, as x-rays can penetrate this material. The physician removes the cast with an electric cast cutter or by making a cut with the plaster knife and plaster scissors. Acetic acid or hydrogen peroxide forced against the cutting line with an Asepto syringe helps to soften the plaster.

The skin that was covered by the cast is flaky, and the muscles and joints are sore and stiff. The skin should be treated gently (no vigorous rubbing). If a second cast is to be applied after the removal of the first, there should be no washing of the skin, as this might be traumatizing. Muscle action is reestablished through prescribed exercise.

Instruments Used

Instruments kept on hand in an orthopedic department for use with a patient in a cast include these:

The hand cast cutter

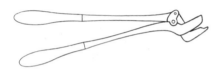

The electric cast cutter

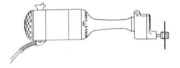

Cast spreaders

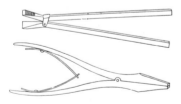

A cast knife

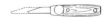

And a cast scissors

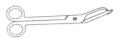

SPLINTS

Splints are used to immobilize and support an extremity in emergencies and in treating some types of fractures, dislocations, and muscular deformities. Splints used in emergencies are usually simple devices such as heavy cardboard, wooden slats, and half-ring traction splints. A pillow and wooden slats are used in the emergency treatment of fractures of the knee, leg, or foot. This splint is applied like this:

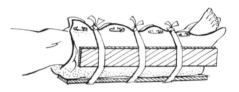

A half-ring traction splint is used for emergency treatment of fractures of the thigh. It looks like this:

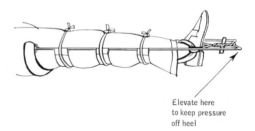

Elevate here
to keep pressure
off heel

For the emergency treatment of fractures of the forearm, wrist, and hand, heavy cardboard or padded board splints are used with a sling.

Splints used for prolonged immobilization may include any of the following:

1. Aluminum splints. These come in an assortment of sizes and shapes contoured to fit entire arms or legs, or parts of them.
2. Plaster of paris splints. These are commercially prepared or can be made by folding plaster of paris bandage back and forth to

make a strip the desired length and width with a thickness of about eight layers. The strip is immersed in warm water like this:

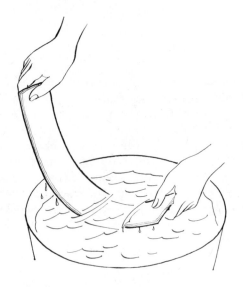

Then the layers are rubbed together with the hand, and the moistened strip is placed next to the extremity and molded to fit the contour like this:

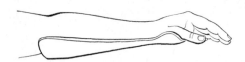

3. Wooden splints. These have seldom been used since the advent of aluminum splints. When they are used, they must be padded on the side that comes in contact with the skin. The padding is fastened to the splint with gauze bandage.
4. Splints that permit some motion are used in treating certain muscular deformities. An example of such a splint is shown here:

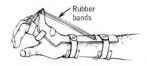

Rubber bands

This splint keeps the wrist in the position of extension, yet allows motion of the fingers.
5. Splints used in providing traction (see p. 185).

Care of the patient wearing a splint includes observation for circulatory impairment and skin irritation due to pressure and friction areas. Bandages holding splints in place are changed as necessary by the physician. If the bandage becomes unsightly, the nurse can cover the soiled portion with another layer of clean bandage.

BRACES

Types of Braces

Braces are designed to support weakened muscles, joints, and bones in rehabilitation and to immobilize specific parts in the treatment of fractures and injuries while permitting a maximum use of the undiseased portion of the body. Braces are usually made of various combinations of leather, metal, and cotton lacing. The types of commonly used braces and the therapeutic uses are as follows:

Leg Braces. These are worn most frequently in muscular deformities when the joint—particularly the knee—buckles with weight bearing. They are also worn for immobilization following fractures of the tibia and fibula when the bone has not healed sufficiently to permit full weight bearing, and for the treatment of clubfoot and foot drop. The leg brace may extend from the foot to the calf, from the foot to the lower portion of the thigh, and from the foot to the upper portion of the thigh. Some braces permit joint motion but not weight bearing. Since there are numerous leg braces manufactured with structural variations, it is impossible to describe every brace. Shown here is a long brace used to support knee and ankle motion:

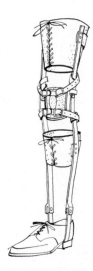

Braces of this type are also made with foot plates to be worn inside a shoe. Shown here is a short leather brace worn for immobilization of the ankle:

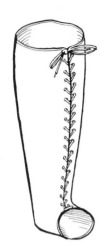

Neck Braces. These are worn to immobilize in the treatment of fractures and diseases of the cervical spine. One type is shown here:

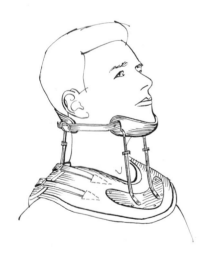

Back Braces. A back brace is worn to immobilize the spine in treatment of fractures or other injuries. A brace used for extensive injury of the lumbar and dorsolumbar spine is shown here:

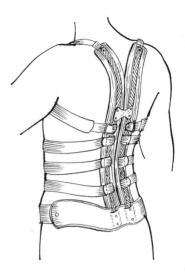

Back braces for less extensive spinal injuries may consist of heavy cloth corsets or belts and short metal-leather braces made on the order of the one just illustrated.

Arm Braces. These are made in sizes corresponding to the leg braces either to support joint motion or to immobilize specific portions.

Care of the Patient with a Brace

In outlining a specific program of rehabilitation, the physician and the physiotherapist prescribe the brace most suitable to the patient's needs and instruct the patient and his family in the functions of the brace, the methods of placing and wearing the brace, the care of the brace, and when the brace should be worn. Depending on the purpose, the brace may be prescribed for use continuously, only during activity, or for a certain number of hours daily.

If the disability is extensive the nurse may be required to assist the patient in putting on the brace. Leg braces extending above the knee, long arm braces, and back braces are put in place with the patient lying flat in bed. Back braces are buckled or laced from the bottom up. Short leg braces and neck braces are put in place while the patient is sitting on a chair. All braces must be fastened firmly in order to fulfill their purpose but must not be fastened so tightly as to cause circulatory impairment. Braces placed while the patient is lying in bed may need adjustment after the patient stands. Any discomfort caused by wearing the brace should be reported to the physician and noted on the patient's records.

The care of braces includes the usual preservative and cleansing treatment of leather, the prevention of rust on metal, and lubrication of metal joints. Cloth corsets are washed by hand. Worn laces must be replaced.

Braces are usually prescribed shortly before the patient's discharge from the hospital or when the patient is being treated as an outpatient. Consequently, the length of time the nurse cares for the patient with a brace is usually brief. The patient who is hospitalized after becoming accustomed to wearing a brace can usually offer helpful suggestions to the nurse in the placement and usage of the brace.

SANDBAGS

Sandbags are used to immobilize portions of the body in specific positions. Sandbags are available in a variety of sizes and shapes. The number and size of sandbags to be used is usually the nurse's decision. The sandbag should be covered with a specially designed washable cover or a face towel before use. Sandbags are useful in all medical and surgical services. Orthopedically they are frequently used to hold a limb in a position of abduction (away from the center of the body) and adduction (toward the center) as shown here:

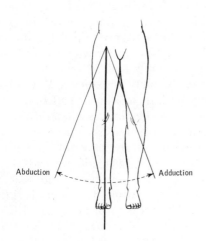

and to prevent outward and inward rotation of the leg as shown here:

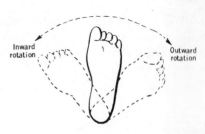

They are also useful in elevating parts of the body.

CRUTCHES

When the patient is ready to start crutch walking he is referred to the physiotherapy department. There the physiotherapist selects the crutches best suited for the patient's needs and teaches the patient how to use them. Occasionally when the patient is going to use crutches for only a brief time, the nurse does the fitting. There are several methods used in measuring for crutches.

1. Measure the distance from the armpit to the sole of the foot with the patient lying flat in bed; then add 6 to 8 inches. The crutches are longer than the body measurement because of the slant away from the body during use.
2. Subtract 16 inches from the patient's total height while the patient is lying in bed.
3. Measure from the axilla to a point 6 to 8 inches out from the side of the heel.

When the patient stands with the crutches, the position of the feet and the crutches should be like this:

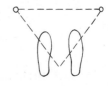

If the crutches are the right length, the arm should be at this angle while standing and resting

In skeletal traction the pulling device is attached to stainless steel tongs, wire, or a pin, which is inserted into the bone. Tongs are generally used only on the skull in promoting traction in the cervical spine. The Crutchfield tongs, designed for use on the skull, is shown here:

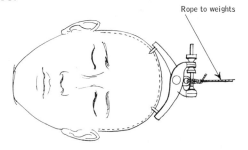

The wire and pin are used on extremities. The Kirschner wire, used most frequently, is placed like this:

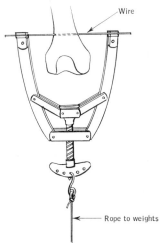

and the Steinmann pin like this:

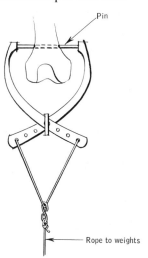

The pulling force in traction is accomplished by the use of weights fastened with a rope on the end of the skin and skeletal traction device. The direction of pull is fixed by placing the rope on one or more pulleys suspended above and/or beyond the frame of the bed. There are a variety of ways to set up traction depending on the condition for which the traction is applied.

Types of Traction

Here are the commonly used types of traction:

Buck's Extension. This is a form of skin traction applied to the leg as temporary treatment for fractures of the upper portion of the shaft or neck of the femur. This traction may also be applied to both legs in the treatment of low back pain. The direction of pull is straight, as shown:

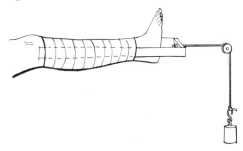

Russell Traction. This is a form of skin traction applied to the leg in treating some fractures of the shaft and neck of the femur. In Russell traction a pulling force in line with the femur is accomplished with the use of a knee sling and the arrangement of pulleys as shown:

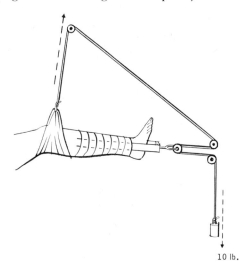

10 lb.

The vertical force at the knee is equal to that of the amount of weight applied. Because of the pulley arrangement at the foot, there are two lines of pull, making the horizontal force twice that of the weight. The pulling force of the two parallel ropes at the foot is illustrated in this diagram:

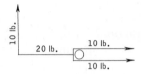

The vertical and horizontal forces combine to produce the resultant force, which, as illustrated below, lies in the direct line of the femur.

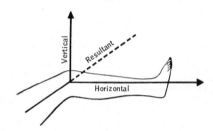

Balanced Traction. Skeletal traction is used with this type traction for the treatment of fractures of the shaft of the femur. The desired flexion of the hip and knee is maintained by the use of the Thomas splint and the Pearson attachment shown here:

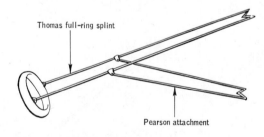

Strips of muslin or face towels are pinned to the metal frame to make a hammock-like support for the leg. The support is held in position by attached weights and ropes suspended on pulleys. Here is one method of applying balanced traction:

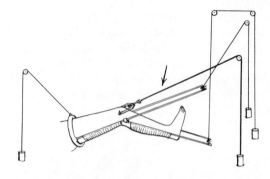

The arrow indicates the weight attachment that creates traction. All other weight attachments serve to hold the leg in the desired position. Note that the muslin support should not extend under the heel in order to prevent the formation of a decubitus.

Arm Traction. Here is a type of skin traction used for fractures of the shaft of the humerus:

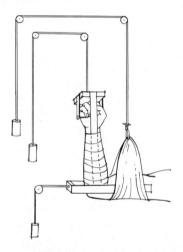

Skeletal traction for some fractures of the lower portion of the humerus may look like this:

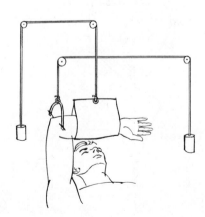

Cervical Traction and Pelvic Traction. For these types the line of pull is straight. The tongs and halter used for cervical traction and the belt used in pelvic traction have already been described.

Setting Up Traction

The surgeon or resident applies traction with the nurse assisting. The nurse is responsible for making certain that all the equipment needed is on hand. When she learns which method of traction is to be used, she can assemble the equipment. Some hospitals have carts with articles such as pulleys, rope, wooden blocks, slings, weights, and frames. In this event the whole cart is brought to the bedside. In other institutions the orderly brings the equipment to the patient's room. If an overhead frame is needed, the nurse and the orderly put it in place. The newer frames are made of aluminum and have the screwing and clamping devices attached in such a way that they cannot be removed and lost. These frames are lightweight and are easy to assemble.

For skin traction the nurse also needs these articles:

Three- or 4-inch wide adhesive or moleskin

Several 2- or 3-inch Ace bandages

Equipment to shave the skin

Tincture of benzoin to paint the skin

The wire and pins used in skeletal traction are usually inserted in the operating room. Occasionally they are inserted in the patient's room. The pin and wire are drilled through the bone with a hand or electrically driven drill. When these are inserted in the patient's room, the nurse needs:

Skin prep tray

Local anesthesia tray

Sterile wire or pin and tongs that hold them

Wire cutters and drill—usually obtained from operating room

Sterile gloves and gown

After the traction device has been applied on the skin or in the bone, the physician fixes the ropes, slings, pulleys, and weights in the manner desired. Weights are never hung over the patient.

Wires protruding from the sides of skeletal traction devices should be covered with cork or rubber bottle stoppers like this:

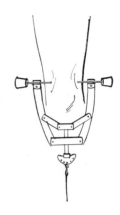

A 2 × 2 inch gauze dressing is slit with sterile scissors and placed around the area where the wire or pin is inserted like this:

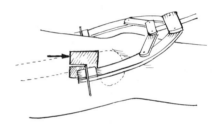

This dressing can be held in place with surgical adhesive (see p. 190).

For every pound of traction applied, an equal amount of force must pull in the opposite direction. The opposite force is called counter traction. In Buck's extension, counter traction is accomplished by elevating the foot of the bed on blocks like this:

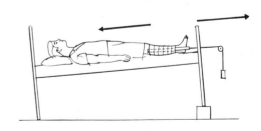

Unless orders are written to the contrary, traction is always continuous. Factors inhibiting traction are: (1) removal of weights; (2)

weights resting on a chair or part of the bed; (3) ropes jammed in pulleys; and (4) improper body alignment that changes the direction of pull. The nurse should check daily to make sure none of these conditions exist.

Care of the Patient in Traction

While in traction, the patient's position must be changed frequently to prevent pressure areas. With a fracture of the lower leg, the patient may sit up as far as he desires. With a femoral fracture the patient may usually assume a semi-Fowler's position, and with fractures of the humerus or clavicle, the head is usually kept flat.

An overhead trapeze bar is used to help the patient move about in bed and on and off bedpans.

To prevent foot drop on the affected leg, a strip of adhesive is placed on the sole, and fastened to weights like this:

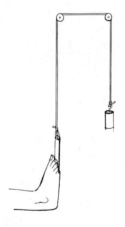

or a special attachment is fastened to the Pearson attachment like this:

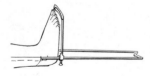

When the leg is in traction, both top and bottom bedding are made up in two sections. The two bottom sheets are overlapped just above the buttocks. The foot-end sheet is placed over the head-end sheet as shown here

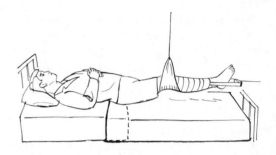

to facilitate easy removal. This section is the one removed most often. The two top sheets are overlapped and pinned together on both sides of the exposed leg like this:

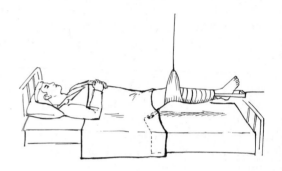

Internal Fixation Devices

Certain devices are used to immobilize fractures internally. Internal fixation devices are made of metal alloys and are commercially prepared in a variety of designs for numerous purposes. The commonly used types and their uses are as follows:

Circular Wiring. This is used in fractures of the mandible. The wire is inserted into the bone and wound around the fractured segments.

Plates and Screws. These are used for short oblique and transverse fractures. They are fastened to the bone like this:

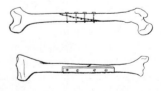

Intramedullary Nails and Pins. These are used in transverse fractures located in the center of bones. There are a number of designs of nails and pins available. Several designs are illustrated here. The Rush medullary pin is inserted like this:

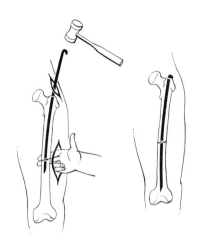

The Hansen-Street pin is inserted in the same manner as the Rush pin. Shown below is a cross section of the Hansen-Street pin, and the pin in place.

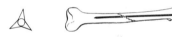

The Smith-Petersen nail is used for fixation of a fracture of the neck of the femur as shown:

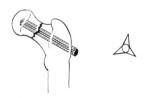

The McLaughlin nail-plate device is used as shown in trochanteric fractures:

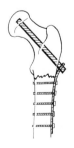

Endoprosthesis or Femoral Head Prosthesis.
A metallic femoral head prosthesis is used when the chances of healing are small in a subcapital fracture of the neck of the femur. In persons over the age of 65, the endoprosthesis is usually the treatment of choice for this type fracture. Shown here is the Moore self-locking femoral head designed to approximate the anatomic outline of the upper portion of the femur:

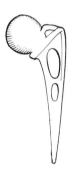

The Minneapolis Orthopedic Society prosthesis looks like this:

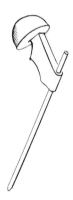

The use of these various types of metal fixation devices has revolutionized the care of many patients. Depending upon the type and location of the fracture, the patient may be ambulatory several days after the fixation. The length of hospitalization is also much shorter. The internal fixation device may be removed after the bony union has taken place, but frequently it is never removed unless symptoms of complication occur. The femoral head prosthesis of course is never removed.

ARTIFICIAL LIMBS

An amputation of an extremity is sometimes necessary in the treatment of gangrene, deformities, tumors, septic wounds, compound fractures, and severe crushing injuries. In considering the amputation site, the physician selects the site most favorable to the utilization of a prosthesis later. The common sites of amputations of the upper and lower extremity are shown here:

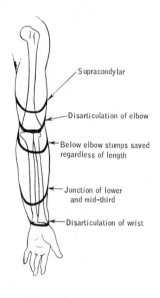

- Supracondylar
- Disarticulation of elbow
- Below elbow stumps saved regardless of length
- Junction of lower and mid-third
- Disarticulation of wrist

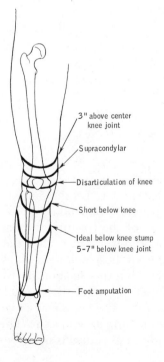

- 3" above center knee joint
- Supracondylar
- Disarticulation of knee
- Short below knee
- Ideal below knee stump 5-7" below knee joint
- Foot amputation

Care of Amputees

When the patient returns from the operating room, vital signs are checked and the dressings are watched for signs of hemorrhage. A heavy tourniquet is always kept fastened to the head or foot of the bed so that it can be applied immediately if sudden hemorrhage should occur.

In all amputations of the arm and those below the knee on the leg, the stump is usually elevated for about a week postoperatively.

After a leg amputation at or above the knee, the stump is usually not elevated for as long, as this causes permanent hip flexure. In these cases it may be necessary to place a sandbag on the leg stump to hold it down. Having the patient lie on his abdomen several times daily also helps to prevent hip flexure.

The stump is bandaged tightly at first to prevent hemorrhage and later to shrink the stump. The nurse is usually responsible for the bandaging after the stump has healed. The method of applying a bandage to the stump is illustrated on page 204. A board or plaster splint is sometimes used to hold the extremity in complete extension in amputations below the knee and elbow. After the wound has healed, the splints are removed, and exercises are started.

The open method of amputation may be used when infection is present. In this type of surgery the skin on the stump end is left open for drainage, and skin traction is applied like this:

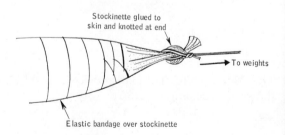

Stockinette glued to skin and knotted at end

To weights

Elastic bandage over stockinette

The stump is closed when edema has subsided, the skin has become well fixed, and drainage has ceased.

Cineplasty is another method being used in arm amputations below the elbow and in amputations above the elbow when the stump is of good length. In cineplasty the muscles of the stump are rebuilt in such a way that they control the prosthetic hand. Shown here is a cineplastic prosthesis controlled by the metal tube placed in the biceps brachii.

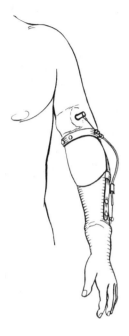

The most radical amputations are the interscapularthoracic amputation in the upper extremity and the hemipelvectomy in the lower extremity. The patient with a hemipelvectomy usually finds this position comfortable.

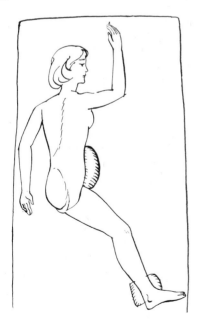

The trunk is supported by a firm pillow tucked tightly under the abdomen.

The artificial limbs used for these radical amputations are currently not too satisfactory. A prosthesis that enables the patient with a hemipelvectomy to sit may be made from felt padding and sponge rubber reinforced with wire such as from a coat hanger. The padding is shaped to fit the patient like this:

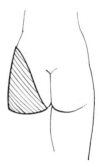

The padding is then fastened inside a binder made with two layers of elastic adhesive tape. The adhesive side is placed next to each side of the padding. The entire binder may be covered with moleskin to prevent wrinkling. The entire binder is made on the patient. After completion the front may be slit and prepared for lacing. The completed prosthesis looks like this:

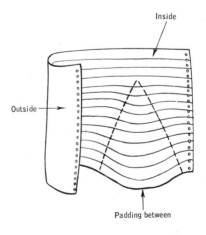

Inside

Outside →

Padding between

ORTHOPEDIC BEDS AND FRAMES

There are various beds and frames available that are designed to make it easier to change the orthopedic patient's position and at the same time keep the fractured part immobile. Beds and frames commonly in use are these:

Fracture Bed. In the newer type fracture bed, the patient rests on suspended canvas strips. Here is a fracture bed with the mattress lowered and a canvas strip loosened for placement of the bedpan:

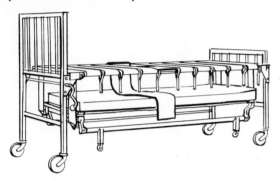

One of the features of the fracture bed is that a bedpan can be given to the patient without disturbing his position.

Ortho-Fit Bed. The mattress of this bed is made in such a way that it does not wrinkle when bent, as shown:

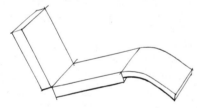

The head-end section of the mattress is moderately firm, the middle section is firm, and the foot section is merely a small pad.

Stryker Frame. The Stryker frame is used for fractures and injuries of the spinal column. With this apparatus the patient is turned from his back to his abdomen and vice versa by turning the whole frame on which he lies. The Stryker frame looks like this:

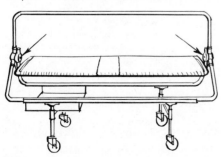

Notice the arrows pointing to the pivots at each end of the frame. These pivots enable the frame to be turned.

To turn the patient, actually two frames are used—one over and one under the patient. The frame on top of the patient is screwed in place like this (arrows):

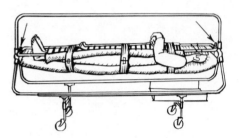

The straps are placed around the frame to prevent the patient from sliding out in the turning process.

An additional feature of this apparatus is that one nurse can turn a patient herself by loosening a locking spring at each end. Steady the frame while you loosen one end, then the other. When both springs are loose, turn it like this:

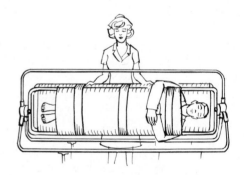

When the frame is turned to the correct position, it is automatically locked in place, signaled by two clicking sounds. Sometimes the frame must be rocked slightly to find the correct position for the locking springs to close. After the patient is turned, the top frame is removed.

The frame on which the patient lies on his abdomen is called the anterior frame and that on which the patient lies on his back is called the posterior frame. Both frames are covered with canvas sections. A small canvas strip across the middle is removed for the use of the bedpan as shown:

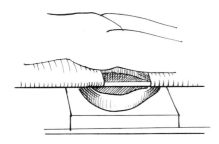

The upper canvas on the posterior frame extends from the top of the frame to the symphysis pubis. The upper canvas on the anterior frame should extend from the shoulder to the symphysis pubis. This allows a space for the head so that the patient can eat and read.

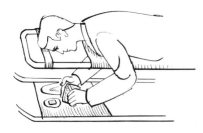

The perineal openings on both frames should extend from the symphysis pubis to about 8 inches below it.

The canvas sections are covered with a bath blanket and a sheet over it. These are brought around the back and pinned in place like this:

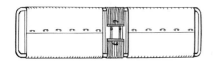

Stockinette is a convenient covering for the perineal sections.

While the patient is on the Stryker frame, his position is usually changed every 1 to 3 hours. While the patient is prone, an arm rest is fastened to the sides of the frame as shown:

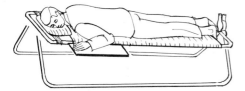

Notice also the small pillow placed above the face opening and the correct length of the bottom canvas, allowing the toes to dangle.

Foster Orthopedic Bed. The Foster bed is used for the same purposes as the Stryker frame. It is similar in design to the Stryker frame but is heavier and more stable and takes up more space. The Foster bed is also more expensive.

CircOlectric Bed. The CircOlectric bed is also used for the same purpose as the Stryker frame. With this bed the position of the patient is changed by electrical operation of the bed. A pushbutton on an electrical switch is depressed to move the patient to "face" and "back" positions. The "back" position on the CircOlectric bed looks like this:

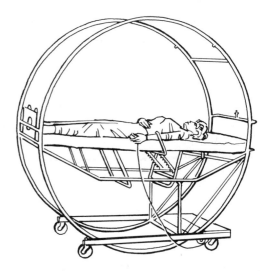

The patient is changed to the prone position by placing a frame on the patient like this:

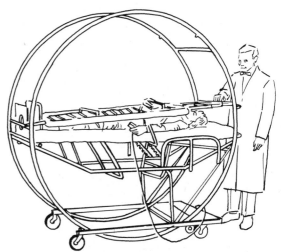

then rotating the bed like this:

Other positions possible with the CircOlectric bed include these:

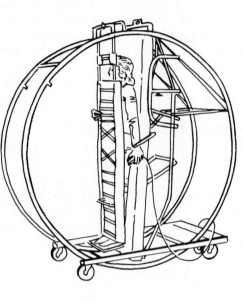

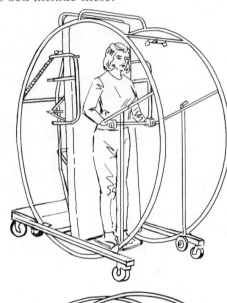

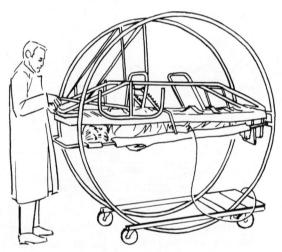

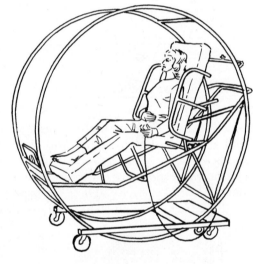

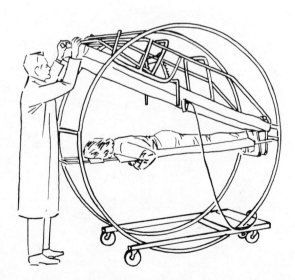

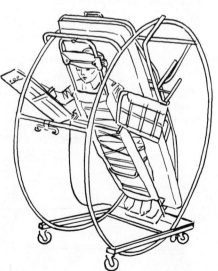

BANDAGING AND BINDING

Bandages have a number of uses in orthopedic nursing. When bandages and binders are used to immobilize fractures, the physician puts the bandage on.

Here are some ways of using various types of bandage materials to immobilize fractures. In the treatment of a fractured clavicle, a heavy muslin bandage, placed over felt or sponge rubber padding, is applied in figure eight fashion like this:

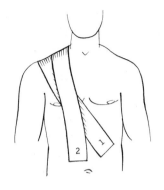

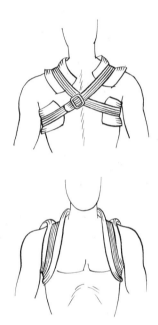

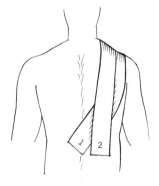

Fractures of the lower ribs are immobilized either with muslin binders or with adhesive strapping. The adhesive strapping may be done over a cotton undergarment like this:

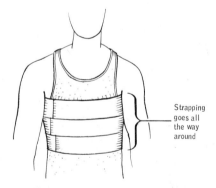

Strapping goes all the way around

Adhesive strapping applied for a dislocated shoulder looks like this:

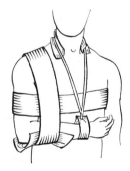

Padding is placed on the arm as shown and in the axilla and between the elbow and chest.

Adhesive strapping for fractures of the upper four ribs is applied like this:

In the emergency treatment of fractures, the swathe and sling are especially useful. For fractures of the arm and elbow, the swathe and sling are used like this:

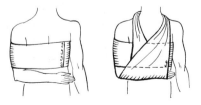

The swathe and sling are also used in the treatment of fractured ribs. The sling, of course, has a number of additional uses, most of which are familiar to everyone.

Most of the bandaging done by the orthopedic nurse is in connection with holding dressings in place preoperatively and sometimes postoperatively. The areas usually presenting the greatest difficulty are the head, neck, shoulder, hands and feet, upper thigh and trunk, and an amputation stump. Here are a few suggestions for handling these problem areas.

Head Dressings. Dressings are best held in place on the head with a gauze drape about 20 inches square. Place the piece of gauze over the dressings like this:

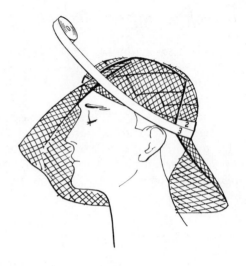

Complete the procedure with several more turns of bandage and a few strips of adhesive as shown:

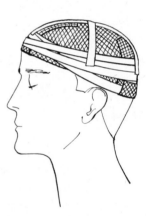

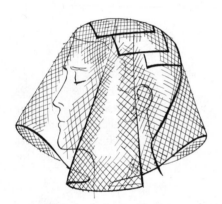

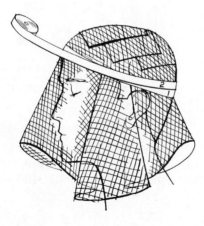

Next put two rows of bandage around the head. On the third time around the head, tuck the gauze up under the bandage as shown:

Neck Dressings. To hold dressings to the neck, a figure eight is applied like this:

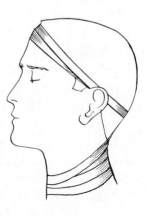

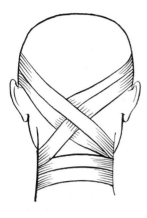

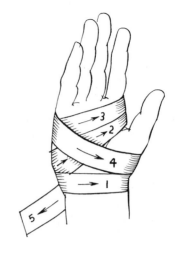

Shoulder Dressings. These are held in place with the bandage applied like this:

A foot bandage should look like this:

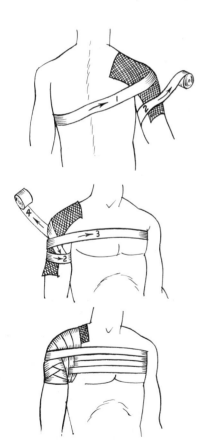

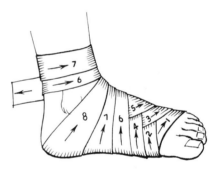

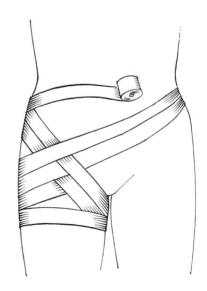

Upper Thigh and Trunk. Dressings on the upper thigh must be anchored around the trunk as shown:

Hand and Foot Dressings. Dressings covering the palmar or dorsal surface of the hand are bandaged like this:

Dressings on the lower trunk should be anchored around the thigh as shown:

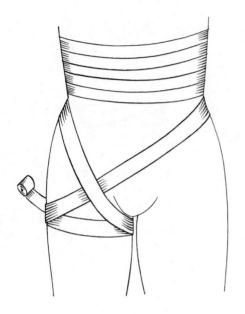

The spiral reverse bandage is used for bandaging all parts, such as the arms and legs, that are conical in shape. The spiral reverse is shown here:

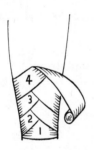

Amputation Stump. The original dressing on an amputation stump is applied tightly to reduce postoperative hemorrhage. As an extra precaution, a tourniquet should also be kept on hand in the event bleeding does occur. The nurse must know how to apply the tourniquet, and if bleeding does occur she does not wait for a doctor's order to use it. Hemorrhage is most likely to occur during the first 24 to 48 hours.

A scant oozing is normally noted on the bottom of the dressing during the first day. It is a good idea to mark the outline of this stain with a pencil so that the rate of drainage

can be closely observed. The dressings are reinforced during this time, not changed. After the wound has healed satisfactorily, the nurse bandages the stump. This bandage must be put on tightly in order to shrink the stump so that it can be fitted into a prosthesis. An Ace bandage is applied like this:

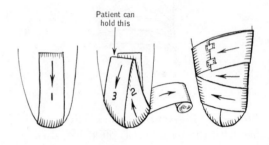

The bandage is applied more tightly around the end of the stump than elsewhere. When the arm or leg stump is short, the shoulder or hip spica must be used to keep the bandage in place as shown:

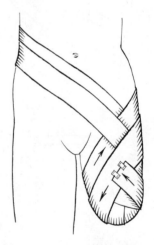

The patient is shown how to apply this pressure bandage before discharge.

PHYSIOTHERAPY

The principles of physiotherapy are applied quite frequently in the treatment of the orthopedic patient. The physiotherapeutic regimen for various conditions may be as follows.

Sprains and Strains. Cold is initially applied to reduce internal hemorrhage. Within 12 to 24 hours, heat may be applied by means of diathermy or hot packs. Massage proximal to the involved joint is frequently helpful, and gentle passive exercise is tolerated beginning on the third or fourth day.

Contusions. Severe contusions are usually treated with cold packs if seen within the first 6 hours. No other physiotherapeutic procedure is performed until the 6-hour period has lapsed. Twenty-four hours after the injury, local heat and gentle massage around but never over the contusion may help to promote resolution.

Dislocations. The application of heat and massage speeds the healing process. These are begun 24 to 48 hours following the injury. Passive exercises are begun within 3 to 4 days. Active exercise to strengthen surrounding muscles is started when healing is complete.

Fractures. Fracture healing can be speeded by the application of physiotherapy. Cold is applied initially to reduce swelling. Mild diathermy and gentle massage may be begun 24 to 48 hours after reduction is completed if the part is not in a cast. Gentle passive exercises of the involved areas except the area over the fracture are useful. Passive exercises of the fracture area may begin within 1 week.

Muscular Aches and Pains. These respond well to measures such as diathermy, infrared lamp, massage, and hydrotherapy.

Bursitis. Although bursitis is treated mainly by cortisone, the applications of diathermy along with passive and active massage also prove helpful.

Arthritis. Osteoarthritis is helped by heating measures such as the infrared lamp, diathermy, and hot packs applied to the involved joint.

Rheumatoid arthritis may be helped by the application of heat followed by massage of the surrounding muscles. Muscular spasms associated with this disease are relieved by mild physiotherapeutic measures.

Traumatic arthritis is treated with diathermy and active exercises designed to increase motion.

THE NURSE'S ROLE IN EXERCISE AND BODY MECHANICS

Since many orthopedic patients are immobilized to some degree for long periods of time, the nurse's role in promoting proper body mechanics and exercise is quite important. As soon as the patient is physically able, he should be encouraged to move all joints that are not immobilized and to help himself in moving about in bed so that muscular atrophy and subsequent loss of function does not develop. Keeping the body in positions of good alignment is also emphasized here because of the increased possibility of developing joint contractures. Measures that can be taken to prevent secondary orthopedic complications are as follows:

FRACTURES

When a form of skin traction is applied to the leg, the nurse must make certain that the leg is not in a position of inward or outward rotation. Sandbags are frequently used to keep the leg in the proper position. When a leg in skeletal traction appears to be rotated outwardly or inwardly, it should be brought to the physician's attention.

Devices to prevent foot drop have been discussed on page 194.

Setting Exercises. When a part of the body is immobilized, setting exercises are done to keep the muscles of that part in condition. A setting exercise is one in which the muscle is contracted without moving the joint. For instance, to exercise the biceps, the arm is ordinarily flexed at the elbow to cause contraction of the biceps. However, by concentrating on the contraction of the biceps, it can be done without flexing the elbow. Try it several times. Setting exercises can be done with all muscles. A setting exercise of the quadriceps femoris is especially important when the leg is immobilized in a cast or other device because this muscle group stabilizes the leg in walking. To exercise the quadriceps femoris, tell the patient to stiffen the muscle and pull the kneecap toward the chest like this:

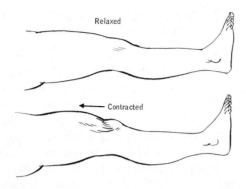

Relaxed

Contracted

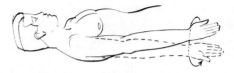

Other Exercises. When a part of an extremity is encased in a cast, the entire extremity need not be immobilized. If, for example, the wrist is immobilized in a cast, there is no reason why the shoulder joint cannot be exercised.

If one arm or leg is immobilized, active exercise of the good arm or leg improves circulation and delays atrophy of the immobilized limb.

PREPARATION FOR CRUTCH WALKING

All patients with leg fractures require the use of crutches during convalescence. Patients with a leg amputation require crutches for indefinite periods of time.

In many institutions the patient who is to use crutches is not referred to the physiotherapist until the actual time of crutch walking begins. In the meantime, while the patient is confined to the bed and wheelchair, the muscles may atrophy, causing a delay in crutch walking. To prevent atrophy of the muscles and to strengthen muscles used in crutch walking, several exercises are important.

While the patient is lying flat in bed, the limbs should be taken through the full range of motion daily. Hand and finger exercises include squeezing a rubber ball, touching the tip of the thumb against each fingertip, and flexion and extension of the wrist.

Because the patient who uses crutches must learn to "walk with his hands," special attention is given to the strengthening of the triceps muscles. This exercise to strengthen the triceps can be done while the patient is lying in bed. Note the two positions of the hand: first pronation, then supination.

After the patient can sit, this exercise is useful:

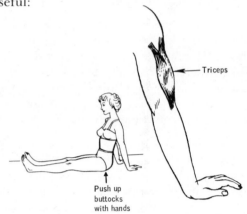

Triceps

Push up buttocks with hands

It is better not to give the patient who will be using crutches an overhanging trapeze bar to assist himself in raising his trunk and in moving from side to side in the bed. With a trapeze bar he will use only the biceps and seldom exercise the triceps.

THE AMPUTEE

Twenty-four to 48 hours postoperatively the patient is encouraged to turn from side to side and to lie on the abdomen to prevent a flexion contracture of the hip. While on his abdomen, a small pillow can be placed under the abdomen and stump.

Exercise is important to the amputee in preparation for the use of a prosthesis. The exercises should be performed on both sides, not only on the amputated side. Exercises for an amputation above the elbow are shown here.

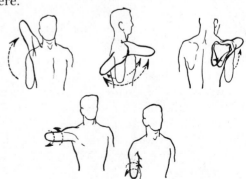

In amputations below the elbow, the biceps muscle must be developed, especially when biceps cineplasty (p. 196) is used. In a leg amputation special attention should be given to the hyperextension exercises as shown:

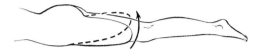

Both legs must be exercised. In a leg amputation the patient should be encouraged to exercise his arms as preparation for crutch walking.

SPINAL COLUMN INJURIES

When the spinal column is to be kept immobilized, the patient is usually placed on a Stryker frame (p. 198) where he can be turned frequently without altering the spinal alignment. If he is not on a Stryker frame, he must be moved like this:

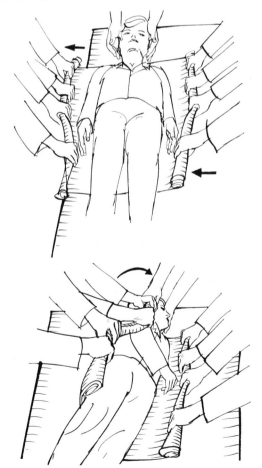

While lying on the back and abdomen, the patient can be instructed to exercise his arms and legs.

ARTHRITIS

The nurse does not encourage the patient with arthritis to exercise the affected joints unless there is a written order to do so, as some types of arthritis are treated by rest. Occasionally the arthritic needs assistance in moving a limb. A weight attached to a rope threaded over pulleys can be used to exercise the arm like this:

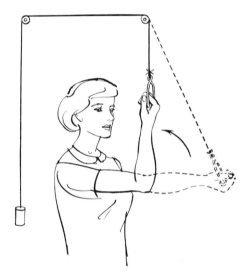

A sling rope and pulley make a simple device to aid in flexing the knee.

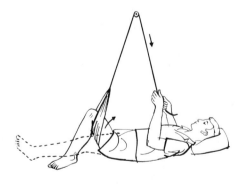

BREATHING EXERCISES

Deep breathing exercises are important to all patients immobilized for lengthy periods. Breathing exercises prevent poor chest expansion and neck flexion deformities. Suitable breathing exercises are illustrated on page 227.

Muscle Relaxants. Soma, Rela, Trancopal, Paraflex, Robaxin, Analexin, Sinaxar

ADDITIONAL PROCEDURES TO REVIEW

Preoperative care (see p. 128)
Postoperative care (see p. 134)
Lifting and moving patients
Good body mechanics for the nurse
Isolation technique (for tuberculosis of bone) (see p. 107)
Application of heat and cold
Feeding the helpless patient
Principles of first aid
Drainage and suction (Gastrointestinal drainage may be used following surgery and in severe accidents. Penrose drains are used in treating osteomyelitis. See p. 156.)

DIETS TO REVIEW

Modifications in proteins, vitamins, carbohydrates, iron, and calcium

MEDICATIONS TO REVIEW

Analgesics. Acetylsalicylic acid, salicylic acid, neocinchophen (Tolysin), cinchophen (Atophan), colchicine, phenylbutazone (Butazolidin)

Anti-infectives. Penicillin (Duracillin, Flo-Cillin, Wycillin, Crysticillin, Ledercillin, Hypercillin, Bicillin), erythromycin (Ilotycin, Erythrocin, Terramycin), tetracycline hydrochloride (Achromycin, Tetracyn, Polycycline, Steclin, Panmycin), oxytetracycline

Hormones. Adrenocorticotropin (ACTH, Acthar, Cortrophin), cortisone (Cortone Acetate, Cortogen Acetate), hydrocortisone (Cortef, Hydrocortone, Compound F), prednisone (Meticorten), prednisolone and metacortandracin (Meticortelone)

BIBLIOGRAPHY

Beeson, P. B., and McDermott, W.: Cecil-Loeb Textbook of Medicine. 12th ed. Philadelphia, W. B. Saunders Co., 1967.

Brown, A.: Medical Nursing. 3rd ed. Philadelphia, W. B. Saunders Co., 1957.

Brown, A.: Medical and Surgical Nursing II. Philadelphia, W. B. Saunders Co., 1959.

Davidsohn, I., and Henry, J. B.: Todd-Sanford Clinical Diagnosis by Laboratory Methods. 14th ed. Philadelphia, W. B. Saunders Co., 1969.

Davis, L.: Christopher's Textbook of Surgery. 9th ed. Philadelphia, W. B. Saunders Co., 1968.

Emerson, C., and Bragdon, J.: Essentials of Medicine. 18th ed. Philadelphia, J. B. Lippincott Co., 1959.

Falconer, M., Patterson, H., and Gustafson, E.: Current Drug Handbook. 1968-1970. Philadelphia, W. B. Saunders Co., 1968.

Ferguson, L., and Sholtis, L.: Eliason's Surgical Nursing. 11th ed. Philadelphia, J. B. Lippincott Co., 1959.

Goodale, R.: Clinical Interpretation of Laboratory Tests. 5th ed. Philadelphia, F. A. Davis Co., 1964.

Harmer, B., and Henderson, V.: Textbook of Principles and Practices of Nursing. 5th ed. New York, The Macmillan Co., 1958.

Hull, E., and Perrodin, C.: Medical Nursing. 5th ed. Philadelphia, F. A. Davis Co., 1956.

Jansen, J.: Introduction to Medical Physics. Philadelphia, J. B. Lippincott Co., 1960.

Krause, M.: Food, Nutrition and Diet Therapy. 4th ed. Philadelphia, W. B. Saunders Co., 1966.

Montag, M., and Swenson, R.: Fundamentals in Nursing Care. 3rd ed. Philadelphia, W. B. Saunders Co., 1959.

Olson, E. V., et al.: The Hazards of Immobility Series. Am. J. Nurs., 67:779, 1967.

Price, A.: The Art, Science and Spirit of Nursing. 3rd ed. Philadelphia, W. B. Saunders Co., 1965.

Sadove, M., and Cross, J.: The Recovery Room. Philadelphia, W. B. Saunders Co., 1957.

Sorensen, K. N., and Amis, D. B.: Understanding the World of the Chronically Ill. Am. J. Nurs., 67:811, 1967.

Stafford, E., and Diller, D.: Surgery and Surgical Nursing. 3rd ed. Philadelphia, W. B. Saunders Co., 1958.

Walikie, B. C.: Rheumatoid Arthritis: the Disease and Its Treatment. Personality Factors; Surgical Intervention. Am. J. Nurs., 67:1420, 1967.

West, J., Keller, M., and Harmon, E.: Nursing Care of the Surgical Patient. 6th ed. New York, The Macmillan Co., 1957.

Williams, M., and Worthington, C.: Therapeutic Exercises for Body Alignment and Function. Philadelphia, W. B. Saunders Co., 1957.

Williamson, P.: Office Procedures. 2nd ed. Philadelphia, W. B. Saunders Co., 1962.

nursing techniques in the care of

Diseases of the Respiratory System

DIAGNOSTIC PROCEDURES

X-RAYS

The most important diagnostic method in diseases of the lungs is the examination of the chest by x-ray.

Routine Chest X-ray

No preparation of the patient is necessary for this.

Fluoroscopy

The movements of the chest, heart, and lungs can be observed during fluoroscopy. No preparation of the patient is necessary for the examination.

Bronchogram

In this procedure small amounts of iodized oil (Lipiodol or Iodochlorol) are injected into the bronchial tubes to visualize the outlines of the tubes and their branches. Breakfast is withheld, and the patient is given a sedative and atropine before being taken for the examination. A local anesthetic is sprayed in the nose and pharynx to prevent coughing and gagging when the tube is inserted for the in-

209

stillation of the oil. Nothing should be administered orally following the examination until the anesthetic has worn off. Postural drainage (see p. 219) is used to drain off the oily dye.

PULMONARY FUNCTION TESTS

The most commonly used tests in determining lung volume, the definition of these tests, and the normal values are as follows:

1. Vital Capacity: The maximal amount of air one can expire after a maximal inspiration. Its normal average value is about 4000 to 5000 cc.
2. Maximal Breathing Capacity: The maximal volume of air that can be ventilated during a 1-minute period with maximal effort. The normal value for the male is 125 to 150 liters per minute, for the female 100 liters per minute.
3. Expiratory Reserve: The amount of air one can expire from the end point of passive expiration. The normal value is about 1000 cc.
4. Residual Volume: The volume of air remaining in the lungs after one has expired all the air he possibly can. The normal value is about 1500 cc.
5. Functional Residual Capacity: The sum of the expiratory reserve and the residual volume.
6. Total Lung Capacity: The sum of the vital capacity and the residual volume. This, in other words, is the total volume of air in the lungs at maximal inspiration. Its normal value is about 5500 to 6000 cc.
7. Walking Ventilation: The volume of air required to walk 1 minute at a rate of 180 feet per minute. The normal is about 25 per cent of the total lung capacity.
8. Walking Index: The walking ventilation divided by the maximal breathing capacity. The value is used in estimating the breathing reserve while walking.
9. Maximal Expiratory Flow Rate: This represents the maximal rate of flow obtained while performing a vital capacity exercise. The normal is usually 4 to 6 liters per second.
10. Index of Intrapulmonary Mixing: The percentage of nitrogen remaining in the alveolar air at the end of 7 minutes' oxygen breathing. This is normally less than 2.5 per cent nitrogen. Disturbances in this value represent uneven distribution of gases within the lungs.
11. Tidal Volume: The amount of air one normally inspires or expires during each respiratory cycle. The normal value is about 500 cc.
12. Oxygen Consumption: The amount of oxygen taken in by the body per minute. The normal values range from 110 to 150 cc. per minute.
13. Carbon Dioxide Excretion: The amount of carbon dioxide given off by the body. Normal values range from 88 to 120 cc. per minute.
14. Alveolar Ventilation: The actual amount of inspired air which enters the alveoli each minute. The normal value is 2.3 liters per minute.
15. Minute Ventilation: This is the total amount of air breathed per minute. The normal is 3.5 liters per minute.
16. Physiological Dead Space: This is the anatomic dead space and the gas ventilating alveoli in excess of that required to arterialize blood. The normal is about 150 cc.
17. Respiratory Quotient: The carbon dioxide excretion divided by the oxygen consumption. The normal value is 0.8.

Rest and Exercise Tests

A series of pulmonary function tests sometimes performed on the patient are called the rest and exercise tests. In these tests a sample of the patient's arterial blood is taken; then breathing tests are performed and a sample of expired air is taken both while the patient is resting and while he is exercising. The patient is usually taken to the pulmonary function lab for these tests. The following nursing procedures should be carried out when the patient is scheduled for a rest and exercise study:

1. Breakfast should be withheld.
2. The patient should not be given a heavy dose of narcotic.
3. The nurse should inform the laboratory in advance if the patient is having severe

pain in the chest or if the patient is experiencing any difficulties that may interfere with the exercise required to perform the study.

4. The laboratory should also be informed if the patient is receiving an anticoagulant medication, as this may interfere with the blood clotting time when the blood is withdrawn from the artery.

5. The patient should be prepared for the test by cleansing the arms. He should wear well-fitted shoes, as the exercise usually consists of stepping on and off a footstool. A warm robe should be worn to prevent chills. If pajamas are worn, the pajama bottoms should be secured well enough around the waist so they do not slide down during the exercise procedure.

In the laboratory the procedures are carried out as follows:

1. A local anesthetic is given in the arm over the area of the brachial artery.
2. Approximately 20 cc. of arterial blood is withdrawn, and a sample of expired air is collected in the spirometer.
3. The patient is instructed to exercise for 1 minute by stepping on and off a footstool. During the exercise another sample of arterial blood is obtained, and while the patient is breathing in the spirometer, another sample of expired air is obtained.

The entire test usually lasts about 2 hours. Following the test the patient is returned to his room where the nurse should observe the following:

1. Check the arm for a hematoma over the brachial artery during the first hour after the test. If a hematoma appears, apply pressure to the area for 20 minutes.
2. Check for numbness in the fingers. Some numbness is expected for a short period from the local anesthetic; however, if numbness persists over a period of time, it may be due to an injury to the brachial nerve.

The tests performed on the arterial blood include those for oxygen content, oxygen capacity, oxygen saturation, carbon dioxide content, and a test for pH. The normal values for these tests are as follows:

Oxygen content (pO$_2$) 17 to 21 vols. per cent
Oxygen capacity 17 to 21 vols. per cent
Oxygen saturation 96 to 98 per cent

Carbon dioxide
  content (pCO$_2$) 46 to 62 vols. per cent
pH 7.38 to 7.42

The lung volume tests calculated during the rest and exercise studies include tests 11 through 17 in the list of lung volume tests mentioned previously.

BRONCHOSCOPY

A bronchoscope is inserted through the pharynx and trachea into the bronchus for the purpose of viewing diseased areas and possible tumors, for obtaining tissue for biopsy, and for the aspiration and study of secretions. The bronchoscope is also used to inject the iodized oil administered prior to a bronchogram. Bronchoscopy is also used therapeutically in removing foreign bodies from the bronchi.

The preparation of the patient is as follows:

1. Nothing by mouth for at least 6 hours.
2. Dentures are removed.
3. Morphine sulfate or a similar drug is administered about one half hour prior to the procedure.
4. The patient is taken to the bronchoscopy room wearing a hospital gown.

Following the procedure nothing should be given orally until the local anesthetic sprayed on the pharynx has worn off.

THORACENTESIS

Chest fluid is aspirated and laboratory studies are made to aid in the diagnosis of some inflammatory and neoplastic diseases of the lungs. Prior to the thoracentesis the patient may be given atropine sulfate. When possible, the procedure is performed with the patient in a sitting position. The two positions used are shown here:

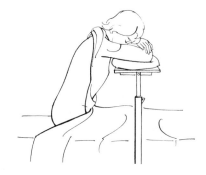

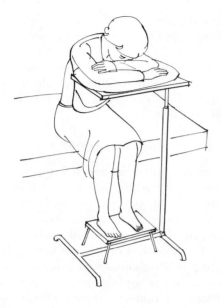

The procedure is performed with sterile technique. The skin is cleansed, and an antiseptic applied. A local anesthetic is given prior to the insertion of the thoracentesis needle. Additional equipment needed includes a 50 cc. syringe, a stopcock and rubber tubing, a Kelly hemostat, sterile gauze dressings, sterile towels, and sterile glass specimen tubes as shown:

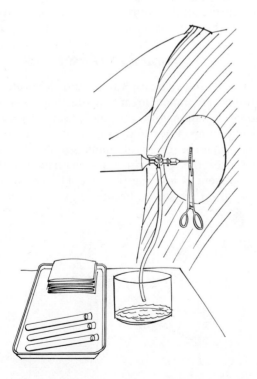

Laboratory studies that may be requested on the thoracic fluid are as follows:

1. Proteins: The normal is 3.0 gm. per 100 cc. In tuberculosis the total protein may be less than 0.5 gm. per 100 cc.
2. Differential Count. The predominating cells are polymorphonuclear leukocytes. In tuberculosis lymphocytes predominate, and only a few monocytes and leukocytes are present.
3. Specific Gravity: This is usually less than 1.018.
4. Papanicolaou Smear: This is done to detect carcinoma cells.
5. Culture: A culture may be requested to determine the kinds of bacteria present or to determine the presence of specific microorganisms. In pulmonary tuberculosis the exudate usually contains *Mycobacterium tuberculosis*. Other organisms found as evidence of disease are hemolytic and nonhemolytic streptococci, pneumococci, staphylococci, *Hemophilus influenzae, Escherichia coli, Pasteurella tularensis, Candida albicans,* and Vincent's organisms, to mention only a few.

Twenty to 30 cc. of chest fluid is usually needed to conduct the studies. Occasionally the physician may prefer to withdraw the entire amount of fluid from the chest and send it to the laboratory. In this event a large sterile receptacle is needed.

EXAMINATION OF SPUTUM

The collection of sputum specimens is a frequently requested procedure in diseases of the respiratory system. The specimen should be collected in the morning before food is taken, as food particles in the specimen may be confusing in the examination. A waterproof, waxed sputum cup is used to collect sputum for a routine examination. A tall glass container is used to observe the layering of sputum. A sterile wide-mouthed bottle with a screw top or a Petri dish is used to collect a sterile specimen for culture.

The patient is instructed to cough up the material from the bronchi or lungs and spit it into the container. Mucus from the posterior nasopharynx and saliva are not satisfactory for the sputum examination. Turning the patient to a lateral position with one arm over the head or turning on the unaffected side with the foot of the bed slightly elevated may help in obtaining a satisfactory specimen. At least one teaspoonful of sputum is needed for the examination. The patient should be advised against contaminating the outside of the container, as this presents a hazard to the personnel who handle it. A 24-hour specimen is needed for a concentration test for Mycobacterium tuberculosis.

The characteristics of sputum and the disease indications are as follows:

CHARACTERISTICS	DISEASE INDICATIONS
Amount	
Progressive increase	Disease is becoming worse
Consistency	
Mucoid, purulent, or mucopurulent	Asthma, bronchitis, rupture of abscess, empyema, pulmonary tuberculosis with cavitation, and bronchiectasis
Serous	Edema of lung
Tenacious	Lobar pneumonia
Layers form when placed in a cylinder	Pulmonary abscess, gangrene, and bronchiectasis
Color	
White to yellow	Large number of pus cells present
Greenish	Bile pigment present as in pneumonia with jaundice
Gray to black	Presence of anthracotic particles
Grayish brown	Ruptured amebic abscess
Blood streaked	Pulmonary tuberculosis and bronchiectasis
Rusty	Pneumonia and pulmonary infarct
Odor	
Sweet	Tuberculous cavities
Foul	Abscess, gangrene, and necrotizing bronchogenic carcinoma
Casts	
Dittrich's plugs	Lobar pneumonia Chronic bronchitis and bronchiectasis

CHARACTERISTICS	DISEASE INDICATIONS
Microscopic Findings	
Curschmann's spirals	Asthma and chronic bronchitis
Elastic fibers	Destruction of alveoli walls as in pulmonary abscess, gangrene, and tuberculosis
Crystals	Bronchial asthma, bronchiectasis, and abscess
Carbon cells	Anthracosis
Eosinophils	Bronchial asthma
Leukocytes	All pyogenic infections and tuberculosis with cavitation

A sputum culture may indicate the same disease-producing organisms as those mentioned in a culture of chest fluid.

NASAL AND THROAT SWABBINGS

Swabbings of the nose and throat secretions are sometimes taken to determine the presence of disease-producing organisms; these are taken with a sterile cotton-tipped applicator in a sterile test tube as shown:

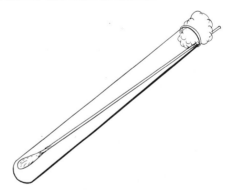

The applicator is removed from the test tube using an aseptic technique. Only the area to be swabbed should be touched by the cotton tip. Two specimens should be collected so that several stains can be made in the laboratory.

EXAMINATION OF GASTRIC CONTENTS

If a sputum specimen cannot be coughed up from the lungs in the diagnosis of pulmonary tuberculosis, a gastric lavage is done. The gastric contents are examined for sputum that has been swallowed. Unlike other organisms, tubercle bacilli are not destroyed by gastric juices. The gastric lavage tube is passed as described on page 153. After the lavage tube is in place, the patient is asked to swallow four ounces of sterile distilled water. Thirty to 50 cc. of the stomach contents is immediately withdrawn and placed in a sterile container. This procedure must be carried out in the morning before any food has been eaten.

SKIN TESTS

Skin tests, used as an aid in diagnosing pulmonary tuberculosis and in determining the causative factor in bronchial asthma, are made in the form of intracutaneous injections, scratch tests, and patch tests. Tuberculin tests include Pirquet's reaction (scratch test), Vollmer's test (patch test), the Mantoux test (intracutaneous), the Sterneedle (Heaf) test, the Tine (Rosenthal) test, and the Mono-Vacc test. In the intracutaneous method, old tuberculin (OT) or purified protein derivative (PPD) is injected intracutaneously. PPD is the most widely used solution. In the Mantoux test, 0.1 cc. of a solution containing 0.0002 mg. of purified protein derivative (PPD I, first test strength) is injected intracutaneously. If there is no reaction within 48 hours, the test is repeated with 0.1 cc. of the solution containing 0.05 mg. of purified protein derivative (PPD II, second test strength). The skin is ob-

served for reaction in a 48-hour period. This test is frequently called the PPD test. The solution must be kept refrigerated.

The Sterneedle, Tine, and Mono-Vacc tests are all newer tuberculin tests. Test kits individually packaged are commercially prepared. A small disc, containing several tiny needles or prongs, is pressed against the skin, causing small punctures. The Tine test and Mono-Vacc test discs are impregnated with OT. The Sterneedle test contains PPD. To give these tests, the patient's forearm is cleansed with acetone or alcohol and allowed to dry. The skin is held taut, and the disc is pressed firmly against the skin. Hold the patient's forearm firmly with one hand because a slight stinging sensation may cause him to jerk his arm, thus causing scratches. It is not necessary to cover the test site with a dressing. The test is read in 3 to 7 days. Inflammation around one or more puncture sites is regarded as a positive reading.

As a rule nurses do not perform tuberculin tests. These are done by the physician.

There are numerous sensitivity tests used in detecting the allergens that cause bronchial asthma.

The procedure for the three types of skin tests is described on page 283.

BLOOD TESTS

Blood tests used in diagnosing diseases of the respiratory system are shown in the table below.

TEST	NORMAL	DISEASE IMPLICATIONS
Blood culture		Used to detect septicemia in any severe inflammation of lungs.
Sedimentation rate	(mm. fall in one hour) 0-8 mm. male 0-10 mm. female (Cutler method)	Increased in pneumonia, lung abscess, and active tuberculosis (the sed. rate parallels the activity of tuberculosis; therefore, periodic tests are helpful in determining progress).
Icterus index*	4-6 units	Used when jaundice is a complication of pneumonia.
Direct van den Bergh*	0.4 mg.	Positive when jaundice is a complication of pneumonia.
Plasma protein*	6-8 gm.	Increased in pneumonia. Slightly increased in tuberculosis.
Nonprotein nitrogen,*† blood-urea nitrogen, uric acid	25-35 mg. 12-18 mg. 2-4 mg.	All are increased when nephrosis and nephritis are complications of pneumonia.

*Withhold breakfast.
†Oxylated tube needed.

TEST	NORMAL	DISEASE IMPLICATIONS
Leukocytes	6-10 thousand	Severely increased in empyema and lung abscess. Slightly increased or subnormal in tuberculosis.
Platelets	250,000 per cu. mm.	Reduced in pneumonia.
Coagulation time	1-7 minutes	Prolonged in pneumonia.
Eosinophils	1-3	Increased in carcinoma of lung and in bronchial asthma.
Cold agglutination test (red cells and serum show agglutination at 0°-5° C.)		Occurs in titers of 1:8 and increasing up to 1:128 in viral pneumonia.

*Withold breakfast.
†Oxylated tube needed.

THERAPEUTIC AND REHABILITATIVE PROCEDURES

ADMINISTRATION OF AEROSOL SPRAYS

Aerosol therapy (see also p. 50) is effective in a number of respiratory conditions. There are a number of inhalant sprays currently on the market (see p. 287). These preparations are usually combinations of several drugs. Specific inhalants are given to liquefy and remove mucopurulent material from the respiratory tract, to relieve irritation of the mucous membrane of the respiratory tract, and to dilate the bronchial tree. Drugs such as penicillin and streptomycin are also given for their antibiotic effect. Frequently two types of solution, such as a bronchodilator and an antibiotic, are used alternately.

The various types of sprays are used for acute inflammatory affections of the respiratory tract and conditions in which there is obstruction of the bronchial lumen due to excessive secretion, muscular constriction, or mucosal swelling.

The inhalant sprays are administered by means of a small nebulizer connected with a continuous blast of air. The solution is converted into a fine mist that can be inhaled deeply into the tracheobronchial tree. An atomizer cannot be used because the droplets in the mist produced by the atomizer are too coarse, and catch in the nose or pharynx, thus not penetrating into the bronchial tree.

The equipment for the aerosol therapy is set up as shown:

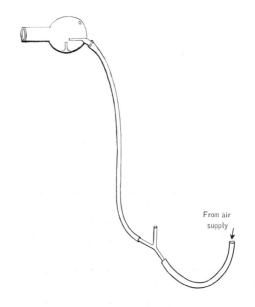

From air supply

A continuous air blast is obtained from an oxygen supply source or from an air pressure pump. When oxygen is used, the liter flow should be set at 4 liters per minute. This flow will use up 1 cc. of solution in approximately 10 minutes.

When possible, the patient can be instructed to administer the spray to himself. It is done like this:

1. The nurse turns on the oxygen supply or air pressure and instructs the patient to sit in an upright position.
2. The open portion of the nebulizer is placed in the patient's mouth. The lips need not

be closed tightly around the nebulizer.
3. The patient is instructed to place his thumb on the open end of the Y-tube and inhale through the MOUTH at the same time. The Y-tube is opened during each expiration.

Placement of the Y-tube in the rubber tubing permits the use of the solution only during inhalation. Requesting the patient to keep his lips open during inhalation will eliminate the tendency to suck on the nebulizer.

Following the treatment the nebulizer should be rinsed with water, as the drugs tend to accumulate in concentrated form over a period of time.

One cubic centimeter of solution is the usual amount given during each treatment, and the patient continues until all of the solution is used. For most conditions the treatment is prescribed two or three times daily. In a condition such as chronic obstructive emphysema, a bronchodilator spray is the mainstay of therapy and may be used as much as five to six times daily. When the inhalant is needed this frequently, the patient is usually instructed to inhale the spray only long enough to relieve respiratory obstruction. From four to twelve deep inhalations will usually provide marked relief. Frequent use of bronchodilator sprays is discouraged because a tolerance to the drug is developed. A local drying and irritation to the mucous membranes also may occur with excessive use of the bronchodilator solution.

An effective routine sometimes used to aid the patient in clearing the air passage is to have the patient sit up; then administer 1 cc. of a bronchodilator inhalant with the nebulizer; then administer an expectorant orally, and request the patient to cough and raise sputum. This is repeated several times daily.

When continuous aerosol therapy is required, the apparatus described on page 50 is used.

THE USE OF TOURNIQUETS FOR PULMONARY EDEMA

Pulmonary edema may develop after obstruction to the air passages, as in severe bronchial asthma or with a tumorous growth in the air passage. The obstruction causes in-creasingly heightened negative pressure in the lungs and, in turn, pulmonary congestion and circulatory embarrassment. The symptoms are dyspnea, orthopnea, cyanosis, coldness and pallor of skin, cold perspiration, cough with blood-tinged foamy mucus, and restlessness. An important procedure in the therapy primarily directed to lowering the intrapleural pressure is that of the application of tourniquets to the extremities, which accomplishes its purpose by slowing down the peripheral circulation, thus preventing blood from returning to the heart and on to the lungs. The blood is kept pooled in the extremities by applying a tourniquet to three extremities at a time. The treatment can be prolonged over a period of time by rotating the tourniquets so that a different extremity is freed about every 15 minutes. This would allow the tourniquets to remain on the other three extremities about 45 minutes. Some system of rotating the tourniquets should be made standard in the hospital department so that everyone who cares for the patient understands the procedure. Also, some physicians prefer to have the fourth tourniquet applied before releasing a tourniquet, whereas others may prefer simply to remove the tourniquet and place it on the extremity that had previously been freed. A suggested procedure is to free the extremities in a clockwise manner (facing the patient), as shown:

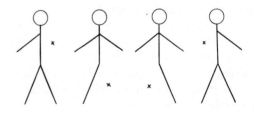

The procedure must be carried out in a systematic manner, so as not to impair circulation further. The frequency of the tourniquets' rotation is prescribed by the physician. The tourniquet is applied as high on the arm and leg as possible. A padding is first fastened around each extremity where the tourniquet is to be applied. After applying the tourniquet, check the arterial pulse. The tourniquet should never be applied so tightly that the pulse cannot be felt. If the ankles are too edematous (as in heart failure) to feel the pulse, try to apply the tourniquet to the leg using the same amount of pressure as was used on the arm.

This treatment causes discoloration, swelling, and discomfort in the extremities. The procedure is not harmful as long as the pulse can be felt while the tourniquet is in place.

There is a special apparatus (Danzer apparatus) designed for this treatment. It consists of four blood pressure cuffs connected to one manometer. The four cuffs are fastened around the arms and legs; then three of the cuffs are inflated to the desired pressure. The pressure in each cuff can be measured separately. The pressure is maintained at a level between the patient's systolic and diastolic pressure. For example, the cuff pressure can be set at about 100 if the blood pressure is around 120/80.

When the tourniquet therapy is to be discontinued, the tourniquets or cuffs should be removed one at a time to prevent overstrain on the heart from the blood returning all at one time.

PARADOXICAL MOTION OF CHEST WALL

In this condition the movements of the chest wall in inspiration and expiration are exactly opposite from the normal movements. The contrast between normal and paradoxical motion is shown here:

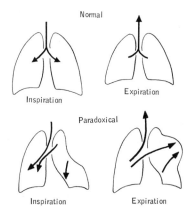

Paradoxical motion of the chest wall is possible whenever the rib cage loses its rigidity such as by resection of two or more ribs or by fractures both anteriorly and posteriorly of two or more ribs. Paradoxical motion renders breathing inefficient, coughing ineffective, and causes the air to shuttle back and forth between the lungs. The latter results in rebreathing the same air, causing anoxia as well as carbon dioxide retention. Symptoms, aside from observation of the abnormal chest movements, are cyanosis, dyspnea, acute pain, and an increase in temperature, pulse, and respiration. Shock is the inevitable end result.

The treatment depends upon the degree of severity. In moderate cases (the usual condition), pressure is applied to the involved side by the use of sandbags or pressure bandages, or by having the patient lie on the involved side. In more severe cases such as in severe injuries to the chest, traction may be applied to the flail chest. Traction is attached to wires or towel clips placed through the skin and under and around the ribs like this:

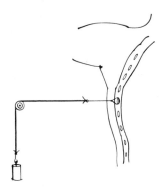

In extreme cases a tracheotomy (see p. 353) is done to reduce the dead space (space not absolutely essential for oxygenation) in the tracheobronchial tree.

ARTIFICIAL RESPIRATION

The technique for artificial respiration by means of mouth-to-mouth resuscitation has been accepted as the most efficient. This procedure is carried out as follows:

Open the airway by removing any obstruction. Since most foreign bodies lodge in the larynx, these can be removed with the finger. When the obstruction cannot be removed with the finger, the victim is placed on his abdomen, and the chest is gently tapped.

In order to resuscitate the victim, the jaw must first be grasped and pulled forward so that the tongue is pulled forward, rendering the air passage open. Unless this step is taken, the treatment is ineffective.

Hold the nose closed with the other hand, and blow air into the mouth like this:

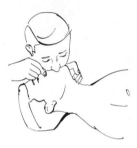

If the nose is not held closed, the air blown into the mouth will go to the pharynx and out the nose. Air is blown smoothly and steadily until the chest walls rise; then the operator removes his mouth from the victim's and allows the lungs to empty like this:

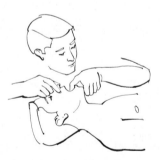

Inflate the lungs three to five times, then check to see if there is a pulse beat. To locate the pulse, always use a large artery such as the carotid or femoral. The carotid is always accessible and is easy to locate. It is located by sliding the fingers gently to the left of the Adam's apple. Do not feel merely with the fingertips, but use a gentle pressure with the fingers flat against the side of the neck. Do not interrupt artificial respiration more than a few seconds to feel the pulse.

If the patient has a pulse, continue lung inflations. The cycle should be continued at a rate of 12 to 20 respirations per minute. The operator should inhale about twice the volume of ordinary respiration. About once a minute he should take a deep breath himself. This procedure may be carried out for about an hour without fatigue to the operator.

If mouth-to-nose resuscitation is given, the victim's mouth is held closed with one hand while holding the jaw forward with the other hand like this:

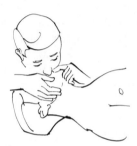

If the patient does not have a pulse beat, external cardiac compression, as illustrated on p. 242, should be incorporated into the cycle like this:

One operator: Give 15 cardiac compressions; then move back to the head and give the lungs two inflations. Continue this cycle.

Two operators: One operator performs cardiac compressions at the rate of one per second without interruption, while the other gives artificial respiration as described previously. The operator administering artificial respiration checks the pulse periodically.

When the pulse reappears, discontinue cardiac compression and continue with artificial respiration.

DRAINAGE METHODS AND DEVICES

In diseases of the respiratory system, drainage methods may be categorized according to the two areas in which they are used: those used to clear secretions from the tracheobronchial tree and lungs and those used to drain secretions from the pleural cavity.

REMOVING SECRETIONS FROM THE TRACHEOBRONCHIAL TREE AND LUNGS

Methods used for this purpose include postural drainage, assisting the patient to cough, and endotracheal aspiration.

Postural Drainage

Postural drainage is sometimes used in inflammatory conditions of the chest to bring up excess secretions. For this procedure the patient is placed in a position that promotes drainage from the chest. The position may be accomplished several ways. There are special postural drainage beds currently available. The Singer postural drainage table is shown here.

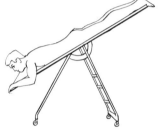

The Nelson postural drainage bed is shown here.

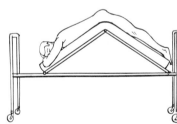

The Nelson bed is more comfortable but is useful only in drainage from the lower zone of the lungs.

When a special bed is not available, the patient is placed in this position on the side of his bed.

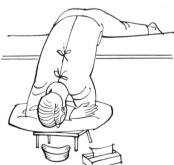

Postural drainage is carried out for periods no longer than 15 minutes three or four times daily. For the first few times the patient may not be able to tolerate this position longer than a few minutes. Usually the discomfort of the position gradually disappears after several treatments. While in the postural drainage position, the patient is instructed to turn slightly from side to side, breathe deeply, and cough. A receptacle is kept available for expectoration. Large amounts of sputum are expectorated during and immediately following the procedure. The sputum is measured, and the amount is recorded. The patient should rest for 30 minutes after the procedure. If the patient is too debilitated to assume any of these postural drainage positions, a Trendelenburg position may be effective.

Assisting the Patient to Cough

One of the most important aspects of postoperative care of the chest patient is to encourage coughing in order to bring up secretions. The complications of retaining secretions are atelectasis and pneumonia. Coughing postoperatively is extremely painful; therefore, the patient is reluctant to cough with enough power to bring up secretions. The importance of the procedure should be explained to the patient.

The patient should sit upright in bed and lean forward to cough. This position promotes better coughing than merely being propped to a sitting position in bed. The nurse supports the chest wound while the patient is coughing. To support the wound, stand on the side opposite the incision, and hold the hands over the dressings like this:

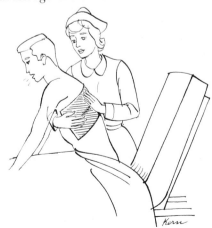

The support will make the procedure less painful. This procedure is carried out every 1 to 3 hours for several days, postoperatively depending upon the physician's preference.

Endotracheal Aspiration

When the patient is unable to cough deeply, it may be necessary to stimulate the cough reflex by endotracheal aspiration. The procedure, when prescribed, is widely becoming a nursing responsibility and is done as follows:
1. A sterile No. 16 rubber catheter (Coudé preferred) is attached to a wall or electric suction apparatus.
2. The patient is instructed to sit upright and protrude his tongue.
3. The tongue is pulled forward with a piece of dry gauze. At the same time the well lubricated catheter is passed through the nose into the pharynx until it reaches the glottis. To place the tube into the trachea, ask the patient to inhale or cough; then quickly advance the catheter. Placement of the tube in the trachea will produce coughing. Inability of the patient to produce vocal sounds will give further evidence that the catheter is in the trachea.

A thumb valve, placed in the aspirating system like this,

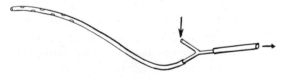

is extremely important in order to prevent a continuous suction during the closure of the glottis. Gentle suction only is used as the tube is moved slowly up and down the trachea.

Aspiration should be adequate but must be done as quickly as possible to prevent prolonged suction and respiratory distress. The postoperative patient's chest must be supported as described previously, while coughing during this procedure.

REMOVING AIR AND FLUIDS FROM THE PLEURAL CAVITY

Methods to remove air and fluid from the pleural cavity include thoracentesis, the use of the pneumothorax apparatus, and open and closed chest drainage.

Thoracentesis

Thoracentesis is used to remove exudate from the pleural cavity in the treatment of the early stages of empyema. A detailed explanation of the drainage methods for empyema is given on page 221.

The procedure for a thoracentesis has been described under the heading "Diagnostic Procedures" in this chapter.

In the event that a thoracentesis must be performed to remove air or fluid from the chest from a postoperative complication, the position shown here:

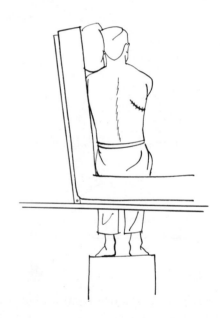

may be better tolerated. The unoperated side is placed next to the elevated head of the bed.

Use of Pneumothorax Apparatus

After chest injuries and sometimes after chest surgery, the physician must determine and readjust intrapleural pressures. For this procedure the patient is placed in the same position as for a thoracentesis. The procedure is carried out using sterile technique. The skin is prepared and a needle is inserted in the pleural cavity using the same equipment and procedure as with the thoracentesis. The equipment ready for use is shown here:

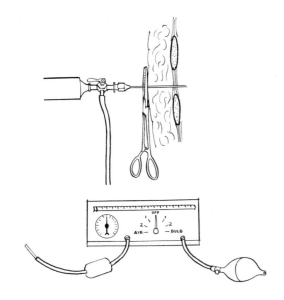

After the needle, stopcock, syringe, and tubing are assembled, the physician will ask the nurse to connect the rubber tubing to the pneumothorax apparatus (the rubber tubing is sterile; the pneumothorax apparatus is unsterile).

For accuracy the manometric readings are taken during even and quiet respirations. Adjustment of intrapleural pressure can be made by removal or injection of air with the pneumothorax apparatus or the syringe. Since small amounts of air are withdrawn or injected, a 10-cc. or 20-cc. syringe is adequate.

Open Chest Drainage

Open chest drainage is used to drain thick pus from the pleural cavity in the treatment of empyema. The term "open" implies that air can enter into the pleural cavity through the drainage wound.

Once the diagnosis of empyema has been made, the physician tries to determine the consistency of the fluid accumulated in the pleural cavity, as the consistency governs the type of drainage to be used. At first the fluid is thin, gradually becoming thicker as the inflammation progresses. While the fluid in the pleural cavity is thin, the treatment consists of draining the cavity either by frequent aspirations by means of a needle (thoracentesis) or by closed chest drainage (see p. 222). After the exudate becomes thick, it can no longer be drained through a needle or small closed

chest drainage tube. In this event open chest drainage is used. In some instances all three methods of drainage are used on the same patient—repeated thoracenteses are done; then closed chest drainage is used. When the exudate becomes thick, the physician resorts to open drainage.

For the placement of the open drainage tube in the pleural cavity, the patient is taken to the operating room, where a section of rib is removed; then a large-diameter soft rubber tube is inserted through the opening into the pleural cavity. If the empyema pocket is large, two or three tubes—each up to $3/4$ inch in diameter—may be inserted.

The open chest drainage tube is either covered by dressings or connected to a suction (Wangensteen type) apparatus depending upon the physician's choice.

The drainage tube is sutured or taped to the patient's skin. When the tube is connected to a Wangensteen suction apparatus, the drainage tube may be fastened in place with a rubber glove fastener made like this:

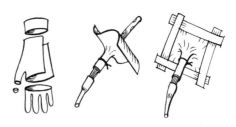

The rubber is cemented to the skin and around the tube. The advantage of this method when suction is used is that it makes the wound airtight, thus allowing for stronger suction.

A number of various solutions are used to clean out the empyema cavity. Some surgeons prefer to irrigate the cavity with normal saline. Others are instillations of Varidase. Varidase is a bacterial enzyme used to remove necrotic tissue, pus, and blood from abscesses. It is prepared in powder form and must be dissolved in normal saline for use.

Irrigation and Instillation through Open Chest Drainage Tube

Irrigation. The patient is turned on the unaffected side. The soiled dressings are removed (see p. 120), and a sterile emesis basin is placed against the chest under the incision. Several ounces of the prescribed solution are instilled through the rubber tube into the cavity with a sterile Asepto syringe, as shown:

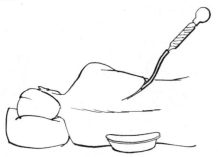

The solution should be at room temperature. The patient is then turned on the affected side to allow the solution to drain from the cavity. This procedure may be repeated two to three times, according to the physician's preference. After the irrigation the skin wound is cleansed with a solution such as benzalkonium chloride 1:1000. Adequate dressings are applied covering the tube and the wound and held in place with Montgomery straps (see p. 170).

Instillation. If an instillation of the empyema cavity is ordered, the prescribed amount of solution is instilled with the Asepto syringe; then the drainage tube is clamped for the length of time given in the order. After this the solution is drained off as explained for the irrigation.

In the case of open chest drainage for empyema, the open thoracotomy does not cause the lung to collapse because the scar tissue around the edges of the pus-filled cavity contracts and pulls the lung back into position against the chest wall.

The open drainage tube is left in place indefinitely until the drainage has subsided. The physician removes the tube.

Closed Chest Drainage

In closed chest drainage the pleural cavity is drained in such a way that air is prevented from entering the pleural space. Closed chest drainage is used to remove large amounts of fluid from the pleural cavity in the early treatment of empyema and to remove fluids from the pleural cavity postoperatively after a thoracotomy.

When closed chest drainage is used to treat empyema, the drainage tube is inserted under local anesthesia either in the patient's own room or in a special treatment room.

Inserting an Intercostal Catheter. When it becomes necessary to insert an intercostal catheter in the patient's own room the nurse assembles the equipment and assists with the procedure. A thoracotomy tray is used or if this is not available, a thoracentesis tray can be used. In addition to the thoracentesis tray, a catheter, scalpel, and trocar are needed.

The equipment on the thoracentesis tray is needed because the physician may first wish to locate a pus-filled cavity and/or withdraw some fluid before inserting the drainage tube. A small incision is then made in the skin and a trocar is inserted through the incision and into the pleural space.

The intercostal drainage tube for closed chest drainage is an ordinary urethral catheter about size 14 French. A whistle tip catheter is usually used (see p. 265). The catheter is inserted through the trocar like this:

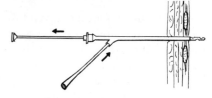

These trocars come in sizes to accommodate catheters from 10 to 24 French.

For the closed chest drainage procedure the patient is placed in the same position as for a thoracentesis (see p. 211) unless he is too ill to sit up. In that event he is placed on his side like this:

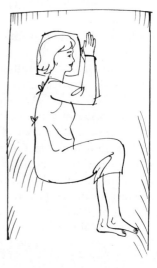

Postoperative closed chest drainage is used to remove the fluid, blood, or air that accumulates in the pleural cavity as a result of surgical intervention. It is now almost universal practice to drain the pleural space after all thoracotomies except after a pneumonectomy. Drainage is essential postoperatively to enable the remaining portion of the lung to expand and fill the hemithorax completely. Prompt filling of the chest cavity by the lung is essential in preventing pleural complications.

The drainage tube for postoperative closed chest drainage is of course inserted in the operating room at the time of surgery. When excessive air leakage or bleeding is anticipated, two tubes are inserted like this:

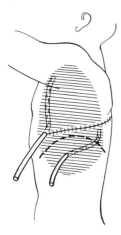

Usually a large bore tube about 28 French is used and secured in place by a suture. After a pneumonectomy, a number of surgeons put a drainage tube in place and keep the tube clamped. The clamp is removed by the surgeon from time to time to observe intrapleural pressures.

When the patient returns to his room from the operating room, he will have one or two drainage tubes in place. The tubes are clamped and remain clamped until the physician sets up the drainage and connects the tube to the drainage setup.

Closed Chest Drainage Setup. In closed chest drainage the drainage system is set up in a manner that prevents air from entering the pleural cavity. Closed chest drainage with or without suction is used. Closed chest drainage is also called water-seal drainage.

Closed Chest Drainage without Suction. Closed chest drainage without suction is used for empyema and sometimes after a pneu-

monectomy. After a pneumonectomy the physician may connect the clamped drainage tube to a drainage setup without suction and KEEP THE DRAINAGE TUBE CLAMPED except on those occasions when he wishes to check the intrapleural pressure.

The closed drainage setup without suction looks like this:

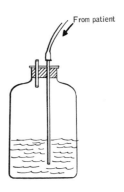

Air is kept from backing up into the drainage tube and entering the pleural cavity by placement of the end of the glass tube under water. With this system the drainage from the chest drains into the water in the bottle. The nurse frequently is called upon to prepare this drainage setup.

When the drainage system is functioning properly, a small amount of water will be drawn up into the tube on inspiration, and bubbles of air or drainage fluid will be seen in the water on expiration as shown:

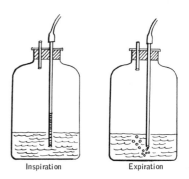

Inspiration   Expiration

This fluctuation of the water up and down the glass tube should be kept in mind when initially putting water in the bottle. The tip of the glass tube must be well enough below water level (about 1 to 2 cm.) so that when the water is drawn up into the tube, the level of the water in the bottle is still high enough to maintain a water seal.

A marker of adhesive tape should be placed on the bottle showing the level of the water and stating the amount of water so that the amount of drainage may be calculated. The same amount of water must then always be replaced in the bottle when it is refilled. The bottle must also be large enough to accommodate about 500 cc. of drainage in addition to the water. Nothing smaller than a gallon jar is used.

Closed Chest Drainage with Suction. Closed chest drainage with suction is sometimes used to treat empyema. It is always used after all thoracotomies except pneumonectomy.

When suction is used with water-seal drainage, an extra bottle must be placed in the drainage system to provide a break in the continuous suction action.

Several methods can be used for the drainage setup. The surgeon uses the method he prefers.

The two-bottle setup is shown here:

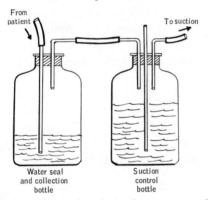

Water seal
and collection
bottle

Suction
control
bottle

In this setup one bottle is the water-seal and collection bottle and the other is the suction control bottle.

The three-bottle setup is assembled like this:

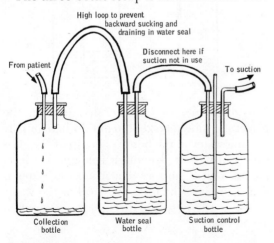

High loop to prevent
backward sucking and
draining in water seal

Disconnect here if
suction not in use

From patient

To suction

Collection
bottle

Water seal
bottle

Suction control
bottle

A number of surgeons prefer the two-bottle setup because there is less danger of air leakage in the system.

When suction is used, every connection including the bottle corks must be airtight (this is unlike the simple one-bottle setup without suction, in which only the connections between the drainage tube and the glass tube need to be airtight.

When two drainage tubes are in place in the chest, each tube is connected to a separate bottle like this:

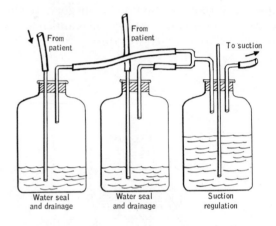

From patient

From patient

To suction

Water seal
and drainage

Water seal
and drainage

Suction
regulation

Keeping the Drainage System in Functioning Order. If the patient is to have suction drainage, the surgeon or resident physician is usually on hand to set up the suction when the patient returns to his room. He connects the drainage tube to the drainage system and the drainage system to the suction pump or wall suction outlet. He also checks to make certain that the proper amount of suction is used. After he leaves, it is up to the nurse to make certain that the suction and drainage are functioning. To tell whether the suction is working, check the suction control bottle. You can always tell which bottle this is because it always has a glass tube with one end in the water and the other end open above the bottle. (Check the drawings again on this page.) Next check the water level INSIDE this glass tube. If the suction is functioning, this glass tube will periodically empty. When the water is emptied out of this glass tube, it causes air to be drawn into the bottle from the outside, and bubbles can be seen in the water. If this tube does not empty and bubbles are not seen periodically, the setup is not functioning properly. The setup may not be functioning properly for these reasons:

1. Something is wrong with the pump.
2. Air is leaking into the drainage setup through loose connectors or bottle tops.
3. Air is leaking into the pleural cavity.

Regardless of the reason causing a malfunction in the suction, it must be corrected. Since the third reason is the most serious, this is the cause to check first. To find out whether or not there is air leakage into the pleural cavity, simply clamp off the chest drainage tube; then check the suction control bottle. If the suction bottle now bubbles, this means there is nothing wrong either with the pump or with the connection system; so air must be leaking into the pleural space. If this is the case, call the physician immediately. If, on the other hand, the drainage tube is clamped off and the suction control bottle still does not give evidence of functioning, there must be something wrong with the drainage connections or the pump. In this event keep the chest drainage tube clamped, and check the system. When the air leaks or whatever else are corrected, the suction bottle will immediately show signs of functioning. Then unclamp the chest drainage tube.

To make sure that the drainage system connections stay in place and keep the system airtight, several things should be done.

All connectors should be secured with narrow strips of adhesive as shown:

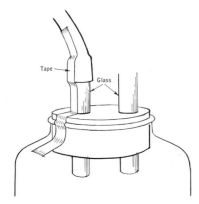

The connection tubing between the patient and the drainage setup should be long enough

to allow free motion of the patient and yet should not be excessive in length, as this causes dead space in the drainage system. Tubing should be secured to the side of the bottom sheet as shown:

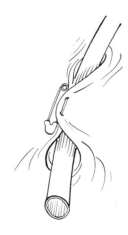

All bottles should be held securely in a specially designed holder or should be fastened to the floor with tape so that they are not accidentally knocked over.

Several hemostat clamps should be kept at the patient's bedside (or taped to the bed) so that they are immediately available to shut off the tubes in the event a disruption in the system occurs.

Another matter of importance is that of making certain that the drainage tube is open and draining. When the drainage tube is first connected to the drainage system, there should immediately be some drainage. The fluid is bloody for the first few hours postoperatively, gradually becoming serous in about 36 hours.

If the patient has a simple water-seal drainage with only one bottle, you can tell whether the tube is open by checking to see if the water is fluctuating up and down the glass tube as shown on page 223. If the patient has a suction drainage setup, the drainage bottle must be checked frequently to see if drainage is taking place. The glass connecting tube in the tubing between the patient and the bottle enables the nurse to check the character of the drainage and whether the tube is open or clogged.

If the drainage tube appears to be clogged, the tube should be milked or stripped as shown:

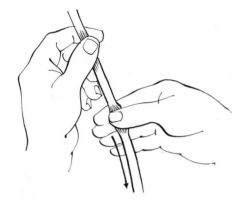

When two tubes are in place, depending upon the patient's position, only one tube may drain fluid from the chest. When the patient is in a sitting position the lower tube drains fluid while the upper tube serves as an escape for air leaking from the resected lung. When the patient is in a recumbent position both tubes may drain fluid.

The patient's position may also affect the behavior of the drainage from the lower drainage tube. With the patient in a semirecumbent position, a remaining lower lobe may fall down and occlude the drainage tube. Placing the patient in an upright position may free the lower tube.

A record is kept of the color, consistency, and amount of drainage. When the drainage bottle is emptied, the chest tube is disconnected in this sequence:

    clamp the chest tube
    disconnect the chest tubing, and empty
      the drainage
    connect the chest tube to the drainage
      system (if suction is used, check the
      suction control bottle to make sure
      there are no leaks)
    unclamp the chest tube

The drainage tube is secured to the patient's skin, but as an extra safety precaution it is advisable to tape the tube to the outside of the dressing like this:

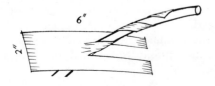

The physician removes the drainage tube when the patient's condition is satisfactory. Postoperatively the tube is removed about the third day. When the tube is used for empyema, it may be left in considerably longer. The equipment required to remove the tube is as shown:

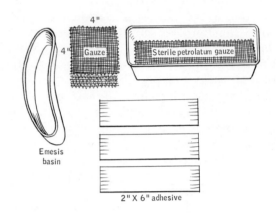

The patient lies on the side opposite the placement of the tubing, and the physician stands at the patient's back. A gauze dressing is placed over the chest opening. The dressing is snugly covered with adhesive tape, thereby making the incision airtight. Some physicians prefer petrolatum gauze dressings. This procedure is moderately painful and is usually preceded by an injection of morphine.

DRESSINGS AND BINDERS

Postoperative Dressings

After chest surgery the dressing covering the thoracotomy incision is usually kept as small as possible so that unusual oozing from the wound will be apparent immediately. A number of surgeons also prefer small dressings so that satisfactory auscultation of the lung field is possible. The thoracotomy incision is usually covered with a thin layer of gauze and several strips of Elastoplast (elastic adhesive). The stab wound for the insertion of the drainage tube is separate from the thoracotomy incision. The tube dressing consists of several adhesive strips. This dressing may overlap the Elastoplast dressing so that it can be removed without altering the thoracotomy incision dressing.

There will be some serosanguineous oozing from the thoracotomy incision. The nurse reinforces the dressings when this occurs. Any bleeding from the chest incision is reported immediately. The thoracotomy incision dressings are left in place at least several days. Some surgeons do not change the dressings until it is time to remove the sutures.

When the chest is flail, larger dressings are used, and they are placed tightly.

Chest Binder

Occasionally the physician will request that a chest binder be applied to relieve pleural pain in some inflammatory conditions of the lung and pleura. An Ace bandage is best suited for this purpose. Several Ace bandages 3 or 4 inches wide are used and applied like this:

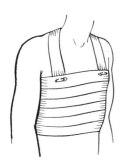

EXERCISE

The aims of exercise in diseases of the chest are to prevent a "respiratory cripple," relieve pain, prevent and correct deformities of the trunk, and prevent restriction of motion of the upper extremity.

PREVENTIVE AND CORRECTIVE EXERCISES

In conditions such as chronic emphysema and asthma, the thorax may remain permanently inflated and become a barrel chest. To prevent this, exercises are prescribed to develop the expiratory phase of breathing and to develop the muscles involved in the compression of the thorax. A simple exercise that may be used to prevent this occurrence is as follows:

1. Lie in the position shown with one hand placed on the upper abdomen.

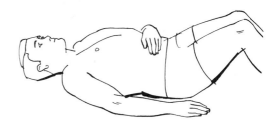

2. Exhale slowly and completely by contracting the abdominal wall. With the hand on the abdomen, feel the depression of the abdomen as it contracts.
3. Breathe in gently and repeat. Continue the exercise for 15 to 30 minutes.

Another exercise to develop expiration with the patient in a sitting position is as follows:

1. Sit, as illustrated, with the hands over the lower ribs.

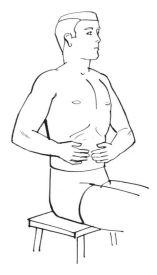

2. Exhale by contracting the abdominal muscles. Feel the narrowing of lower rib cage.
3. With the hands exert pressure at the end of the exhalation to get as much air as possible out of the lungs. Repeat the exercise for about 15 minutes.

Exercise for thoracic surgery patients both pre- and postoperatively has become an important part of the surgical program. Scar formation after surgery and the tendency of the patient to guard the affected area against painful movement may result in permanent structural and functional deformity. An exercise carried out to develop expansion of the chest after surgery is this:

1. Instruct the patient to lie in the position shown and flex one arm to vertical while taking a deep breath.

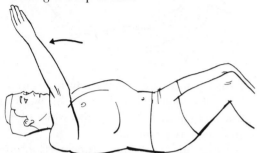

2. Lower the arm while exhaling.
3. Repeat with the other arm.

After the patient has mastered this exercise, he may progress to raising both arms together vertically and finally overhead while inhaling. He exhales while returning both arms to the side.

The aforementioned exercise to develop expiration is also preferred by some for use postoperatively.

Shoulder exercises include an active rotation of the shoulder.

Postoperative exercises are started as soon as the patient is able to cooperate. These exercises are done as often as a few minutes every hour.

POSTOPERATIVE POSITIONING OF THE PATIENT

The best thing we can say about the routine for positioning the postoperative thoracotomy patient is that nothing definite can be said. Every surgeon seems to have a different theory about which position is best. In doing some research on the subject, the following variations in opinion were noted:

Keep the patient turned with the operative side down to stabilize the chest incision, minimize pain, and permit expansion of the dependent lung.

Don't place the patient with the operated side down because it prevents expansion of the lung on that side.

Placing the patient on the operated side causes too much discomfort.

Never place the patient in Trendelenburg position because it elevates the diaphragm and interferes with ventilation.

Place the patient in Trendelenburg position to combat shock and facilitate postural drainage.

The best advice we can give is to check with the surgeon responsible for the patient.

The important point is that regardless of the side the patient is permitted to turn on, he must be turned from his back to his side about every hour. A number of surgeons have no rules and feel that the patient can be turned on both sides.

When the patient is turned on his operated side, the drainage tube must be checked to make certain that it is not kinked. If the placement of the drainage tube interferes with lying on the operated side, make a little trough in which the tube can lie between two small pillows. Most surgeons who want the patient to lie on the operated side place the drainage tube at a point far enough forward that it does not interfere with positioning. In most instances as soon as the blood pressure is stabilized, the patient's head is elevated 30° to 45°.

The patient is usually gotten out of bed to stand on the first postoperative day and to walk on the second day. A patient can walk a few steps from the bed even with chest tubes in place.

POSTOPERATIVE CONVALESCENT ACTIVITY

Convalescent activity of course must be tailored to the nature of the disease. Under normal circumstances the patient is usually instructed to gauge his degree of activity by his feeling of fatigue. For a period of several weeks after surgery, light activities aside from automobile driving are usually recommended. The breathing exercises are continued during the convalescent period.

MANAGEMENT OF PATIENT FOR CHEST SURGERY

Having read the discussion on the procedures thus far in the chapter, you already have some idea of what the pre- and post-operative care in chest surgery entails. Here we are giving an outline of the usual management so that a composite picture can be obtained.

PREOPERATIVE MANAGEMENT

Many of the diagnostic studies mentioned in the beginning of the chapter are made.

The preparation for surgery may include these:

1. Administration of blood when blood volume is diminished
2. Use of intermittent positive pressure breathing apparatus
3. Use of parenteral or nebulized antibiotics and bronchodilators
4. Use of digitalis-like drugs prophylactically for arrhythmias frequently noted following chest surgery
5. Exercise and coughing instructions
6. Preoperative medication, a barbiturate, morphine, and atropine or scopolamine about 75 minutes before surgery
7. Anesthesia by the endotracheal route.

POSTOPERATIVE MANAGEMENT

In hospitals that have a recovery room and intensive care unit, the patient is kept in the recovery room until conscious and in the intensive care unit until the chest tubes are removed.

In hospitals where these facilities are not available, the immediate care of the patient includes these aspects:

Measuring Status of Patient
1. Blood pressure and pulse rate are checked frequently. Both apical and radial pulses may be taken 2 to 3 days.
2. Intake and output are recorded. Weight may be measured daily to further determine fluid imbalance. In presence of hypotension, hourly urinary output may be recorded (see p. 268).
3. Chest x-rays are taken with the portable machine on first postoperative day and periodically thereafter.

Positioning of Patient
1. Varies with surgeon; see page 228.
2. Change every hour.
3. Start exercises when conscious (see p. 227).
4. Out of bed first day.

Blood and Fluid Replacement
1. Careful tally of blood loss is kept during surgery. Blood is administered as needed.
2. Vasopressors may be required for short periods of time.
3. Patient is usually kept on "dry" side. Around 2000 cc. parenteral fluids are given first day at 50 to 60 drops per minute. Oral fluids given after first 24 hours.

Dressings (see p. 226)
1. Tube and incision dressings are separate.
2. Check for hemorrhage.
3. Some oozing usually occurs.

Drainage of Pleural Space
1. Two-bottle water seal with suction used most often (see p. 224).
2. Following pneumonectomy KEEP DRAINAGE TUBE CLAMPED (see p. 223).
3. Fluid draining from chest cavity is bloody during first few hours, then becomes serous in 36 to 48 hours.
4. Tubes are usually left in place several days.

Management of Airway
(Unless constant vigilance is maintained to insure prompt evacuation of tracheobronchial secretions, pulmonary complications are likely to occur after any intrathoracic surgery.)
1. Patient must cough every hour (see p. 219).
2. Endotracheal suction aids coughing reflex (see p. 220).
3. Heavily misted oxygen by tent or nasal catheter given for 1 or 2 days. Oxygen is used only to insure adequate oxygenation and is not given after the patient can accomplish this by breathing room air.
4. Bronchodilators such as Imprel may be given in aerosol form several times daily if patient has bronchospasm (see p. 215). After oral intake is tolerated, potassium iodide may be given.
5. In presence of heavy tracheobronchial

secretions and ventilatory insufficiency, a tracheotomy is done.

6. In cases of atelectasis, laryngoscopy and bronchoscopy may be used to pass tracheal suction tube.

7. NEVER USE A BLOW BOTTLE following chest surgery.

Antibiotics

1. Usually given prophylactically for several days postoperatively.

Relief of Pain

1. Small doses of narcotics given closer together than for general surgery to prevent depression of respiratory functions.

2. Control of pain is important. Uncontrolled pain causes muscular spasms of chest wall and in turn limitation of chest movements.

Gastrointestinal Function

1. Transient depression of gastrointestinal system may be present for first 24 to 36 hours.

2. Thirty to 60 cc. clear liquid may be given every hour on first postoperative day to see if it is tolerated.

3. Liquid diet usually started second day.

4. In seriously ill patient, gavage may be necessary.

ADDITIONAL PROCEDURES TO REVIEW

Oxygen therapy (Chap. 4)

Controlling the spread of disease (Chap. 7)

Preventing and relieving abdominal distention, a frequent occurrence in pneumonia (Chap. 11)

Special mouth care (see p. 159) is necessary when the patient is febrile and the sputum is purulent

Comfort measures to patient and environment

Use of side boards when patient is orthopneic

Use of restraints when patient is in toxic confused state as occurs occasionally in pneumonia

Measuring fluid intake and output

Intramuscular and intravenous injections (Chap. 6)

Gastric intubation for nutritional purposes (see p. 161)

Cooling sponge baths in temperature elevation

Use of suction apparatus (see p. 136)

Radiation therapy in the form of x-rays used occasionally for metastatic tumor of lungs (see p. 18)

Administration of allergens from atmosphere in bronchial asthma

Use of respirator (Chap. 5)

Use of blow bottles for emphysema (p. 216)

DIETS TO REVIEW

Proteins and caloric content increased to counterbalance increased metabolism and nitrogen loss in febrile illnesses

Fluid intake increased (eliminate those which cause distention)

Vitamin B-complex and C supplements given during inflammatory illness

Liquid to soft consistency used in inflammatory illnesses and postoperatively

Proteins, vitamins, and minerals increased in chronic inflammatory diseases

Elimination diet used in diagnosis and treatment of bronchial asthma

MEDICATIONS TO REVIEW

Antibiotics. Penicillin (Duracillin, Flo-Cillin, Wycillin, Crystacillin, Ledercillin, Hypercillin, etc.) streptomycin, Chloromycetin, Aureomycin, Seromycin, erythromycin, kanamycin, oleandomycin (Matromycin), Terramycin, tetracycline hydrochloride (Achromycin, Tetracyn, Polycycline, Stecline, Panmycin)

Anti-infectives Specific for Tuberculosis. Paraaminosalicylic acid (PAS), isonicotinic acid (Isoniazid Hydrazide, Rimifon, Nydrazid, Isoniazid, Cortinazin, Ditubin, Armazide, Dinacrin, Isolyn, Tisin, Tyvid, INH), pyrazinamide

Antihistamines. Parabromdylamine maleate (Dimetane), chlorothen citrate (Tagathen, Alerin-td, Chestamine, Chloramate, Histitrin, Teldrin), chlorpheniramine maleate (Chlor-Trimeton), clemizole hydrochloride (Allercur, Reactron), diphenhydramine hydrochloride (Benadryl), diphenylpraline

(Hispril), promethazine (Phenergan), tripelennamine hydrochloride (Pyribenzamine), pyrilamine maleate (A-H Tob, Antamine, Antihist, Antopic, Copsamine, Diaminide, Enrumay, Histabort, Histacap, Histacin, Histalon, Minihist, Nasaval, Pyramal, Stangen, Statomin, Thylogen)

Stimulants. Carbon dioxide gas

Nebulae and Sprays. Alevaire, Aludrin, Isuprel, epinephrine, Clopane Hydrochloride, Norisodrine, Isonorin

Expectorants. Ammonia, potassium iodide, terpin hydrate elixir

Sedative Cough Medicines. Benzonatate (Tessalon), Brown's mixture, codeine (Cotussis, Cosadein, Cheracol), dihydrocodeinone (Hycodan, Mercodol)

BIBLIOGRAPHY

Beeson, P. B., and McDermott, W.: Cecil-Loeb Textbook of Medicine. 12th ed. Philadelphia, W. B. Saunders Co., 1967.

Brown, A.: Medical and Surgical Nursing II. Philadelphia, W. B. Saunders Co., 1959.

Brunner, L. S., et al.: Textbook of Medical-Surgical Nursing. Philadelphia, J. B. Lippincott Co., 1964.

Chapman, J. S.: The Atypical Mycobacteria; Their Significance in Human Disease. Am. J. Nurs., 67:1031, 1967.

Davidsohn, I., and Henry, J. B.: Todd-Sanford Clinical Diagnosis by Laboratory Methods. 14th ed. Philadelphia, W. B. Saunders Co., 1969.

Davis, L.: Christopher's Textbook of Surgery. 9th ed. Philadelphia, W. B. Saunders Co., 1968.

Falconer, M., Patterson, H., and Gustafson, E.: Current Drug Handbook. 1968-70. Philadelphia, W. B. Saunders Co., 1968.

Friedman, R. M.: Interferons and Virus Infection. Am. J. Nurs., 68:542, 1968.

Goodale, R.: Clinical Interpretation of Laboratory Tests. 5th ed. Philadelphia, F. A. Davis Co., 1964.

Harmer, B., and Henderson, V.: Textbook of Principles and Practices of Nursing. 5th ed. New York, The Macmillan Co., 1958.

Krause, M.: Food, Nutrition and Diet Therapy. 4th ed. Philadelphia, W. B. Saunders Co., 1966.

Larson, E.: The Patient with Acute Pulmonary Edema. Am. J. Nurs., 68:1019, 1968.

Nett, L.: Acute Respiratory Failure: Principles of Care. Am. J. Nurs., 67:1847, 1967.

Price, A.: The Art, Science and Spirit of Nursing. 3rd ed. Philadelphia, W. B. Saunders Co., 1965.

Sadove, M., and Cross, J.: The Recovery Room. Philadelphia, W. B. Saunders Co., 1956.

14

nursing techniques in the care of
Cardiovascular Diseases

DIAGNOSTIC PROCEDURES

LABORATORY TESTS

Blood Tests

TEST	NORMAL	ABNORMAL INDICATIONS
Antistreptolysin titer		400 U or higher is consistent with, but not diagnostic of, rheumatic fever
Blood cultures	Negative	Positive in bacterial endocarditis
Blood serum protein†	6 to 8 gm./100 ml.	Measured in heart disease because edema sometimes results when protein content is low
Blood sugar*†	70 to 110 mg./100 ml.	Used because of susceptibility of diabetic to arteriosclerosis
Blood urea nitrogen† BUN	10 to 20 mg./100 ml.	Elevated when heart disease disturbs renal circulation
Calcium†	9 to 11 mg./100 ml.	Increased in heart failure

232

BLOOD TESTS (*Continued*)

TESTS	NORMAL	ABNORMAL INDICATIONS
Coagulation tests		
Bleeding time	1 to 5 minutes	
Calcium clotting time (CaT)	90 to 130 seconds	
Clot retraction	78%	
Clot retraction time	33 minutes	
Clotting time (Lee-White),	6 to 10 minutes	All coagulation tests are used in diagnosis
(capillary method)	3 to 5 minutes	of hemorrhagic disorders
Fibrinogen	200 to 400 mg./100 ml.	
Fibrinolysis	No lysis in 24 hours	
Partial thromboplastin		
time (PTT)	40 to 100 seconds	
Prothrombin index	70 to 100%	
Prothrombin consumption		
test	16 seconds	
Prothrombin time	14 to 18 seconds	
Thrombin time (TT)	11 to 14 seconds	
Thromboplastin generation		
test (TGT)	Less than 12 seconds	
C-reactive protein	Negative	A protein substance, not normally present, is found in active rheumatic fever, myocardial infarction, and pulmonary infarction
Differential count of cells		
Basophils	0 to 200 per cu. mm., 0 to 2%	
Eosinophils	25 to 400 per cu. mm., 0.5 to 4%	Decreased in congestive heart failure
Lymphocytes	1250 to 3500 per cu. mm., 25 to 35%	
Monocytes	200 to 1000 per cu. mm., 4 to 10%	
Neutrophils	3000 to 8000 per cu. mm., 53 to 80%	Increased in rheumatic heart disease, acute bacterial endocarditis
Enzymes†		
Lipase	0 to 400 units	
SCPK—serum creatine phosphokinase		
SGOT—serum glutamic transaminase	5 to 7 units	All increased in myocardial infarction
SHBD—serum hydroxy-butyrate dehydrogenase	50 to 150 units	
SLDH—serum lactic dehydrogenase	60 to 250 units per cc.	
Erythrocytes	4 to 5.5 million	Decreased in rheumatic fever and subacute endocarditis. Increased in many forms of chronic heart disease as in some types of congenital heart disease and in heart disease with pulmonary complications
Hematocrit	Females: 37 to 47% Males: 40 to 54%	Rises considerably in shock
Hemoglobin	Females: 12 to 15 gm./100 ml.	See comments for erythrocytes
Leukocytes	5 to 10 thousand	Increased in coronary infarction and rheumatic heart disease
Lipids†		
cholesterol		
esters	50 to 65% of total	
free	40 to 50 mg./100 cc.	Increased in hemorrhage and arteriosclerosis
total	150 to 280 mg./100 cc.	Decreased in pernicious anemia
fatty acids	350 to 450 mg./100 cc. ⎫	
neutral fat	0 to 370 mg./100 cc. ⎬	Increased in anemias and leukemia
phospholipids	220 to 400 mg./100 cc.	Increased in anemia from hemorrhage; decreased in other anemias
total	400 to 600 mg./100 cc.	

BLOOD TESTS *(Continued)*

TEST	NORMAL	ABNORMAL INDICATIONS
Mucoproteins†	8 to 14 mg./100 cc.	Increased in leukemia, myocardial infarction, rheumatic fever
Nonprotein nitrogen*† (NPN)	15 to 35 mg./100 ml.	
Platelets	200 to 500 thousand	
Reticulocytes	0.5 to 2.0% red cells	
Sedimentation rate	2 to 20 mm. in 1 hour (depends on method)	Abnormal always higher. Useful in following the course of acute rheumatic fever and acute myocardial infarction
Serological tests for syphilis	negative	Used because syphilis is a common cause of aortic aneurysm

*Oxylated collection tube needed.
†Withhold breakfast.

URINALYSIS

Albuminuria, hematuria and casts occur in kidney impairment due to heart failure. Albumin and erythrocytes are found in the urine in rheumatic heart disease. Specific urine tests are discussed in Chapter 15.

OTHER TESTS

VENOUS PRESSURE

Venous pressure is measured with a glass manometer tube connected to a needle in the vein. The procedure is carried out as follows:
1. The patient is kept at rest for at least 15 minutes before the test.
2. The right arm is supported at a position level with the right auricle.
3. The forearm is prepared as for an intravenous injection (see p. 85).
4. The needle attached to a three-way stopcock and a 10-cc. syringe containing 5 cc. of sterile 3 per cent sodium citrate solution is injected as shown:

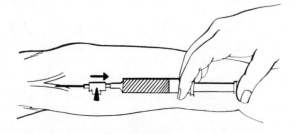

5. The tourniquet is released as soon as the needle is in the vein or an accurate reading will not be obtained.
6. A few cubic centimeters of blood are withdrawn into the syringe.
7. The manometer is attached as shown and the blood and citrate in the syringe are injected into the manometer.

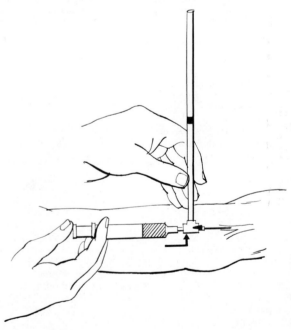

8. The mixture is then allowed to run into the veins. As the fluid level falls, it becomes stabilized at a definite level. The manometer reading at that point is recorded.

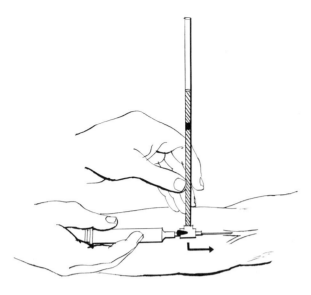

Normally the venous pressure is low in comparison with the arterial pressure. The venous pressure is elevated abnormally in patients with congestive heart failure due to myocardial or valvular disease, fluid accumulation in the pericardial sac and compression of the heart by a scarred inelastic pericardial membrane.

CIRCULATION TIME

Circulation time is obtained by measuring the time interval between the intravenous injection of a solution and the moment the solution is tasted or smelled. Systemic circulation time is the time from the injection of a solution (calcium gluconate or sodium succinate) to the detection of its taste on the tongue. The normal range of time is 10 to 16 seconds. The pulmonary circulation time is the time from the injection of a solution to the detection of its smell on the breath. A stop watch is needed to measure the time. Circulation time is lengthened in congestive heart failure and is shortened in advanced anemia.

REGITINE TEST

Tests are sometimes used to distinguish between high blood pressure caused by the adrenal gland and that of essential hyper-

tension. Regitine (phentolamine), an adrenergic blocking drug, neutralizes the action of epinephrine, thus reducing an arterial pressure elevated due to the hormone. The Regitine test is conducted as follows:

1. The patient is placed flat on his back in bed and the blood pressure is checked and recorded.
2. Five milligrams of Regitine is dissolved in 1 cc. of sterile water and injected intravenously.
3. Thereafter the blood pressure is taken and recorded at 30-second intervals for 3 minutes; then at 1-minute intervals for 7 minutes.

If hypertension is due to adrenal malfunction, the blood pressure will fall between 25 and 35 mm. of mercury. No effect is caused in cases of essential hypertension UNLESS the patient is receiving rauwolfia (reserpine, Serpasil, Reserpoid, Rauwiloid) or phenobarbital. These drugs must be withheld about a month before the test can be conducted.

Other drugs given to perform similar tests are those stimulating a sudden rise in blood pressure in patients with adrenal disease. These drugs include histamine, methacholine (Mecholyl) and tetraethylammonium chloride (Etamon Chloride). The test is conducted in the same manner with these drugs as with Regitine. If the hypertension is essential, there will be no change in blood pressure. If the hypertension is due to adrenal malfunction, the blood pressure will suddenly rise.

TOURNIQUET (CAPILLARY FRAGILITY) TEST
(Quick's Method)

A blood pressure cuff is applied above the elbow, and the pressure is maintained at a point just above the diastolic pressure for a period of 5 minutes. The blood pressure cuff is removed. Fifteen minutes after the cuff is removed, petechiae are counted in a 5 cm. circle just below the elbow pit. A count greater than five denotes increased capillary fragility. The patient should be told that everyone develops some petechiae after this test. This test is also sometimes called the Rumpel-Leede test.

TRENDELENBURG TEST

This test provides information concerning the superficial veins. The patient is placed flat on his back, and the leg is elevated until the veins are fully collapsed. A tourniquet is placed around the thigh, and the patient is requested to stand. If the saphenofemoral valve is the sole source of incompetency, the veins will remain empty for a minute or two before filling from below. Rapid filling of the veins from below indicates that there are more perforating veins below the level of the tourniquet.

PERTHES' TEST

This is performed to test the patency of the deep veins. A tourniquet is placed around the patient's thigh, and he is requested to exercise his leg by kicking it vigorously back and forth or by rapid walking. With exercise the blood should go into the deep veins, causing the varicosities to empty. If the deep veins are not functioning properly, the varicosities will not empty.

BONE MARROW TEST

An examination of bone marrow is necessary in the diagnosis of numerous blood diseases. The bone marrow specimen is obtained by aspiration from the sternum. The nurse assists the physician in performing the procedure as follows:
1. The skin over the midsternum is shaved if necessary and sterilized with an antiseptic. Aseptic technique is observed throughout the procedure.
2. A local anesthetic (1 per cent solution of procaine) is administered into the skin, subcutaneous tissue and periosteum.
3. A short-beveled 18-gauge needle with a guard and stylet is inserted vertically into the middle of the sternum between the second and third ribs.
4. When the needle is in place the stylet is removed and a 5-cc. syringe is attached. Suction is applied and marrow pulp is pulled into the syringe.

5. After removal of the needle a sterile bandage is placed over the wound.

The normal values of bone marrow cells are as follows:

PERCENTAGES OF CELLS IN BONE MARROW OF NORMAL ADULTS		
Myeloblasts	0.3	to 5.0
Promyelocytes	1.0	to 8.0
Myelocytes:		
Neutrophilic	5.0	to 19.0
Eosinophilic	0.5	to 3.0
Basophilic	0.0	to 0.5
Metamyelocytes ("juvenile" forms)	13.0	to 32.0
Polymorphonuclear neutrophils	7.0	to 30.0
Polymorphonuclear eosinophils	0.5	to 4.0
Polymorphonuclear basophils	0.0	to 0.7
Lymphocytes	3.0	to 17.0
Plasma cells	0.0	to 2.0
Monocytes	0.5	to 5.0
Reticulum cells	0.1	to 2.0
Megakaryocytes	0.03	to 3.0
Pronormoblasts (macroblasts)	1.0	to 8.0
Normoblasts (basophilic, poly-chromatophilic, and acidophilic)	7.0	to 32.0

Attention in evaluating the bone marrow smear is given to the M. E. (myeloid:erythroid) ratio. The normal ratio is usually 0.56:1. If the proportion of myeloid cells to erythroid cells is increased leukemia may be suspected. An increased proportion of erythroblasts may be due to red cell loss and/or destruction. The presence of tumor cells, which are normally not present, may indicate carcinoma or Hodgkin's disease. Other changes in bone marrow cells are too numerous to mention in this context.

GRAPHIC DEVICES

Electrocardiogram

The electrocardiogram is used to determine the mechanism of rhythmic disturbances of the heart and to distinguish types of myocardial damage. The electrocardiogram is a sensitive instrument that records a picture of the passage of electric currents through the heart. The graphic picture depends on the connections between the machine and the patient's body. There are a variety of connections used to the arms, legs, and chest. Each connection is called a lead and is designated by Roman numerals or letters such as I, II, III, IVF, CF, V, AVR, AVL, and AVF. The title of each lead signifies the arrangement of the electrodes for that particular lead. In heart disease, only one lead of the total number of leads taken may be abnormal. For this reason it is customary to take as many as 10 to 12 leads at a time.

An electrocardiogram showing the cardiac cycles is as shown:

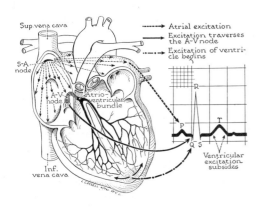

The cardiac cycle is designated by a series of waves called P, Q, R, S, T, and sometimes U. The letters indicate the electric activity of the heart in the following order:

P wave—contraction of auricles.

PR interval—time it takes to go from auricle to ventricle.

QRS complex—contraction in ventricle.

T wave—retreat of excitation wave as it passes up the pulmonary conus. This wave attracts a great deal of attention in heart disease because it is sensitive to disease and drugs.

U wave—a small wave of obscure origin which occasionally occurs following the T wave. In potassium depletion a U wave may make its first appearance.

By an examination of each lead, many diseases of the heart may be identified. Since the electrocardiogram is sensitive to the action of drugs, especially digitalis, mention should be made of any drugs taken by the patient when he is referred for an electrocardiogram.

In coronary artery disease where there is no organic disease of the heart, the electrocardiogram would appear normal. In this case the physician may prefer to conduct "stress' tests to determine deviations from normal. Two stress tests used are the anoxia test and the two-step or Master test. In the anoxia test, tracings are taken before, during and after the patient inhales a 10 per cent oxygen concentration. In the two-step test the tracings are taken after the patient walks up and down steps for a prescribed time. Both tests are used only rarely, since serious reactions sometimes occur in patients with heart disease. These tests are also not 100 per cent valid in the diagnosis of coronary artery disease.

Ballistocardiogram

The ballistocardiogram affords information concerning the efficiency and quality of myocardial contraction. It gives a measurement of cardiac output and tells whether the heart is performing its function easily or with difficulty.

When a ballistocardiogram is taken, the patient lies on a board and the ballistocardiograph records the movements that the thrusts of the heart and the pulsations of the artery send to the entire body. A great majority (but not all) of the patients with coronary artery disease have abnormal ballistocardiograms. Many patients have abnormal tracings before symptoms develop. Ballistocardiography is also believed to be helpful in the diagnosis of mitral stenosis and chronic constrictive pericarditis.

Plethysmography

The plethysmograph measures the volume of blood flow in a specific part. These studies are extremely important in detecting occlusive vascular disease. For instance, when the device is attached to the foot and calf of the leg, the physician can determine whether or not there is arterial occlusion causing insufficient circulation in the limb. No preparation of the patient is necessary.

Phonocardiograms

Electrical instruments measuring and recording the heart sounds and murmurs are called phonocardiographs or stethocardiographs. The phonocardiograph amplifies the heart sounds so that even the faintest sound may be detected. Heart sounds simultaneously registered with electrocardiograms make possible the placement of each heart sound in its exact position in the cardiac cycle. This prevents an erroneous diagnosis of a systolic murmur as a diastolic murmur and vice versa.

X-RAY EXAMINATIONS

Fluoroscopy

Fluoroscopy shows the heart in action and is used more often than other x-ray methods in cardiologic examinations. Fluoroscopy is used to look for abnormal configuration, tumors, and calcifications in the heart, aorta, and pulmonary vessels, to find congestion of the lungs, and to detect pleural or pericardial effusions. During examination of the heart under fluoroscopy, barium is given by mouth so that the outline of the esophagus can be seen. An enlarged left auricle pushes the esophagus aside as it becomes larger. There is no preparation of the patient for this examination.

Orthodiagraphy

Orthodiagraphy is a type of fluoroscopy in which pictures are recorded of the contour of the heart.

Intravenous Angiocardiography

This is a procedure in which an opaque medium is injected into a vein followed by a rapid series of x-ray pictures taken of the course of the medium through the heart, to the lungs, back to the heart, and out through the aorta. Commonly used organic iodide media include Hypaque Sodium, Cardiografin and Ditriokon. The dosage of contrast media is calculated according to the kilograms of body weight (1 cc./kg.). The solution is injected through a large bore (12-gauge) needle held in position in the vein, usually by a "cutdown." Speed of injection is imperative, since the solution must pass through the heart in a large bolus to make possible a good examination. The solution is injected after the patient has been instructed to inhale deeply.

The inspiration is held for the entire series of x-rays.

This diagnostic method is unexcelled for precision in detecting congenital cardiac defects. Individual chambers of the heart are visualized, pathways for the blood stream are demonstrated, and chamber enlargement can be seen.

The opaque medium may cause a flushing sensation as it flows through the body. If necessary, the studies may be conducted under mild anesthesia. After one complete circulation, the opaque media is so diluted that it is no longer visible by x-ray.

No special preparation of the patient is necessary unless anesthesia is to be given. In that event, food may be withheld prior to the studies. A record of the patient's weight should be sent to the x-ray department with him.

Aortogram

The aorta and its branches are studied by the injection of a contrast medium through a plastic catheter or with a needle directly into the aorta. Terms used in connection with the aortogram are retrograde aortogram (retrograde meaning against the direction of blood flow) and translumbar aortogram (meaning the injection is made below the twelfth rib and to the left of the spine in back). No preparation of the patient is necessary.

Cardiac Catheterization

This is a procedure in which a radiopaque catheter is manipulated under fluoroscopic observation through the heart. The exterior end of the catheter is connected by a three-way stopcock to a saline-filled regulated drip system that also contains a pressure gauge (strain gauge) and a camera. During the procedure the blood pressures within the heart are automatically transmitted to the strain gauge, which in turn transmits the pressure to the camera recording the findings on photographic film. Samples of blood are also withdrawn from the heart chambers and great vessels and analyzed for oxygen content.

The pressures within the heart indicate any existing strain placed on individual heart chambers. The oxygen content indicates whether the blood is circulating directly through the heart or whether the blood is being shunted because of an anatomical defect.

During the entire procedure an electrocardiograph and an electrocardiotachometer are recording readings on photographic paper. The electrocardiotachometer is connected by leads that operate as do those of the electrocardiograph and instantaneously records the heart rate. It also contains a small light that flashes on with each heartbeat, thus enabling the physician to observe in the dark the condition of the patient.

There are several routes used for the catheter approach to the heart. Not long ago only the right side of the heart was studied by catheterization. The cardiac catheter was inserted by means of a "cut-down" into the antecubital vein of either arm, then manipulated through the innominate vein, superior vena cava, right atrium, tricuspid valve, right ventricle, semilunar valve and pulmonary artery.

Several studies also include the left heart. The approach is made directly to the left atrium by means of an 18-gauge, 6-inch needle with a stylet through the patient's back directly into the heart. After the tip of the needle is placed in the left atrium, the stylet is removed and the catheter is manipulated into the left atrium, left ventricle and the ascending aorta.

Here is an anatomical sketch showing how this approach (posterior percutaneous or transthoracic left atrium puncture) is possible.

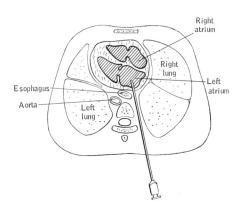

Since this method has been successfully used, the direct approach is also being used to study the right heart. Studies now also include the examination of both sides of the heart simultaneously through the transthoracic introduction of two needles, one in each atrium.

The patient is taken to the fluoroscopy or cardiology department for the study. The entire procedure may last from 1 to 3 hours. The procedure is a painless one. The patient is prepared as follows:

1. Solid foods are withheld. Liquids are permitted up to 3 hours prior to the procedure.
2. Nembutal and morphine may be given 30 minutes prior to the procedure.
3. A systemic antibiotic is administered to prevent infection.

After the procedure the patient is returned to his room, remaining flat in bed for 24 hours or more. The pulse rate is checked every 10 minutes during the first hour, then every 30 minutes for 3 hours. The patient may be nauseated following the procedure.

A systemic antibiotic is continued several days following the procedure to prevent thrombophlebitis.

MEASURING THE BLOOD PRESSURE

Although taking the blood pressure is one of the first procedures learned by nurses, there are a few points about this procedure which are worthy of mention in this context. These points are as follows:

1. With extremely obese patients the application of the cuff around the forearm and auscultation over the radial artery may give a truer measurement of blood pressure than does the ordinary method.
2. In patients with slight hypertension or in those suspected of having congenital heart disease, the blood pressure is measured in both arms and in one or both legs. A higher pressure in the arms than in the legs is a sign of coarctation of the aorta. In aneurysms the pressure of the two arms differs. When taking the blood pressure on the leg, the cuff is placed above the knee and the stethoscope is placed over the popliteal artery shown on the following page.
3. The small pulse pressure in severe aortic stenosis and the paradoxical pulse in peri-

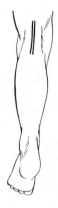

cardial disease are best detected with a blood pressure apparatus.

OPHTHALMOSCOPIC EXAMINATION

Examination of the eye by means of an ophthalmoscope is a valuable diagnostic aid in that it provides the only way of looking at an artery (retinal artery). This gives direct information concerning the condition of a patient's arteries.

THERAPEUTIC AND REHABILITATIVE PROCEDURES

ANTICOAGULANT THERAPY

Anticoagulant drugs, heparin and Dicumarol (see p. 255) are used extensively in the treatment of thrombosis. In a patient under treatment with anticoagulants, the coagulation time, prothrombin time and prothrombin index are important in guiding the dosage of drugs administered. The effect of heparin is almost immediate while that of Dicumarol takes about 48 hours. Some physicians start treatment with heparin and Dicumarol together and stop heparin at the end of 48 hours so that no time is lost in establishing effective treatment.

The techniques of anticoagulant therapy vary somewhat with the use of the two drugs. In heparin therapy the clotting time is first determined; then heparin is administered intramuscularly in a dosage of 50-100 mg. Four hours later the coagulation time is determined once more and if the time is pro-

longed the test will be repeated again in 2 hours. If at the end of 4 hours no appreciable effect is noted, a larger dosage of heparin is administered and the clotting time is again checked in 4 and 6 hours. When the dosage shows the desired effect at the 4- and 6-hour intervals, this dosage is established as suitable for continuous treatment.

In Dicumarol therapy, the prothrombin time is first determined and a dosage of from 200 to 300 mg. is administered orally. A second considerably smaller dose is administered the following day. The prothrombin time is determined daily and subsequent doses of Dicumarol are adjusted accordingly. The average daily dose is usually 50-100 mg. Phenindione or Hedulin is another drug similar to Dicumarol and is sometimes substituted for Dicumarol. The nurse should have some understanding of the tests used, the normal values, and the optimal therapeutic values in the use of the two drugs. These facts are shown in the table:

ANTI-COAGULANT	TEST	NORMAL VALUES	OPTIMAL VALUES DURING TREATMENT
Heparin	Coagulation time (modification of Lee-White method)	9 to 15 minutes	45 to 60 minutes
Dicumarol	Prothrombin time (Quick method)	12 to 20 seconds	35 to 80 seconds
Dicumarol	Prothrombin index	70 to 100 per cent	20 to 60 per cent
Dicumarol	Per cent of prothrombin activity (Quick)	70 to 100 per cent	15 to 25 per cent

Anticoagulant drugs are also used in the preventative therapy of thromboembolic diseases.

The principal complication of anticoagulant therapy is spontaneous bleeding anywhere in the body. The earliest evidence of hemorrhage is microscopic hematuria observed in a routine urinalysis. Because of this a routine urinalysis is performed frequently during anticoagulant therapy. The treatment of hemorrhage in heparin therapy consists of an intravenous injection of protamine sulfate. In Dicumarol therapy the treatment of hemorrhage is more difficult because of the lasting effects of the drug. The administration of whole blood and injections of vitamin K_1 (Mephyton) is usually the treatment of choice in this case.

OSCILLATING BED

In peripheral vascular disease, some of the vessels of the extremities may be partially occluded, leading to the formation of ulcerations. Great benefit is derived from the use of an apparatus that draws blood into and forces blood out of the extremity. Nearly normal circulation may be re-established by increasing the capacity of collateral vessels in this manner.

An apparatus used to accomplish this is the oscillating bed, also called the rocking bed. The patient is placed on the bed, which, as the name implies, rocks up and down as shown here:

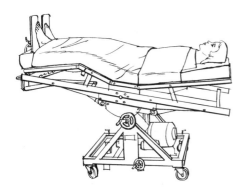

The degree of tilt and the length of the cycle can be regulated. This treatment may be prescribed for periods of 6 hours or longer. Some patients have adjusted so well to the device that they are able to sleep during the treatment.

Other methods for improving circulation include specific wet dressings (see p. 244), the use of drugs (see p. 240), and Buerger's exercises (see p. 243).

PERICARDIOCENTESIS

Occasionally an accumulation of fluid is removed from the pericardial sac to relieve pressure on the heart. The pericardial sac normally holds a few cubic centimeters of fluid. In chronic disease the amount may accumulate to several hundred cubic centimeters and in extreme cases to several thousand. When the fluid is excessive there is pressure on the heart, lungs, bronchi, trachea and esophagus. The patient is placed in a position that best facilitates breathing and the puncture is made in the fourth or fifth left or right intercostal space. The equipment required for the procedure and the technique is the same as for a thoracentesis (see p. 211), except that it does not require as large a receptacle for the fluid. Antibiotic therapy has greatly reduced the need for this procedure.

CARDIAC ARREST AND RESUSCITATION

Cardiac arrest is the general designation for the sudden cessation of an effective heartbeat. Whenever cardiac arrest is a sharp deviation from the course of progress that would ordinarily be expected from the patient's state of health or disease, resuscitative efforts are used. Causes of cardiac arrest amenable to successful resuscitation are coronary occlusion, drug poisoning, hemorrhage, shock, electrocution and heart surgery.

The absence of peripheral pulses and heart sounds is all that is necessary to make the diagnosis. Respiration may not be absent at first but may continue to be jerky or gasping for a minute or so after heart sounds and pulse have disappeared. Time should not be wasted taking the blood pressure. If the patient is to survive, treatment must begin within 4 minutes after the heart has ceased to function as a pump.

Resuscitation requires that two basic functions be restored simultaneously: blood must be pumped through the body, and there must be a gaseous exchange of oxygen and carbon dioxide. Restoration of one system without the other is not adequate and will lead to failure.

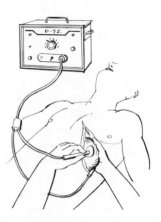

RESTORING THE HEARTBEAT

Several methods are used to start the heart, depending upon the facilities available: direct heart massage through an emergency thoracotomy may be done, external compression by striking the chest may be done, and a cardiac pacemaker may be used to start the heart by electrical stimulation.

Direct Heart Massage

For direct massage through an emergency thoracotomy, only one instrument is needed, the scalpel. In some hospitals a small sterile cardiac arrest kit has been made available in all departments. The kit consists of a scalpel handle fitted with a No. 10 blade and a notched aluminum tube approximately 10 cm. in length for holding the ribs apart.

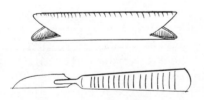

The thoracotomy is made by the physician without preparation of the skin and without gloves. Drugs such as epinephrine, procaine or Xylocaine, Isuprel, calcium chloride, digitalis, quinidine and Pronestyl may be needed during the resuscitation. When ventricular fibrillation is present, it may be stopped by the use of an electrical defibrillator. The electrodes are applied as shown:

External Compression

External compression of the heart has been successfully accomplished by forcefully striking the lower end of the sternum. It was discovered that this rhythmic external force can compress the heart to sufficiently pump enough blood to the brain to supply some oxygen. Although the amount of blood circulated in this manner is much less than that circulated normally, it can sustain life for some time. To apply external heart compression, place the heel of one hand on the sternum and place the heel of the other hand over the first hand as shown:

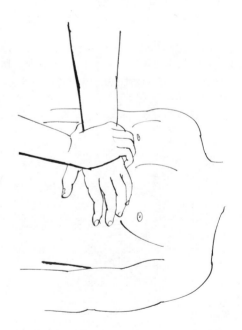

One inch of the sternum should extend below the heel of the hand. When compressing, use only the heel of the hand. Hold the fingers up off the chest.

During this procedure the patient must be lying on a rigid surface such as a stretcher or on the floor so that there is no "give" in the vertebral column. The strokes should be given at a rate of 60 per minute and forcefully enough to depress the rib cage 1 to 2 inches.

WARNING! Please note that external cardiac compression should be used only by those specially trained in the procedure. There are complications of external cardiac compression. If the hands are placed too low, the liver or other abdominal organs may be ruptured. If the hands are placed too high, the breast bone may be fractured. If they are placed too far to the right or left, severe rib fractures and damage to the lungs may result.

The Cardiac Pacemaker

Many hospitals now have electrical pacemakers kept on hand in strategic areas. In some hospitals the nurses are instructed in the use of the pacemaker in an emergency situation. One type of pacemaker looks like this:

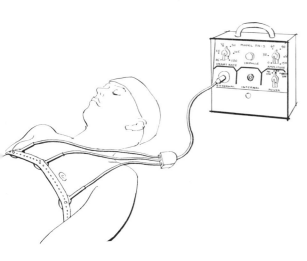

KEEPING THE PATIENT BREATHING

When the heart stops, oxygen administered with a positive pressure mask (see p. 41) will in most instances prove adequate to keep the patient breathing. If breathing stops, mouth to mouth resuscitation (see p. 217) may be necessary. When possible, an attempt is made to inflate the lungs by administering oxygen through an endotracheal tube.

The nurse's role in cardiac arrest is of extreme importance in saving a life, since the nurse may be the first one to observe the emergency. It is expedient to keep a well planned course of action in mind at all times in the event that this emergency should arise; knowing whom to call for help and where to locate all of the necessary equipment is essential. It may also be necessary for the nurse to apply mouth to mouth resuscitation and external cardiac compression (if the hospital's policy permits) until the physician arrives.

Care after successful resuscitation requires constant attention to all systems. Any patient who remains comatose shows signs of central nervous system damage. The treatment for this consists of placing the patient on hypothermia (see p. 10) and maintaining the rectal temperature at 32° to 33° C.

EXERCISE AND BODY MECHANICS

The physical activity of the patient with heart disease is limited according to the functional capacity of the heart and the influence of the activity on the heart. Activity may not be limited in any way or it may be limited in degrees from a slight disability to complete disability. The amount of exercise permitted following heart surgery is discussed later in this chapter.

In peripheral vascular diseases in which there is occlusion of the vessels exercise may be prescribed to improve circulation. Patients may be advised to walk short distances each day, providing the exercise does not cause pain in the legs. Buerger's exercises are sometimes prescribed to improve circulation. These exercises consist of elevating the limb for a peroid of 1 minute, lowering the limb for 2 minutes then leveling the limb for 2 minutes as shown:

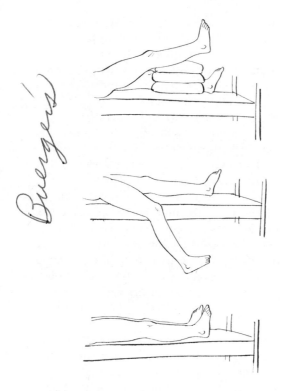

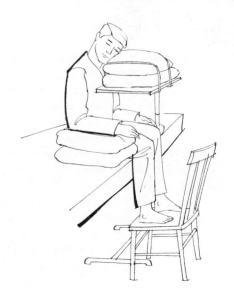

A special board, pillows, or an overbed table is used to hold the limb in the elevated position. The limb is placed in the "down" position by allowing it to hang over the side of the bed. Active exercises to develop leg muscles are prescribed in the treatment and prevention of thrombophlebitis. Active contraction of muscles raises venous pressure and forces venous blood out of the legs stimulating the development of more competent collateral venous channels.

The position of the patient resting in bed is extremely important to the patient with cardiovascular disease since various positions affect the circulation in different ways. In addition to knowing good body mechanics and comfort measures to the patient, the nurse should be aware of certain factors concerning the positioning of the patient with various cardiovascular diseases. These factors are as follows:

1. The patient with congestive heart failure may have to be propped straight up in bed, or may find comfort in sitting on the side of the bed with his feet dangling as shown:

When the head of the bed is elevated, the knee rest must be raised slightly to prevent the patient from sliding down in bed.

2. In peripheral vascular disease with occlusion of the blood vessels, the legs should never rest higher than the heart. The recommended position is to elevate the head of the bed about 10 inches by elevating the legs of the bed. This elevation places the feet about 6 inches below the level of the heart, which is the recommended position for prolonged rest periods. When ulceration or gangrene results from occluded circulation, sitting on the side of the bed with the feet resting on a chair should be discouraged since this position causes edema formation, which in turn prevents healing and promotes a spread of infection.

3. For thrombophlebitis, elevation of the legs during rest is necessary from both prophylactic and therapeutic standpoints.

DRESSINGS AND BANDAGES

Special Wet Dressings

Wet dressings or soaks are usually prescribed when gangrene develops as a result of peripheral vascular disease. The wet dressings or soaks are applied to remove crusts from lesions and promote healing. Solutions that are used include plain water and various antiseptic solutions. Wet dressings are applied for periods of 20 to 30 minutes several times daily. The temperature of the solution should be around 95° to 100°F. It is extremely important that the dressings be maintained at this temperature by the use of hot water bottles, because if the dressings become cool, vasoconstriction, the very condition one is trying to prevent, will occur. For this reason, soaks are preferred to wet dressings, since wet dressings require constant attention in order to maintain the desired temperature.

After the wet dressings are removed the lesions are cleaned and allowed to dry, then covered with dry sterile gauze.

Unna's Paste Boot

The treatment of chronic ulcers caused by varicose veins sometimes includes the application of Unna's paste. Unna's paste is a mixture of 150 cc. water, 400 gm. gelatin, 800 cc. glycerin, and 200 gm. zinc oxide. Heat the water; then add the gelatin and stir until it dissolves. Mix the glycerin and zinc oxide; then add it to the gelatin mixture and boil for ½ hour. The mixture is allowed to cool to lukewarm before application.

The leg is cleansed, dried and elevated for one hour before the dressing is applied. A layer of gauze bandage is applied to the foot and entire leg below the knee. A layer of paste is applied over the gauze; then a second layer of gauze and paste until three or four layers have been applied. (For bandaging techniques see page 203.) The boot is removed and replaced every week or two. The paste mixture will harden when cooled and must be reheated to apply.

An Unna paste bandage is now commercially available.

Pressure Bandages

Bandages applied for the purpose of providing pressure are used frequently in peripheral vascular disorders. Elastic bandage is the material best suited for this purpose. The bandage is applied with an even firmness over the extremity. If the bandage is applied too tightly the patient will complain of severe pain.

In this case the bandage must be removed and reapplied.

When pressure bandages must be worn daily for long periods of time as a preventive measure, the patient is usually advised to use elastic stockings.

HEART SURGERY

During the past 25 years heart surgery has passed through several vast phases of development. The first phases were concerned with operations such as the closure of patent ductus arteriosus, resection of coarctation of the aorta and systemic-pulmonary arterial anastomosis for the correction of the tetralogy of Fallot. These advances were followed by closed surgical procedures carried out on the beating heart such as the mitral commissurotomy and pulmonary valvotomy. The most striking advances followed the introduction of techniques in visual intracardiac surgery, namely "open heart" surgery.

Operative procedures for the heart can be classified under closed surgery or open surgery. Closed heart surgery refers to those surgical procedures that can be carried out without direct visualization of the defects within the heart. Open heart surgery refers to those procedures performed under direct vision within the heart.

The techniques employed in the complexities of open heart surgery demand a large team trained in many areas. The nursing care of the patient undergoing intracardiac surgery has indeed become a specialty.

ADVANCES IN OPEN HEART SURGERY

The advances making open heart surgery possible are as follows:

Extracorporeal Circulation

Extracorporeal circulation (also called cardiopulmonary bypass) is accomplished by use of the artificial heart machine (also called the pump-oxygenator). With this machine, the blood bypasses both the heart and lungs. The blood that returns to the heart through the vena cava is directed through a catheter to the pump-oxygenator where it is artificially oxygenated and returned to the body through a catheter placed in an appropriate systemic artery, usually the femoral artery.

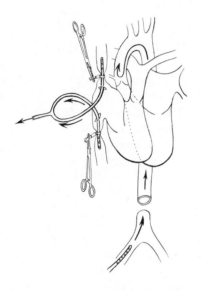

The aorta is perfused in retrograde fashion; the aortic valve, if normal, remains closed, and a coronary circulation is maintained. Thus the heart continues to beat during cardiopulmonary bypass at normal body temperature. The cardiac cavities are not completely empty because of the return of myocardial venous blood to the right atrium and bronchial venous blood to the left atrium. It is now universal practice to insert a catheter into the left atrium, to apply suction and return the blood to the extracorporeal circulation. The combination of a moving heart and a continuous flow of coronary venous blood in the field of operation makes accurate surgery sometimes difficult. This can be overcome by the use of hypothermia and cardiac standstill.

There are several pump-oxygenators currently on the market. These include the Gibbon (first developed), DeBakey, Sigma, Daval and McNeil. The mechanisms of these machines vary slightly.

Hypothermia

Surface hypothermia as described in Chapter 2 seemed at first to provide the answer to cardiac standstill during open heart surgery.

It was soon learned, however, that below 30° C. (86°F.) the human heart may develop irreversible ventricular fibrillation, and the tolerance of the brain to cardiac standstill at this temperature is limited to only 8 to 10 minutes. For this reason surface hypothermia at present plays a minor role in surgical procedures on the heart. It is almost entirely confined to the closure of a simple atrial septal defect.

It has been discovered, however, that if the function of the heart is taken over by an artificial heart machine with a heat-regulating unit, it is possible to cool a patient to a very low temperature. The heat regulator attached to the pump-oxygenator produces general hypothermia by cooling the blood.

With this method the body may be cooled to 8° to 10°C. (46-50°F.), a temperature at which the metabolic requirements of the body are so low that the heart and respiration ceases and the pump-oxygenator may be turned off while the intracardiac defect is repaired in a bloodless, motionless field. This period of suspended animation may be safely extended to periods up to 55 minutes, which is time enough for most operations. This method of hypothermia is termed "profound" hypothermia.

Heart surgery, then, may be performed with the aid of either the pump-oxygenator or surface hypothermia or both. In addition, as is the recently preferred procedure, surgery may be performed using extracorporeal circulation and profound hypothermia by use of a pump-oxygenator with an attached heat-regulating unit.

Other methods employed during open heart surgery include the use of the electrocardiogram and electroencephalogram to monitor changes in the heart and brain and the use of electrical manometers, attached to catheters placed in blood vessels, that continuously record changes in blood pressure.

During the operation frequent measurements are made of blood electrolyte and acid base changes. As a rule, the anesthetist is responsible for the observations and maintenance of the blood balance.

In order for the reader to have a better understanding of the nursing responsibilities involved in cardiac surgery, a brief summary of the cardiac defects currently being corrected is given as follows:

Congenital defects corrected during childhood by open heart surgery include atrial and ventricular septal defects, tetralogy of Fallot, transposition of the great vessels and aortic stenosis. Mitral stenosis is corrected by either the closed or open method.

Conditions encountered and corrected in the adult patient are as follows:

1. Simple atrial septal defect. The congenital opening in the atrial septum is closed with sutures.
2. Mitral stenosis. The mitral valvulotomy, also called the mitral commissurotomy, is the most frequently performed of all heart operations. In most instances this is a closed heart procedure. Open heart surgery is used when the entire valve is extremely scarred and partly destroyed.
3. Aortic stenosis. This condition is treated mainly by open heart surgery. The rigid valve is repaired by cutting and suturing.
4. Mitral and aortic insufficiency. In many ways the surgical techniques are the same for both valves. If the valve is not calcified, the valve ring, which is usually dilated, is narrowed by suturing. A valve cusp may be repaired by an Ivalon or silicone rubber patch as shown:

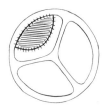

When a serious deformity of a single cusp is present, the cusp may be removed and replaced by a prosthetic cusp sutured in place as shown:

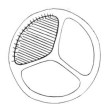

When the entire valve is beyond repair, the entire valve may be removed and a prosthetic valve may be sutured in place. There are several types of prosthetic valves currently being used. One is a caged ball valve containing a solid silicone ball in a seating ring padded with Teflon felt.

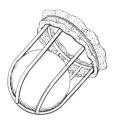

Cases have recently been reported in which a patient had both the mitral and aortic valves replaced with prosthetic ones. Evaluation of this surgical procedure is not yet definite.

PREOPERATIVE NURSING TECHNIQUES

Specific procedures that may be prescribed prior to heart surgery are as follows:

1. The medical evaluation in preparation for surgery may take a few days. This evaluation will include many of the diagnostic tests mentioned earlier in this chapter.
2. The blood pressure and pulse are taken and recorded several times daily.
3. The patient is usually weighed daily.
4. A special diet (see p. 254) may be prescribed depending upon the diagnosis.
5. Medications such as diuretics, digitalis and anticoagulants (see p. 254) may be administered.
6. Coughing and deep breathing exercises are encouraged.
7. Preoperative orders may include the following:
   a. Prepare the skin as ordered. (Many surgeons prefer to have the whole trunk prepared.)
   b. Prepare arms and legs for intravenous cut-down or placement of intra-arterial cannulas.
   c. Type and crossmatch blood.
   d. Sedative such as Seconal at bedtime.
   e. Nothing by mouth after midnight.
   f. Give tap water enema the evening before surgery.

g. Medications such as Demerol and atropine to be given one hour before surgery.

h. Antibiotics such as Crysticillin to be given the night before and the morning of surgery.

POSTOPERATIVE TECHNIQUES IN OPEN HEART SURGERY

The care of the patient after closed heart surgery is similar to that after a thoracotomy (p. 229); therefore, only the care of the patient after open heart surgery will be discussed here.

It should be stressed that the success of cardiac surgery depends as much upon the postoperative care of the patient as on the skill employed during the operation. Postoperative care must be carried out in an intensive care unit especially equipped for the open cardiotomy patient. The unit should contain the following:

1. Equipment to meet any respiratory emergency such as outlets for oxygen and suction (see p. 30), a respirator or intermittent positive pressure apparatus (see p. 55), an anesthesia machine, laryngoscope, airways, endotracheal tube, a tracheotomy set (p. 353), croupettes and drugs (see p. 254).
2. Equipment to meet any cardiac emergency, such as a defibrillator, pacemaker (discussed later in this context), and drugs.
3. Monitoring devices such as the electrocardiograph, electroencephalograph, and devices to register intra-arterial and venous pressures, the pulse rate and the rectal temperature.

The nurse must be specially trained to meet the needs arising from specific problems usually related to open heart surgery. These problems are concerned with the following:

1. Ventilation and tracheobronchial secretions
2. Blood and fluid replacement
3. Circulatory failure
4. Disturbances of cardiac rhythm
5. Cerebral damage
6. Disturbances of acid base balance
7. Sedation
8. Infection
9. Elevation of temperature

Ventilation and Tracheobronchial Secretions

After open heart surgery patients have increased pulmonary secretions. Cyanosis, the presence of shallow rapid respirations, flaring nostrils and tachycardia are all warning signals. Steps to maintain adequate ventilation are:

1. A chest x-ray is taken in the operating room, on the evening of the operation and daily for the next 3 days.
2. The thoracotomy tubes are checked and the function is maintained as described in Chapter 13.
3. The patient is placed in an oxygen tent with high humidity (see p. 44).
4. He is turned from side to side and is made to sit up, take a deep breath and cough every 30 minutes. Voluntary coughing is painful and difficult; therefore, persistence is necessary. When the patient is unwilling or unable to cough, endotracheal suction (see p. 220) is employed as frequently as necessary. Bronchoscopy is not used in the care of postoperative cardiac patients. A tracheotomy is a rare necessity.

Blood and Fluid Replacement

1. Restoration of the clotting mechanism is a fundamental requirement because Heparin is administered to prevent blood clotting during extracorporeal circulation. Polybrene is administered after surgery in the operating room; therefore bleeding due to defects in the clotting mechanism is rare.
2. Blood loss during surgery is estimated by weighing sponges and measuring all blood aspirated. In addition, all blood introduced into the extracorporeal circulation is measured, and the amount remaining at the end of the perfusion is again determined. The patient returns from the operating room in blood balance.
3. The thoracotomy jugs are calibrated and drainage into the jugs is measured hourly. The blood is replaced volume for volume by fresh whole blood. Any sudden increase of blood in the thoracotomy jug is cause for immediate attention. Drainage from the thoracotomy tube usually becomes

serous in 12 hours, and the tube may be removed the morning after surgery. (For removal of tube see page 226.)

4. The patient may be weighed before and after surgery to detect abnormalities of blood volume.

5. Laboratory studies to determine erythrocyte and plasma volumes may be made before and after surgery (see pp. 232 and 233).

6. Blood pressure, pulse and respirations are taken and recorded every 15 minutes for the first 8 hours, then every 30 minutes for 8 hours, then hourly. During the first few hours postoperatively, the arterial and venous pressure and the pulse rate may be measured by direct monitoring devices. Intra-arterial pressure is measured by means of the polyethylene catheter inserted in the femoral artery at the beginning of the operation. Intravenous pressure is measured by means of a polyethylene catheter inserted into the antecubital vein and threaded into the superior vena cava. This catheter is also the main route for intravenous therapy. The pulse rate can be measured on a tachometer. The pulse beat is displayed as a flashing red light. Any change in these signs should be reported immediately.

7. Limitation of fluid intake reduces the significance of postoperative pulmonary and cardiac complications. The fluid intake is usually limited to 40 to 50 ml. per kilogram of body weight for 18 hours postoperatively. The orders for intravenous fluid are usually quite specific including the rate of flow desired. Ice chips by mouth are allowed immediately after surgery, and these are followed by small amounts of water or juice. The nurse should be aware that after open heart surgery the patient may exhibit unusual thirst and wish to drink large quantities of fluid. An accurate record must be kept of the intake of oral fluids, intravenous fluid and blood administered.

8. The patient will void a small amount of urine on the day of surgery. The first voided specimen occasionally contains hemoglobin, especially after a long per-

fusion. Subsequent urine specimens will be clear. There is diuresis the day after surgery, and the urinary output after that should be normal. Specific gravity (see p. 258) is determined to measure kidney function. Temporary renal failure is rarely seen.

Circulatory Failure

Observation of the state of the patient's peripheral circulation is one of the most important phases of care after cardiac surgery.

The best place to observe the patient's peripheral circulation is on the feet. Since the patient is receiving oxygen under high humidity by tent, it will be difficult to observe his face through the tent. Opening the tent frequently defeats the purpose of the tent. If the feet are pink and warm and if the dorsal veins are filled, the peripheral circulation is good.

Venous distention in the neck may occur as the patient is regaining consciousness. This may simply be caused by straining due to the presence of an endotracheal tube and to chest discomfort. One should be aware of the presence of venous distention, as more serious implications may be cardiac failure, inflow obstruction to the right side of the heart, herniation of the heart through the pericardial incision and pressure pneumothorax.

Circulatory failure is most common in patients with pulmonary hypertension and tetralogy of Fallot.

Disturbances of Cardiac Rhythm

Complete heart block is no longer a serious problem following heart surgery. If atrioventricular dissociation occurs during surgery, a transistor pacemaker is attached to electrodes implanted directly within the myocardium. Frequently by the time the chest is to be closed, a normal sinus rhythm will be present. If the atrioventricular dissociation persists, the myocardioelectrodes are left in place several days or longer. If necessary, the patient can be discharged with the pacemaker in place. Most patients discharged with heart block revert to normal cardiac rhythm within a month. Several cases have been reported in which the patient continued using the pacemaker for 15 months.

The transistor pacemakers designed for continued use are battery operated. The pacemaker stimulus (about 8 volts in intensity) is delivered directly to the heart by means of electrodes implanted in the ventricular myocardium. The electrodes consist of stainless steel needles about 3 cm. long, which are imbedded in the myocardium. These needles are attached to two wires that are in turn attached to the pacemaker.

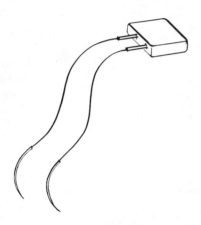

An *external* or *internal* pacemaker may be used. The external pacemaker is about the size of a package of cigarettes and is worn in a leather case strapped to the body.

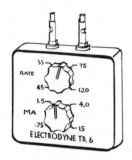

The internal pacemaker is encased within an envelope of Teflon mesh and is 6.5 × 1.7 cm. in size. This pacemaker is implanted subcutaneously on the left anterior chest, slightly below the nipple line.

The pulse rate on the pacemaker is fixed at about 70 per minute. The battery life for both types is estimated at 5 years.

(This equipment is also used for nonsurgical patients incapacitated by complete heart block with low cardiac output.)

For the emergency treatment of cardiac arrest, see page 241.

Cerebral Damage

Cerebral damage is sometimes caused by an air embolism trapped in the heart upon closure. It occurs when the left side of the heart is opened directly. The air embolism may cause mild symptoms such as hallucination and incoherence immediately after surgery. These usually clear within a day or two. More severe symptoms are due to focal neurologic damage and may persist several weeks.

1. Before the patient has recovered from anesthesia, the facial expression, size of pupils and state of muscle tonus in the extremities may be observed for an indication of cerebral damage.
2. Surface hypothermia is used for several days if there is evidence of cerebral damage. The rectal temperature is maintained at 30° to 40°C. See Chapter 2.

Disturbances of Acid-Base Balance

The changes in acid-base balance after open heart surgery are similar to those after any thoracotomy. During surgery there is respiratory alkalosis and metabolic acidosis. This condition corrects itself within 24 hours postoperatively if there is normal oxygenation and adequate peripheral circulation. Careful observations by the nurse in these two areas are important once again.

Sedation

The patient must remain alert enough to cough voluntarily. Relief of chest pain, however, will improve ventilation and make the patient's efforts to cough more effective.

1. Relief of pain without oversedation is achieved by the administration of small doses of narcotics.
2. Morphine or Demerol is given in about one half the usual amount as often as every 3 hours.
3. Narcotics are given routinely, and the patient's condition is carefully assessed before the administration of sedation.
4. Restlessness may be due to hypoxia or other complications rather than pain.
5. Morphine or Demerol is discontinued in 2 or 3 days, and codeine is substituted.

Infection

Since all portions of the extracorporeal equipment can be sterilized, infections are rare. Antibiotics are administered before surgery and continued for 1 week after surgery.

Unexplained Fever

Many patients have an elevation of temperature for 3 to 4 days following open heart surgery. The rectal temperature may range from 100 to 102°F. (38° to 39°C.). The cause of the fever is not clearly understood.

1. Aspirin is administered and the temperature of the oxygen tent is lowered for temperatures up to 101° F. (38° C.).
2. Hypothermia by means of a mattress placed beneath the patient is used for elevations higher than this. The use of hypothermia may produce some peripheral vasoconstriction, and the resulting cyanotic extremities may be misleading when the patient's condition is evaluated.

Convalescence

The activity of the patient following heart surgery is determined on an individual basis. The patient may be allowed to dangle his feet and get out of bed within 5 to 7 days postoperatively, then gradually reach full mobilization around the fourteenth day. During this period the patient is frequently encouraged to move his left arm actively by combing his hair and reaching for objects, etc., in order to prevent a "frozen left shoulder." As a rule the patient has a tendency to keep the left arm inactive because of left shoulder pain.

The entire convalescence period usually requires about 8 weeks. Upon discharge from the hospital, the patient receives detailed instructions regarding rest, activity and the diet. An unrestricted diet is usually prescribed. In instances where only partial improvement is achieved, salt restriction may be necessary for several months or longer.

HEART TRANSPLANTS

The newest procedure in heart surgery is the heart transplant. Several terms that the reader must know to bring her up to date in the field of tissue transplantation include these:

Autograft—A transplant in which the donor is also the recipient (skin grafts).

Isograft—A transplant between two individuals identical in histocompatibility antigens (see p. 252).

Allograft—Previously called a homograft, this is a transplant between members of the same species, such as two humans.

Xenograft—Previously referred to as a heterograft, this is a transplant between different species, such as monkey to man.

Factors important in tissue transplantation include a program for the removal and preservation of donor organs and the suppression of the rejection reaction which occurs in the recipient.

Removal and Preservation of the Donor Organ

The ultimate goal in transplants is to set up a bank of organs which could be stored and used as needed. The ideal sources of organs are healthy persons who have died as the result of an accident, for in such a situation there would be no infection or other disease which would prevent the usefulness of the organ.

Currently, as soon as the donor patient is declared dead, the following procedures are carried out to preserve the organ while it is still in the body. (These procedures are the same for any organ.)

1. Heparin and adrenalin are injected into the heart.
2. Artificial respiration by means of an endotracheal tube and respirator is given.
3. External cardiac massage is given.
4. The entire body—especially the organ to be transplanted—is cooled rapidly. Currently, the organ is cooled by intraperitoneal, intrapericardial (for the heart), or intrapleural infusion of cold saline at 2° to 4°C. through several 16-gauge needles.

As soon as possible, the body is taken to the operating room, and the organ is removed under a surgically aseptic technique. Ideally, the organ should be transplanted immediately. If this is not possible, the organ can be preserved for a few hours. Organs can be preserved up to 24 hours by placing them in a pump oxygenator system which is filled with various fluid media at normal body temperature.

At present, experimentation on the long-term preservation of organs is being accomplished by the combination of hypothermia, hyperbaric oxygenation (see p. 50), and perfusion. A chamber has been built for this purpose; whether it will successfully preserve organs for long periods of time is indefinite.

Rejection Reaction in the Recipient

Another factor important to the success of a heart transplant is the prevention or suppression of the rejection crisis which occurs after the patient receives a transplanted heart. The theoretical basis of this rejection is too complex to discuss here. Basically, the process is due to the body's reaction to foreign antigens. Normally, it is the desire of medical science to increase the body's immunity to antigens. With tissue transplants the immunity must be suppressed. Hence, the terms "immune responses," "immune suppression," "immunosuppressive techniques," and "histocompatibility" are used frequently in a discussion on the subject of tissue transplants.

Immunosuppressive Techniques

Currently, the most successful immunosuppressive techniques include the administration of Imuran, Actinomycin C, and prednisone. Another technique includes a thymectomy (the thymus is the regulatory center for the body's immune responses).

Histocompatible Transplants

The ideal goal in transplants is to set up a bank in which the donors and recipients can be typed and crossmatched for antigen compatibility (histocompatibility), as is done currently for blood. Three types of tests are under investigation for this purpose: two tests deal with the interaction of lymphocytes, and one is serological testing of leukocytes. Authorities report that these tests look very promising.

Heart Transplant Techniques

The heart transplant was first performed by Dr. J. D. Hardy in 1964. Since then the technique has been changed. One successful technique is the Shumway technique, in which the posterior walls of the recipient's atria are left in place. The heart transplant is then inserted by suturing the walls and septum of the atria, the aorta, and the pulmonary artery.

PERIPHERAL VASCULAR SURGERY

Various changes in former operative techniques and the incorporation of new surgical techniques have recently enlarged the scope of the surgical treatment of diseases of the peripheral vascular system. In general, these changes are mentioned as follows:

Vascular Prostheses

The use of synthetic material for blood vessel replacement is now usually preferred to the use of homografts. Materials from which prosthetic blood vessels are made include Vinyon "N," Nylon, Orlon, Dacron and Teflon. The use of each material has its own particular advantages and disadvantages. In one type of prosthesis the yarn is woven, then crimped, as shown, to afford flexibility.

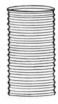

In another type prosthesis, one of the aforementioned yarns is interwoven with Helanca stretch yarn to provide a longitudinal stretch.

The grafts are soaked in fresh whole blood before use so that fibrin is deposited between the woven threads, thus eliminating the porosity of the material. When the prosthesis is sutured in place, the passage of blood across the inner surface of the tube results in the formation of a second layer of fibrin, which lines the inner surface and smooths out many of the depressions and rough spots.

Vascular prostheses in various diameters can be sutured in a variety of patterns as illustrated.

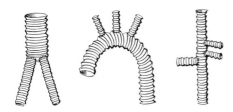

Some of the conditions involving blood vessels now being treated surgically with the use of the vascular prostheses are coarctation of the aorta, aortic (abdominal and thoracic) aneurysms, popliteal aneurysms, chronic occlusive disease of the femoral artery, aorto-iliac obstruction, bypass grafting in both renal and cerebral arterial disease and bypass grafting on intestinal arterial insufficiency.

Thrombectomy and Endarterectomy

The treatment of an arterial thrombus may consist of the removal of the thrombus (thrombectomy) and the removal of the diseased innermost coating of the blood vessel from which the blood clot originated (endarterectomy). Since both of these procedures are usually carried out in the same surgical procedure, the term "thromboendarterectomy" is commonly used. In some instances of clot formation, the diseased portion of blood vessel is removed and replaced by a prosthetic one. A thrombectomy is also used occasionally in venous thrombosis.

Vein Stripping

The standard surgical procedure for varicose veins consists of the ligation and separation of the great saphenous vein at the saphenofemoral junction and the removal (stripping) of the entire length of the great saphenous vein from the groin to the ankle.

Sympathectomy

In some forms of arterial occlusive disease, such as chronic occlusive disease of the femoral artery, Raynaud's disease and Buerger's disease, the sympathetic nerves are excised to relieve symptoms and check further vasoconstriction. A lumbar sympathectomy is performed for vascular insufficiency in the legs. Cervicodorsal sympathectomy is performed for vascular insufficiency of the arms.

The excision for the lumbar sympathectomy is as shown:

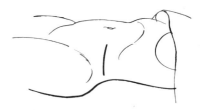

Several areas of incision are used for the cervicodorsal sympathectomy; the axillary approach is the most recent.

Still another procedure is the superior cervical sympathectomy sometimes indicated in the treatment of cerebral vascular disease.

Coronary Artery Surgery

A number of surgical procedures are currently being employed in the treatment of coronary artery disease. Not all of these operations have as yet been widely accepted. They are summarized as follows:

1. A dorsal sympathectomy is done only to reduce anginal pain.
2. Formation of collateral blood supply. A foreign substance such as asbestos powder or talcum powder is placed in the pericardial sac to create adhesion. Blood flow through adhesions is presumed to increase according to this concept; as the blood flow through the diseased coronary artery decreases, a collateral blood flow is established from the pericardium.
3. Providing a new source of blood supply. Arteries such as the internal mammary, intercostal, carotid and subclavian are transplanted directly into the myocardium.
4. Endarterectomy of coronary arteries. This appears to be the most promising of the surgical procedures.
5. Direct anastomosis between a systemic artery and a coronary artery. Arteries such as the internal mammary and intercostal are anastomosed to the proximal portion of the coronary artery.

Special factors in postoperative nursing care of the peripheral vascular system:

1. After venous ligation and stripping, elastic support is worn for several months (see p. 245).

2. The immediate postoperative care after the repair of an abdominal aneurysm is of critical importance. Vital signs are taken frequently, and any drop in systolic blood pressure below 110 is reported immediately.

   Urinary output is measured hourly (see p. 268), and meticulous care must be taken to maintain an open tracheobronchial airway. Nasogastric suction, frequent rectal flushes, and pantothenic acid derivative drugs are used to combat a sluggish ileus during the first 2 to 3 postoperative days.

3. In operations involving a thoracotomy, the care is as discussed previously.

4. In surgery of the great vessels, hypothermia is sometimes used. The postoperative care when hypothermia is used is discussed in Chapter 2 and mentioned again earlier in this chapter.

5. After coronary artery surgery the patient is usually kept on his back for 48 hours. Patients with artery transplants should not be turned on their left side because of the possibility of herniation of the pericardial sac. After 48 hours they may turn from the back to the right side every 2 hours.

6. Amputations are sometimes necessary in arterial disease. The postoperative care of the amputee is discussed in Chapter 12.

ADDITIONAL PROCEDURES TO REVIEW

Oxygen therapy (Chapter 4)

Preventing and relieving abdominal distention (Chapter 11)

Special mouth care (see p. 159)

Comfort measures to patient and environment: Maintenance of an atmosphere free from distractions and excitement. Diversional therapy as indicated

Use of side boards if patient is orthopneic or comatose

Measuring fluid intake and output

Intramuscular and intravenous injections (Chapter 6)

Cooling sponge bath for temperature elevation

Use of suction apparatus (see p. 136)

Use of bedside commode (many physicians feel that more effort is needed to use bedpan than to use the commode)

Daily weight check

Use of bed cradle—heated or unheated—for vascular disorders

Review and understanding of the term "absolute bed rest"

Gastric suction (p. 161) used postoperatively

DIETS TO REVIEW

Consistencies affording easy digestion and preventing intestinal distress

Low caloric to prevent obesity

Small quantity and frequent servings to prevent gastric distress

Low salt or salt-free to prevent edema and treat hypertension. Karell-Kempner or rice diet

Low cholesterol as prevention for arteriosclerosis

Liquid to soft consistency following surgery

MEDICATIONS TO REVIEW

Vasodilators (Antihypertensive). Azamethonium bromide (Azamethone); azapetine phosphate (Ilidar); bretylium tosylate (darenthin); chlorisondamine chloride (Ecolid); hexamethonium bromide (Bistrium Bromide); hexamethonium chloride (Methium Chloride); hydralazine hydrochloride (Apresoline); Isoxsuprine hydrochloride (Vasodilan); Khellin (Khelloyd); mecamylamine hydrochloride (Inversine); nitrites (amylnitrite, nitroglycerine, Tolanate, Isordil, Nitranitol, Metamine); nylidrin hydrochloride (Arlidin); papaverine, phenoxybenzamine hydrochloride (Dibenzyline); rauwolfia (Rauwiloid, Harmonyl, Raudixin, Moderil, Reserpoid, Serpasil, Singoserp, Serpate, Serfin); tetraethyl-ammonium chloride (Etamon Chloride); thiocyanate; tolazoline (Priscoline).

Cardiotonics (Indirect Heart Stimulants). Digitalis preparations include Digalen, Digilanid, digipoten, digitalin, Digitan, Digitol, digitoxin (Purodigin, Digitaline Nativelle), digoxin (Lanoxin), gitalin, and deslanoside (Cedilanid-D). Other preparations include squill (Scillaren, urginin) and strophanthus (Strophanthin Ouabain).

Cardiac Depressants. Procainamide hydrochloride (Pronestyl) and guinidine.

Anticoagulants. Anisindione (Miradon); bishydroxycoumarin (Sintrom, Dicumarol, Cumopyran, Tromexan, Liquamar); fibrinolysin (Actase, Hydrolysin, Thrombolysin); heparin sodium, phenindione (Hedulin, Eridone, Danilone); warfarin sodium (Coumadin Sodium, Panwarfin, Warcoumin).

Coagulants. Calcium lactate, calcium chloride, carbazochrome salicylate (Adrenosem, Adrestat), ceanothyn, hexadimethrine (Polybrene), protamine sulfate, tolonium chloride, vitamin K (Synkayvite, Hykinone, Kayquinone, Thyloquinone, Ido-K, Mephyton).

Cardiac Stimulants (Used in Emergency Cardiac Arrest). Epinephrine (Adrenalin, Suprarenaline, Suprarenin); isoproterenol hydrochloride (Aludrine, Isuprel).

Vasoconstrictors (Hypertensive). Clopane, ephedrine, epinephrine, Isuprel, Levophed, Wyamine, Aramine, Vasoxyl-P, Oenethyl, Neo-Synephrine.

Diuretics. The inorganic salts are ammonium acetate, calcium chloride, potassium acetate, sodium acetate and sodium chloride. The mercurials are Neohydrin, Mercuhydrin, Thiomerin, Cumertilin, Mercupurin, Dicurin and mersalyl (Salyrgan, Mercusal). The xanthines are aminophylline, theobromine and theophylline. Synthetics include Diamox, Naturetin, Diuril, Esidrix, Hydro-Diuril, Oretic, Saluron, Cardrase, Aldactone, Naqua, and Travinol.

BIBLIOGRAPHY

Abram, H. S.: Psychological Problems of Patients after Open Heart Surgery. Hosp. Topics, 44:111, 1966.

Austin, H.: After Cardiothoracic Surgery—The Use of Hypothermia. Nurs. Times, 60:754, 1964.

Barker, W. F.: Surgical Treatment of Peripheral Vascular Disease. New York, McGraw-Hill Book Co., 1962.

Beeson, P. B., and McDermott, W.: Cecil-Loeb Textbook of Medicine. 12th ed. Philadelphia, W. B. Saunders Co., 1967.

Berger, M. H.: New Vistas in Heart Valve Surgery. RN, 28:75, 1965.

Brown, A.: Medical and Surgical Nursing II. Philadelphia, W. B. Saunders Co., 1959.

Brunner, L. S., et al.: Textbook of Medical-Surgical Nursing. Philadelphia, J. B. Lippincott Co., 1964.

Butler, R. O.: Induced Hypothermia in Cardiac Surgery. Nurs. Times, 60:296, 1964.

Cartwright, R. S., et al.: Combined Replacement of Aortic and Mitral Valves. J.A.M.A., 180:6, 1962.

Circulatory System in Surgery. Surg. Clin. North America, 41:265, 1961.

Clarke, C. P.: What Is Involved in Open Heart Surgery. New Zealand Nurs. J., 58:8, 1965.

Cochrane, C., and Atkinson, J.: Surgical Treatment of Aortic Stenosis by Valve Replacement. Nurs. Mir., 121:1, 1965.

Coleman, D.: Surgical Alleviation of Coronary Artery Disease. Am. J. Nurs., 68:763, 1968.

Davidsohn, I., and Henry, J. B.: Todd-Sanford Clinical Diagnosis by Laboratory Methods. 14th ed. Philadelphia, W. B. Saunders Co., 1969.

Davis, L.: Christopher's Textbook of Surgery. 9th ed. Philadelphia, W. B. Saunders Co., 1968.

Drew, C. E.: Advances in Cardiac Surgery. The Practitioner. 187:513, 1961.

Elizabeth, M.: Occlusion of the Peripheral Arteries; Nursing Observations and Symptomatic Care. Am. J. Nurs., 67:562, 1967.

Falconer, M., Patterson, H., and Gustafson, E.: Current Drug Handbook. 1968-1970. Philadelphia, W. B. Saunders Co., 1968.

Flitter, H. H.: An Introduction to Physics in Nursing. 5th ed. St. Louis, C. V. Mosby Co., 1967.

Goodale, R.: Clinical Interpretation of Laboratory Tests. 5th ed. Philadelphia, F. A. Davis Co., 1964.

Hanks, E. C., et al.: A Special Care Unit for the Postoperative Open Cardiotomy Patient. Am. J. Cardiol., 6:778, 1960.

Harmer, B., and Henderson, V.: Textbook of Principles and Practices of Nursing. 5th ed. New York, The Macmillan Co., 1958.

Idriss, F. S.: Whole Organ Transplantation. Surg. Clin. North America, 47:29, 1967.

Jones, B.: Inside the Coronary Care Unit. Am. J. Nurs., 67:2313, 1967.

Kennedy, M. J.: Coping with the Emotional Stress in the Patient Awaiting Heart Surgery. Nurs. Clin. North America, 1:3, 1966.

Krause, M.: Food, Nutrition and Diet Therapy. 4th ed. Philadelphia, W. B. Saunders Co., 1966.

Larson, E.: The Patient with Acute Pulmonary Edema. Am. J. Nurs., 68:1019, 1968.

Pitorak, E.: Open-Ended Care for the Open Heart Patient. Am. J. Nurs., 67:1452, 1967.

Pre- and Postoperative Management of the Patient with Heart Disease. Modern Concepts of Cardiovascular Disease, 479. September, 1958.

Price, A.: The Art, Science and Spirit of Nursing. 3rd ed. Philadelphia, W. B. Saunders Co., 1965.

Sadove, M., and Cross, J.: The Recovery Room. Philadelphia, W. B. Saunders Co., 1965.

Safer, P., et al.: Ventilation and Circulation with Closed Chest Cardiac Massage in Man. J.A.M.A., 176:574, 1961.

Sloan, H., and Stern, A.: Problems in the Care of Patients Following Open Heart Surgery. Surg. Clin. North America, 41:1245, 1961.

Sorensen, K. M., and Amis, D. B.: Understanding the World of the Chronically Ill. Am. J. Nurs., 67:811, 1967.

Stephenson, H. E., Jr.: Cardiac Arrest and Resuscitation. 2nd ed. St. Louis, C. V. Mosby Co., 1964.

Vernick, J., and Lunceford, J.: Milieu Design for Adolescents with Leukemia. Am. J. Nurs., 67:251, 1967.

Zimmerman, H. A.: Intravascular Catheterization. 2nd ed. Springfield, Charles C Thomas, 1966.

15

nursing techniques in the care of
Urological Diseases

DIAGNOSTIC PROCEDURES

EXAMINATION OF URINE

THE COLLECTION OF SPECIMENS

Routine Examinations

1. It is important to use absolutely clean specimen containers.
2. The patient should void directly into the specimen bottle. When this is not possible, the patient should void in a clean basin. The construction of bedpans and urinals makes it almost impossible to be certain that they are clean.
3. Feces must not be mixed with urine. Make certain the patient understands this.

4. Send the specimen to the laboratory as soon as it is obtained.
5. Frequently it is most desirable to collect a single voided specimen from the male in three separate bottles. Ninety to 100 cc. is collected in the first bottle, and without stopping the flow of urine, the remaining urine is collected in a second and third bottle. The first bottle contains cells and exudate from the urethra, the second contains uncontaminated bladder urine, and the third may contain material expressed from the prostate at the completion of the urination.
6. Vaginal discharge should be avoided in

collecting specimens because of false findings in the sediment.

7. For 24-hour specimens, the specimen must be kept cool on ice or in a refrigerator. A preservative such as toluol is added to check the growth of bacteria. Enough toluol (a liquid) is added to form a film over the surface of the urine.

Bacteriological Examinations

Urine for culture is obtained with sterile precautions. In women this is usually done by catheterization. In collecting the specimen, first allow an ounce of urine to flow from the catheter, then collect the specimen in a sterile test tube as shown:

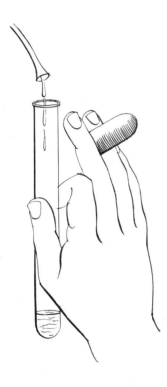

Do not allow the end of the catheter to become contaminated, as this will also contaminate the specimen.

A voided specimen is usually collected from the male. The foreskin is drawn back, and the head of the penis is cleansed with soap and water, then sponged with an antiseptic solution. The patient then voids about an ounce into another receptacle before voiding into a sterile test tube.

LABORATORY FINDINGS

The normal characteristics and constituents of urine and the disease implications are shown in the table on page 258.

In some instances when the patient's urine must be tested frequently for specific findings, the nurse does the test. Tablets and other devices currently used by the nurse in testing the urine are as follows:

Clinitest: These are tablets used to determine the presence of sugar in the urine.

Ictotest: These tablets are used to test the urine for bilirubin.

Occultest: This is also a tablet used to test for the presence of blood in the urine.

Acetest: These tablets test for ketone bodies.

Uristix: These are small flat strips of heavy paper used to test for sugar and albumin.

Phenistix: These are strips of paper used to test for phenylketone.

The tablets are placed in a urine-water mixture and the strips of paper are simply dipped in urine. If abnormalities exist color changes occur. The complete directions for use and description of the color changes occurring in all of these tests are supplied by the manufacturer.

KIDNEY FUNCTION TESTS

Kidney function tests fall in three categories:

1. The ability of the kidneys to concentrate and dilute urine
2. The ability of the kidneys to excrete certain chemicals
3. The ability of the kidneys to excrete urea.

CONCENTRATION AND DILUTION TESTS

The kidneys normally excrete urine that differs markedly in volume and specific gravity at different periods within a day. Damaged kidneys excrete urine with almost the same specific gravity throughout the day.

Mosenthal Concentration Test
Preparation of Patient
1. No food or fluids other than those given at mealtime are permitted from 12 mid-

night on the day of the test until after 8 A.M. the following morning.

2. On the day of the test, three meals are served as usual with 500 cc. of fluid given at each. Fluid must be taken at mealtime within a half-hour period.

3. At 8 A.M., immediately before breakfast, instruct patient to empty bladder and discard urine.

4. Collect 7 urine specimens as follows, saving all urine voided. Bladder must be emptied completely each time. The time intervals must be exact.

No. 1 — 8-10 A.M.
No. 2 — 10-12 A.M.
No. 3 — 12- 2 P.M.
No. 4 — 2- 4 P.M.
No. 5 — 4- 6 P.M.
No. 6 — 6- 8 P.M.
No. 7 — 8 P.M.-8 A.M. following day
             (before breakfast)

URINE LABORATORY TESTS AND INTERPRETATIONS

CHARACTERISTIC AND/OR CONSTITUENT	NORMAL	DISEASE IMPLICATIONS
Volume	1000-1500 cc. daily	Nocturia (more than 500 cc. of urine at night with a specific gravity of less than 1.018) occurs in nephritis. Oliguria in acute nephritis, nephrosis and poisoning by agents that damage the kidneys. Anuria in extensive kidney damage.
Color	Yellow or amber	Smoky red to brown in hemorrhage from urinary tract. Dark when concentrated.
Turbidity	None	Presence is caused by pus cells and alkaline urine. Pink turbidity caused by salts of uric acid.
Odor	Aromatic	Ammoniacal odor due to urine standing. Foul odor in presence of pus cells.
Chlorides*	10-16 gm. in 24 hours	Decreased in nephritis and nephrosis.
Creatinine*	1-1.25 gm. in 24 hours	Increased in uremia.
Phosphates*	3 gm. in 24 hours	Increased in alkalosis. Decreased in nephritis with acidosis.
Proteins:		
albumin	None	Present in all urinary tract infections, all stages of nephritis, nephrosis and nephrosclerosis and systemic diseases that injure the kidney tubules (diabetes mellitus, jaundice, fever, hyperthyroidism, and some blood diseases). Albuminuria also caused by calculi of ureters and bladder.
proteoses	None	Present in atrophy of kidneys.
mucin and mucoid	None	Present in urinary tract infection.
nucleoprotein	None	Present in pyelonephritis, pyelitis and cystitis.
Reaction	pH of 6.0	Urine becomes alkaline on standing. Strongly acid in acidosis and chronic nephritis.
Specific gravity	1.010 to 1.030	See kidney function tests (p. 257).
Urea	20 to 35 gm. in 24 hours	Decreased in severe kidney disease (see urea clearance test p. 261).
Sediment:		
epithelial cells	Few	Present in increased amounts in tumors of urinary tract and nephrosis.
erythrocytes	Occasional	Hematuria occurs in glomerulonephritis; infarction; tuberculosis of kidneys; pyelonephritis; tumors of kidneys, ureters and bladder; polycystic kidneys; and calculi.

*24-hr. specimen needed

Urine Laboratory Tests and Interpretations

CHARACTERISTIC AND/OR CONSTITUENT	NORMAL	DISEASE IMPLICATIONS
leukocytes	Few	Also present in contamination by menstrual blood and catheter trauma. Increased in urethritis, cystitis, prostatitis, pyelitis, pyelonephritis, seminal vesiculitis and tuberculosis of kidneys. Also present in contamination of urine by vaginal discharge (leukorrhea) and catheter trauma.
casts	None	Hyaline casts suggest glomerulonephritis, nephrosis, and arteriosclerotic nephritis. Granular and fatty casts occur in nephrosis and some types of glomerulonephritis.
Crystals	None	Uric acid crystals suggest a calculus. Sulfanilamide crystals may occur following administration of the drug and are of concern to the physician.
Pathological organisms	None	Organisms most commonly found in urinary tract infections are staphylococci, streptococci, *Proteus vulgaris* and *Escherichia coli*. *Mycobacterium tuberculosis* is found in secondary tuberculosis.

*24-hour specimen needed.

Interpretation of Laboratory Findings. A night volume of over 750 cc. suggests kidney impairment. The specific gravity of the night specimen should be 1.018 or higher. The specific gravity of the day specimens should not vary more than 10 points.

Fishberg Concentration Test

Preparation of Patient

1. A high protein diet is given at the evening meal on the day before the test. No fluid is given. No other food is allowed.
2. Before bedtime the bladder is emptied. Discard this urine and all urine passed during night.
3. Collect a specimen of urine at 6 A.M., 7 A.M., and 8 A.M.
4. Breakfast may be served.

Interpretation of Laboratory Findings. With an intake of high protein and no fluids, the normal kidney will produce concentrated urine. Specific gravity of at least one specimen should be 1.025. Less than this indicates disease.

Volhard's Concentration Test

Preparation of Patient

1. Nothing by mouth after evening meal the day before the test.
2. 8 A.M.—Empty bladder and save specimen; serve breakfast of dry cereal with syrup, one egg, toast and butter—no fluids.
3. 11 A.M.—Collect urine specimen.
4. 12 noon—Serve lunch of roast beef, steak or chops, boiled or baked potatoes and bread with butter or jam.
5. 2 P.M.—Collect urine specimen.
6. 5 P.M.—Collect urine specimen. Serve supper of two eggs, bread with butter or jam.
7. 8 P.M.—Collect urine specimen.
8. 8 A.M. next morning—Collect all urine from 8 P.M.
9. Allow nothing by mouth during entire test except what is given with meals.

Interpretation of Laboratory Findings. The specific gravity should be from 1.025 to 1.030. In severe kidney disease it will be near 1.010.

Urea Concentration Test
Preparation of Patient

1. Withhold food and water 12 to 18 hours prior to test.
2. 8 A.M.—Empty bladder. Discard urine.
3. Give orally 15 gm. of urea dissolved in 100 to 150 cc. water.
4. 9 A.M.—Collect urine specimen.
5. 10 A.M.—Collect urine specimen. If this specimen exceeds 150 cc., collect another specimen in 1 hour.

Interpretation of Laboratory Findings. Damaged kidneys have a decreased ability to concentrate urea. A concentration of 2 per cent urea or more is normal. In kidney impairment the concentration is 1.6 to 1.8 per cent.

Pituitrin or Pitressin Concentration Test
Preparation of Patient

1. Empty bladder and save specimen.
2. Give 10 units of Pituitrin or Pitressin (whichever drug is being used) subcutaneously.
3. One hour later collect a urine specimen. At the end of another hour collect a second specimen.
4. Give nothing by mouth during test.

Interpretation of Laboratory Findings. A specific gravity below 1.020 indicates kidney impairment.

Dilution Test
Preparation of Patient

1. On the day of the test, withhold breakfast.
2. 8 A.M.—Empty bladder and discard specimen. Give 1500 cc. water.
3. Collect specimen of urine every half hour at 9:00, 9:30, 10:00, 10:30, 11:00, 11:30, 12:00.
4. Give usual diet for dinner and supper. Allow one glass of water after supper.
5. Collect urine from 12 noon until 8 A.M. the next day in one container.

Interpretation of Laboratory Findings. A normal first specimen is usually 400 cc. with a specific gravity of 1.001-1.003. After this, the volume decreases, and the specific gravity increases until after the fourth hour, when the volume is 100 cc. and the specific gravity 1.012-1.016. In renal impairment the output in the first hour is 200 cc. or less with a specific gravity of 1.010 or higher.

EXCRETION TESTS

Phenolsulfonphthalein Test (P.S.P. test)
Preparation of Patient

1. Give two to four glasses water.
2. Twenty minutes later have patient empty bladder and discard urine.
3. 1 cc. of phenolsulfonphthalein is injected intramuscularly or intravenously (this route of injection is preferred). I.V. injection is usually given by the doctor.
4. One hour and 10 minutes later, collect urine specimen.
5. One hour after this, or 2 hours and 10 minutes after injection, collect another urine specimen. Make certain the exact time in minutes is labeled on the specimen bottle.

Interpretation of Laboratory Findings. The dye output in the first hour is normally 40 to 60 per cent; in 2 hours, 55 to 80 per cent. A total output below 55 per cent is abnormal.

Phenolsulfonphthalein Test of Kidneys Separately
Preparation of Patient

1. With ureteral catheters in place, 1 cc. of dye is given intravenously.
2. Each catheter is placed in a separate test tube containing a few drops of 10 per cent sodium hydroxide.
3. The time of the first appearance of dye is noted for each tube.
4. Four specimens of urine are collected for periods of 15 minutes, the total extending to 1 hour. The test tubes are labeled "left" and "right."

Interpretation of Laboratory Findings. Normally the dye appears in 3 to 5 minutes. The excretion of dye is normally

    15 min.—35-45%
    30 min.—50-60%
    1 hour—65-80%

Delayed appearance of the dye and a reduced total excretion indicate impairment of function.

Urea Clearance Test
Preparation of Patient
1. Omit breakfast.
2. Give a glass of water and have patient empty bladder. Discard specimen but record the time of voiding.
3. One hour later, collect urine specimen and note exact time.
4. At the same time a sample of blood is collected in an oxalated tube for determination of urea nitrogen.
5. Give another glass of water.
6. One hour later have patient empty bladder and save all urine. The exact time must be noted because in the laboratory the volume of urine output per minute is calculated.

Interpretation of Laboratory Findings. Normal standard clearance is around 54 cc. Clearance is decreased in kidney disease.

Other Clearance Tests
These include the creatinine, insulin and Diodrast tests. Since they are rarely used, the normal clearance only will be given here:

creatinine: 148 cc. per minute
insulin: 125 cc. per minute
Diodrast: 700 cc. per minute

X-RAY EXAMINATIONS

The kidneys, ureters and bladder may be outlined by any one of several techniques used singly or in combination depending upon the situation. A radiopaque material (such as Urokon, Diodrast, sodium iodide and Neo-Iopax) is used to fill the hollow portion of the urinary tract. The radiopaque substance may be injected several ways.

Intravenous Urogram
In this examination the radiopaque substance is injected intravenously. This method finds its greatest usefulness in the study of patients with pain of suspected renal origin who have no other evidences of urinary tract abnormality. The preparation of the patient is usually as follows:
1. Nothing by mouth 12 to 18 hours prior to the test. It is essential that the patient have no fluids whatsoever in order to concentrate the urine.
2. A laxative is given the evening before and an enema the morning of the examination.

Retrograde Pyelogram
In this examination the radiopaque dye is injected into the kidney through ureteral catheters. The retrograde method is used when knowledge of the function and state of each kidney is needed. The preparation of the patient is the same as for a cystoscopy.

Aortography
Aortography is sometimes used to delineate the vascular pattern of the urological system. A translumbar injection of radiopaque iodine is made into the aorta. (See p. 238.)

CYSTOMETRIC EXAMINATIONS

Bladder function can be evaluated by a cystometric examination. By this means the physician can distinguish between neurogenic and obstructive urinary retention. For instance, is urinary retention due to hypertrophy of the prostate or to a neurogenic bladder? The different types of incontinence can also be determined. In the female patient, for example, is stress incontinence due to a lack in sphincter control, or is it due to a defect in the renal system?

The cystometric examination is usually done in the urology laboratory. No preparation of the patient is necessary. The examination is conducted as follows.
1. The patient is requested to void. The time taken to initiate micturition and the size, caliber and continuity of stream are noted.
2. A catheter is passed, and the volume of residual urine recorded.
3. Sixty cubic centimeters of cold water, and then 60 cc. of warm water are instilled through the catheter to test exteroceptive sensations.
4. The urethral catheter is connected to a water manometric cystometer, and water is instilled at the rate of 60 drops per min-

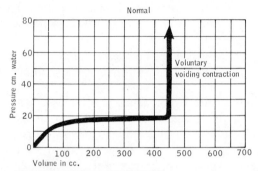

EXTEROCEPTIVE SENSATION
  HEAT — PRESENT
  COLD — PRESENT
PROPRIOCEPTIVE SENSATION
  FIRST DESIRE — PRESENT AT 175 CC. VOL.
  FULLNESS — PRESENT AT 450 CC. VOL.
CAPACITY — 500 CC. VOL.
UNINHIBITED CONTRACTIONS — NONE
VOIDING STREAM — UNINTERRUPTED
RESIDUAL — 0 CC.

ute. The patient tells the operator when he becomes conscious of the desire to void and when the bladder feels full.

5. When the bladder is full, the catheter is removed, and the patient voids. Observations, as before, are made during micturition.

Cystometrographs of a normal and neurogenic bladder are indicated above.

The symptoms of the patient with the uninhibited neurogenic bladder are hesitancy, increased frequency of urination, urgency and incontinence. The sensation of filling is not disturbed, and the bladder empties completely upon micturition. This type of bladder is seen frequently in cerebrovascular accidents. There are several other types of neurogenic bladders.

CYSTOSCOPIC EXAMINATIONS

The cystoscope is an instrument that makes possible visual inspection of the lumen of the bladder and the ureteral orifices. With the cystoscope, tissue may be taken for biopsy, catheters may be passed into the ureters, and ureteral or vesicular calculi may be removed. A retrograde pyelogram is frequently obtained during cystoscopic examination. The preparation of the patient for a cystoscopy may include the following:

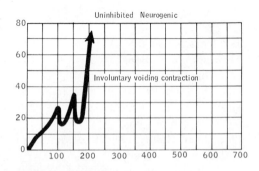

EXTEROCEPTIVE SENSATION
  HEAT — PRESENT
  COLD — PRESENT
PROPRIOCEPTIVE SENSATION
  FIRST DESIRE — PRESENT AT 75 CC. VOL.
  FULLNESS — PRESENT AT 175 CC. VOL.
CAPACITY — 175 CC. VOL.
UNINHIBITED CONTRACTIONS — PRESENT
VOIDING STREAM — UNINTERRUPTED
RESIDUAL — 0 CC.

1. If the ureters are to be catheterized, the oral fluid intake is increased to provide an abundant secretion of urine during the examination.
2. If retrograde pyelograms are to be made, a laxative and enema are necessary as for an intravenous urogram, but fluids are not withheld.
3. Some urologists prefer to give morphine just prior to cystoscopy.
4. The patient is taken to the cystoscopy room for the examination.

After the examination the patient may have a brief reaction with frequent and painful urination, pain in the region of the bladder or kidneys, fever and chills and nausea and vomiting. The physician may prescribe the use of hot water bottles and a drug such as codeine for relief of pain. When the patient returns from the cystoscopic examination, the nurse should check to see whether ureteral and/or urethral catheters are in place. Factors regarding the use and care of catheters are discussed later in this chapter.

URETHRAL CALIBRATION

Various instruments are utilized in determining the presence and size of a urethral stricture. The instruments used for this purpose include a variety of semirigid catheters and bougies and rigid sounds. Since these devices are sometimes used at the patient's bedside, especially for the patient with prostatic hypertrophy, the nurse should be familiar with their identity and use.

1. Coudé tip catheters: the coudé tip is the one most used. The coudé derives its name from the French word *(coude)* meaning elbow.

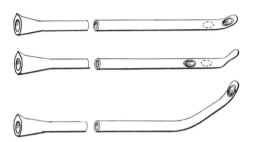

2. The straight and curved olive tip catheters:

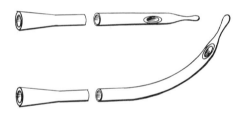

3. Phillips one-piece and two-piece screw-on filiform urethral catheters:

4. Urethral bougies are semirigid dilating instruments. The bougie à boule (acorn and olive tip) shown here is used to locate strictures.

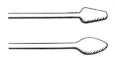

The dilating bougies have a conical tip as shown:

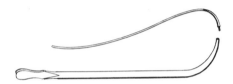

Notice that the bougies have no lumen; therefore, they cannot be used to dilate and drain urine as can the semirigid catheters.

5. Urethral sounds are made of metal. The most commonly used sound is the follower sound with a screw-on filiform guide as shown here:

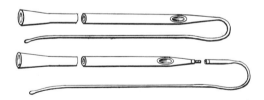

Urethral sounds come in sets of varying sizes. The sets should always be kept together so that the physician can select the size or sizes he prefers at once.

Other equipment the nurse will need when the physician uses these urethral instruments in the patient's room includes a catheterization tray and possibly a bladder irrigation set. Aseptic technique is used for all bladder instrumentation. When filiform devices are used, the bladder must be full so that the filiform has ample space to coil. In this event an irrigation set (see p. 276) is used for the instillation of a sterile solution.

BLOOD TESTS

The blood tests most frequently used in urological nursing include those carried out to determine the nitrogenous compounds in the blood, namely, the nonprotein nitrogens (urea, uric acid, creatinine, ammonia, amino acids) and plasma proteins (albumin, globulin, fibrinogen).

These and other tests sometimes used are listed here:

TEST	NORMAL	INTERPRETATION
Base*	145-155 mEq./L.	The alkali reserve is decreased in kidney disease and prolonged obstruction of lower urinary tract.
Calcium*	9-11 mg./100 ml.	Increased in uremia. Decreased in chronic glomerulonephritis with hypertension and nephrosis.
Chlorides* (sodium)	570-620 mg./100 ml.	Increased in obstruction of urinary tract, acute glomerulonephritis without excessive loss of fluid and chronic glomerulonephritis with low protein and high salt intake. Decreased in severe vomiting, some types of nephrosis and advanced chronic nephritis, particularly in uremia.
Cholesterol, total plasma*	150-280 mg.	Increased in chronic glomerulonephritis and lipoid nephrosis.
Complement fixation test (Wassermann)	negative	Positive in syphilis.
Creatinine serum*†	0.7-1.7 mg./100 ml.	Increased in those conditions where nonprotein nitrogen is increased. There is frequently a lag in the increase of creatinine; consequently, when it is increased, the disease is more severe.
Flocculation test (Kahn)	negative	Positive in syphilis.
Nonprotein nitrogen*†	15-35 mg./100 ml.	Increased in nephritis (all forms), toxic nephrosis, tuberculosis of the kidneys, pyelonephritis, pyelonephrosis, and urinary obstruction anywhere in the urinary tract.
Phosphatase, serum acid*	0.2-0.8 units/100 ml. (Bodansky method)	Increased in prostatic carcinoma.
Phosphatase, serum alkaline*	1-4 units/100 ml. (Bodansky method)	Decreased in severe chronic nephritis.
Phosphorus, inorganic*	3-4.5 mg./100 ml.	Increased in renal disease.
Proteins, total*	6.5-8.0 gm./100 ml.	Decreased in diseases of kidneys involving prolonged albuminuria.
Proteins* albumin globulin	58% 4.5-5.5 gm. 38% 1.5-3.4 gm. /100 ml.	Albumin: globulin ratio is decreased in diseases of kidney involving albuminuria.
albumin globulin ratio	1.5 to 2.5:1	
Urea nitrogen*	10-20 mg./100 ml.	Increased in same conditions as nonprotein nitrogen.
Uric acid*†	2.0-6.0 mg./100 ml.	Increased in acute and chronic nephritis before a rise appears in nonprotein nitrogen.

*Done on fasting.
†Oxylated specimen tube needed.

MISCELLANEOUS DIAGNOSTIC TESTS

Examination of Spermatozoa

This is done in investigating the male partner of a sterile marriage. The specimen is collected in a condom. The condom is washed and dried before use, as the powder in it may kill or inhibit the motility of the sperm. The specimen should be examined as soon as possible but may be kept under refrigeration for a short period of time without harm. The examination includes the total sperm count, motility and a stained smear for the determination of abnormal forms.

Smear and Culture Examination

A smear and culture may be made of a lesion to determine whether or not it is syphilitic. The specimen is obtained on sterile cotton-tipped applicators placed in a sterile test tube.

The Frei Intradermal Test
    This is carried out in the diagnosis of lym-

phopathia venereum, a venereal disease found mostly among Negroes in the South. An intradermal injection of infected yolk sacs is made and read in 48 hours. Redness, swelling and central necrosis indicates that the test is positive.

THERAPEUTIC AND REHABILITATIVE PROCEDURES

INTUBATION METHODS AND TYPES OF TUBES

Urethral Catheters
    The urethral catheters commonly used are the solid-tip

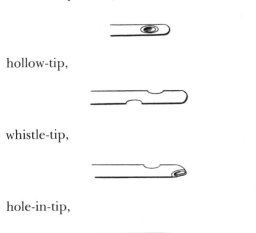

hollow-tip,

whistle-tip,

hole-in-tip,

and the various coudé-tipped catheters pictured on page 263. The whistle-tip seems to be the easiest for female catheterization and the olive-tipped coudé the most satisfactory for male catheterization.
    Retention catheters include the mushroom-tip (Pezzer),

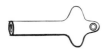

four-wing tip (Malecot),

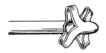

Foley,

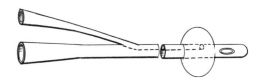

and Foley-Alcock.

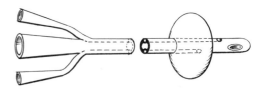

The third outlet on the Foley-Alcock is for the purpose of irrigation.
    The mushroom and four-wing-tip catheters are put in place with the use of a flexible metal stylet shown here.

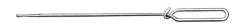

    The stylet is placed inside the catheter, and the catheter is pulled back tightly as shown.

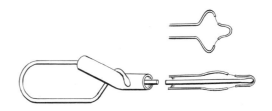

    The Foley is the only catheter effectively retained when the patient can move about in bed freely and ambulate.

Ureteral Catheters

Ureteral catheters, of course, are much smaller in diameter and longer than urethral catheters. Ureteral catheters may be plain, radiopaque or graduated. The radiopaque catheters are impregnated with lead or bismuth salts to make them visible under x-ray. The graduated catheters have a line every centimeter along the length so that the physician can tell by inspection through the cystoscope how far the catheter has been inserted into the ureter. The ureteral catheter is made in a variety of tips, namely, the solid tip, whistle tip, and olive tip. Ureteral catheters are more rigid than urethral catheters and are usually made of plastic.

All catheters are manufactured in sizes calibrated to the French scale, ranging from No. 1 to No. 30. Ureteral catheters range in sizes between No. 4 and 10. Numbers 5, 6 and 7 are the most commonly used. Numbers 18 and 20 are the sizes used for ordinary bladder catheterization.

Foley catheters are identified by the size of the retention bag in addition to the diameter size. The 5 cc. No. 18F is the most commonly used Foley.

Cystostomy Tubes

These tubes are placed directly in the bladder through an incision made into the bladder through the abdominal wall. The cystostomy tubes, also called bladder drains, are made of rubber. In order to prevent kinking during use, they are made either with a right-angle curve or are connected to a right-angle glass adapter as shown:

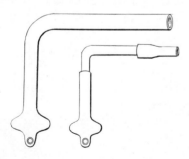

Cystostomy tubes then are either right-angled or straight. Both forms also come in a variety of tips. The mushroom tip, whistle tip and four-wing tip have already been identified in the discussion of urethral catheters.

The Marion bladder drain has an attached tube for irrigation as shown here:

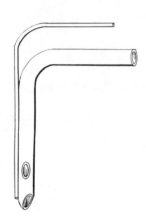

GRAVITY AND DECOMPRESSION DRAINAGE

The nurse is well aware of the importance of the maintenance of urinary drainage in urological nursing. The objectives of an effective urinary drainage system are (1) to maintain or restore the normal physiological functions of the urinary system, (2) to prevent trauma and infection in the urinary tract, and (3) to keep an accurate record of the urinary output. If one keeps these objectives in mind while comparing many of the nursing techniques encountered in urinary drainage, one will conclude that there are many practices used which should be abandoned. It is hoped that the following discussion will cause the reader to become aware of the common areas of negligence in urological nursing.

THE INDWELLING CATHETER

The Foley catheter is the only catheter effectively used as an indwelling catheter. The inflation balloon should be tested before insertion. With a 5 cc. bag, 2 to 3 cc. of sterile solution or air, is sufficient to hold the catheter in place. Always make certain that the catheter is in place in the bladder before inflating the balloon. If the balloon is inflated with the catheter-tip in the urethra, it will be painful to the patient.

After inserting the Foley catheter, inflating the balloon, closing the inflation tube and connecting the catheter to a sterile tube, the catheter should be gently withdrawn until the balloon strikes the bladder outlet. The catheter is then pushed inward about 2 cm. This is the point at which the patient will be most comfortable with the catheter indwelling; the inflated balloon does not impinge on the bladder outlet and create the desire to urinate.

The catheter must be anchored to prevent any tension or pulling on the urethrovesical segment. The only effective way to anchor the catheter is to fasten it to the upper thigh. The most satisfactory method of doing this is with Montgomery tapes placed as shown:

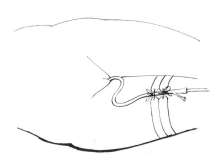

The tapes are tied in solid knots. The catheter or catheter connector is laid over the knots. Tie a single knot over the tubing; wrap the tape around a second time and tie a single knot, then a bow as shown:

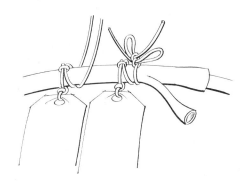

The bows tied in this manner will not loosen.

It is best to allow enough play in the catheter so that a washcloth may reach all parts of the genitals.

If for some reason Montgomery tapes are not available, use 2-inch adhesive to anchor the catheter. Place the tape around the catheter to form a loop, thus holding the catheter up off the skin as shown:

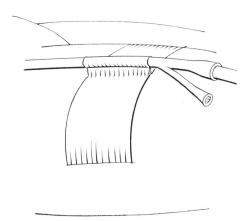

The adhesive should be long enough to cover a large portion of the thigh on both sides.

The catheter should always be attached to a drainage system on the side of the patient nearest the bedside table. This makes unnecessary any uncomfortable stretching by the patient.

The Connecting Tube

All too frequently the nurse has difficulty in finding a connecting tube that will fit both the catheter and the drainage tube. The first impulse may be to use an adaptor tube smaller at one end than at the other. This type should never be used. Always use a connector tube that has the same diameter throughout as shown:

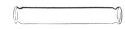

This tube is not apt to become clogged.

The tube should be replaced frequently enough to prevent sediment from coating the inner surface of the tube.

Disconnecting the Catheter

When for various reasons the catheter must be disconnected from the drainage system, the connector should be secured in a clean, germ-free place. A test tube, filled with an antiseptic solution, taped to a convenient location on the bed, best serves this purpose as shown:

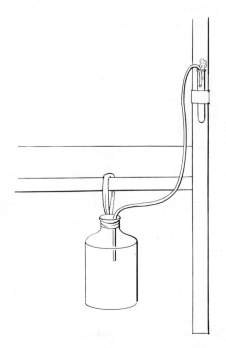

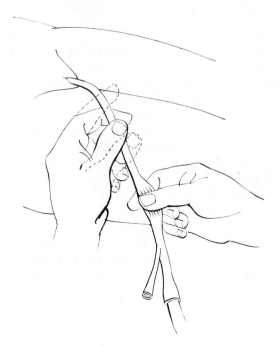

The catheter plug should also be kept in a small jar of antiseptic solution that can be conveniently fastened to the bed:

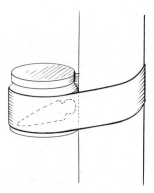

Measuring the Urinary Output

It is the nurse's responsibility to check the drainage system frequently to make certain there is no obstruction in the flow of urine. An obstructed drainage system is worse than none. If the catheter appears to be clogged, pinch it about 6 inches from the body with one hand while rapidly squeezing and releasing the tube at a point closer to the body with the other hand as shown:

The physician may prefer to have the catheter irrigated at designated intervals to keep the drainage system open. Never irrigate a catheter unless there is an order for such. For the techniques of bladder irrigation, see page 275.

The total urinary output is usually measured every 4 to 6 hours. The simplest method of emptying the drainage bottle is to have two collection bottles labeled for each patient. A clean labeled bottle may be carried to the bedside and exchanged for the drainage bottle in use. The filled drainage bottle already labeled with the patient's name is removed to the utility room, where the urine is measured and the bottle is cleaned with an antiseptic solution. When there are a number of patients requiring this treatment, a cart may be used to carry all the bottles back and forth at one time.

There are many clinical situations in anuria or oliguria in which the physician desires an hourly record of urinary output. The setup shown here will provide an accurate account and at the same time save the nurse many steps.

The size syringe needed may be taped to a bedside rail or to an intravenous pole. At any established interval the urine measurement is read and the clamp below the syringe is released, allowing the urine to enter the

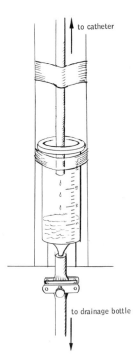

main collection bottle where the total output is stored. Specific gravity of each urine collection may be obtained by means of a hydrometer placed directly in the syringe.

When frequent urine specimens are needed for laboratory analysis, a **Y** tube may be placed in the setup as shown:

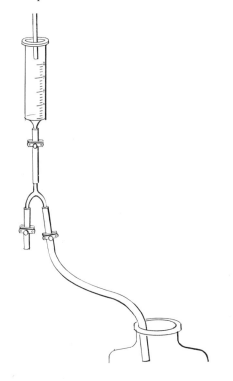

Keeping the Drainage System Clean

When the indwelling catheter is left in place for periods longer than several days, some schedule is needed for keeping the total drainage system clean. The physician may prescribe daily irrigations, as shown on page 276, and leave an order to change the catheter every 4 to 7 days. A closed drainage system that includes an attached container of irrigation solution, as described on page 276, may also be used. In addition, it is the nurse's responsibility to keep the connecting tube, drainage tubing and collection bottles clean by using aseptic techniques when handling these devices and by replacing the connection tubing and bottles as often as necessary. Plastic disposable drainage tubing is now used most frequently for this purpose.

THE URETERAL CATHETER

The physical characteristics of the ureteral catheter have already been described. When a ureteral catheter is left in place, it is connected to a connection tube by means of a sterile rubber bulb from an ordinary medicine dropper as shown:

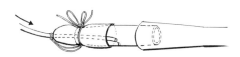

The opening in the medicine dropper bulb is made with a sterile hypodermic needle.

The flow of urine may be observed through the glass connector tube. When the ureteral catheter is functioning properly, there will be a continuous dripping of urine from the catheter opening. The nurse should observe this flow at least once or twice hourly and report immediately any obstruction. The catheter is kept open by frequent irrigation, the techniques of which are described on page 276.

Keep the ureteral catheter in place by tying it with heavy thread to the indwelling urethral catheter as shown:

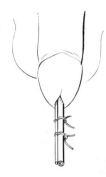

When the patient leaves his bed, as during transportation to the x-ray department, etc., the ureteral catheter is removed from the rubber bulb and placed in a sterile test tube or small jar with a cork top. The receptacle may be held upright between the patient's legs or taped to the outer side of the upper thigh.

The urinary output from the ureteral catheter and that from the bladder are recorded separately.

Cystostomy Drainage

Drainage from a cystostomy tube is employed following operations on the bladder such as for removal of calculi and tumors and following surgery involving the urethra such as the suprapubic prostatectomy when it is necessary to direct the passage of urine by another route.

The types of tubes used for cystostomy drainage have already been illustrated. A Foley catheter is also used for this purpose.

The cystostomy tube must be held in place exactly at the level of insertion selected by the physician. If the tube is allowed to pull out, drainage will be inadequate. If the tube is pushed in farther, it will touch the base of the bladder, causing pain and spasm. The surgeon sutures or tapes the tube in place. The nurse makes certain the anchors are left in place.

Dressings are placed around the cystostomy tube and changed as described on page 277.

The cystostomy tube is usually removed 4 to 10 days postoperatively. The wound is left to heal by granulation. In some instances the physician may find it necessary to apply suc-

tion to keep the wound dry. A sump drain or similar device as illustrated on page 160 is used for this purpose.

When for some reason it is impossible to restore the normal passage of urine through the urethra, the cystostomy drainage is a permanent arrangement. In this event a cystostomy tube is left in place or a commercially made cup is held in place with a belt over the opening. Both devices are connected to a plastic bag worn as shown:

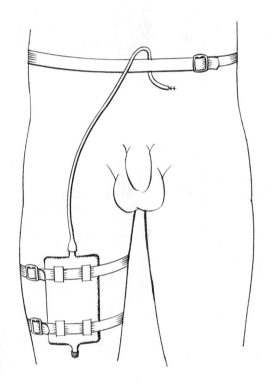

The general considerations and care of the patient who must wear a device such as this are the same as for the patient who has a permanent colostomy or ileostomy (see p. 171). A few crystals of thymol placed in the receptacle will prevent odors.

Nephrostomy Drainage

After a nephrotomy, pyelotomy, or kidney resection, a drainage tube is secured in place by sutures and is either connected to a collecting bottle or left to drain in the dressings, according to the surgeon's preference. The drainage through these tubes is quite bloody for the first 24 to 48 hours postoperatively. Irrigations, if necessary, are usually given by the physician. The care of dressings is discussed on page 277.

URETEROSTOMY DRAINAGE

After a ureterotomy a tube may be left in place to act as a splint as well as to afford a passageway for urine as shown:

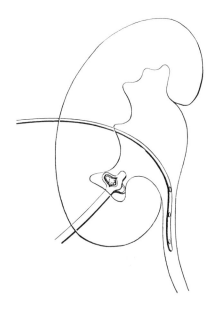

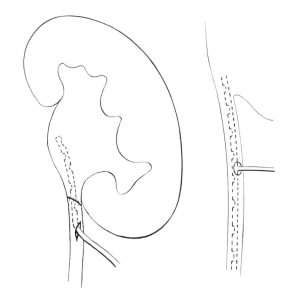

Sometimes the surgeon places the splint tube in the ureter through a nephrostomy opening. In this event, the nurse may encounter two nephrostomy tubes: a larger one for drainage from the kidney pelvis and a small polyethylene tube serving as the ureteral splint.

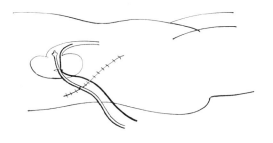

A ureteral catheter is also used occasionally for a ureteral splint. The ureteral splint is removed several days postoperatively.

URETERAL TRANSPLANTS

Other methods of draining the urine directly from the ureters include those used following transplantation of the ureters. After removing the diseased bladder, the surgeon may transplant the ureters in the sigmoid colon, skin, or ileum.

Ureterosigmoid Transplant

In this method the urine drains into the colon and is eliminated with the feces. The intention for this operation is to establish elimination of urine through trained control of the anal sphincter. After this surgical procedure, a large rectal tube is kept in place from 2 to 10 days. The rectal tube should have additional holes perforated in the tip so that there is less chance of the tube becoming clogged.

The rectal tube is connected to a drainage bottle which should be draped with a face towel because of the unsightly drainage. The rectal tube must be held securely in place. This can be done with the use of 1-inch adhesive and strings as shown:

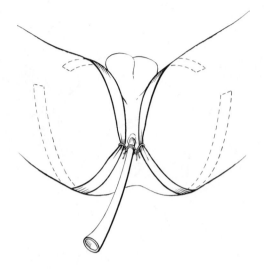

The physician may prefer to use a large Foley catheter or a mushroom catheter instead of the rectal tube for drainage. Another type tube designed especially for this purpose is shown here. This tube has a solid acorn bulb.

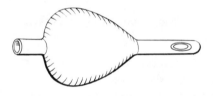

The physician may request that the tube be irrigated occasionally to dislodge small particles of feces. In this case, 30 cc. of sterile water or saline is instilled. Under no circumstance should the intestine be allowed to become distended with gas or feces. If there is no drainage from the rectal tube for as long as an hour, the physician must be notified.

Electrolyte imbalance, resulting from intestinal absorption of urine, and nephritis, resulting from intestinal contamination, are two of the complications of the ureterosigmoid transplant. After surgery, continuous rectal drainage is maintained until the patient is able to remain in electrolyte balance without it. This is often a weaning process, and periodic resumption of the drainage may be required to restore balance. When the patient is not using rectal drainage, he is instructed to empty his rectum frequently. After continuous drainage in the immediate postopera-

tive period, rectal drainage may be maintained during the night, but discontinued during the day. The patient may be instructed to continue this routine when he goes home.

To prevent infection, the bowel is kept as bacteria-free as possible by the administration of intestinal bacteriostatic drugs preoperatively and postoperatively. The bacteria-free stool is soft and odorless. A low-residue diet is administered before and after surgery to aid in proper urinary and fecal drainage.

An entirely different type of ureteral transplant involving the colon is the operation that diverts the urine to an isolated rectal segment. In urinary diversion to a rectal segment, the colon is resected and the upper portion is attached to the abdominal wall forming a colostomy for the elimination of feces. The ureters are transplanted to the lower portion of the rectum, and urine is eliminated through the anus. The advantages to this operative technique are that no drainage devices need be worn by the patient, since elimination of feces can be controlled through the colostomy, and elimination of urine can be controlled by the anal sphincter. Urine and feces are also kept separate, permitting a more accurate account of output. Following this operation, no urinary drainage devices are used. The care of the colostomy is discussed in Chapter 11.

Cutaneous Ureterostomy

When transplantation of the ureters to the skin seems desirable, a urinary fistula is made as shown:

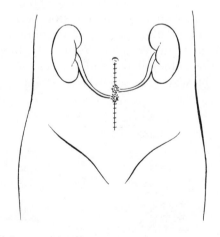

Immediate postoperative drainage is provided by passing a catheter within each ureter with the tip resting in the renal pelvis. A straight urethral or a 5 cc. Foley catheter may be used for this purpose. The catheters are secured to the skin by sutures. They are connected to separate drainage bottles so that the function of each may be observed. The catheters should be labeled "left" and "right" so there is no mix-up in urinary output records.

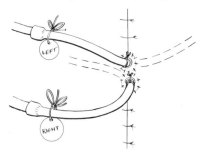

The drainage bottles are also labeled "left" and "right." The catheters are left in place 7 to 12 days postoperatively. After the removal of the catheters, a specially designed collection bag is cemented in place over the stoma. An ileostomy bag (see p. 171) may be used for this purpose. An ordinary rubber balloon may also be used. A hole is cut in one side of the balloon so that the edges will fit closely around the urinary fistula. The entire side of the balloon is cemented to the skin. Cement is applied to the skin only. Cement applied to the balloon causes puckering and prevents a smooth application.

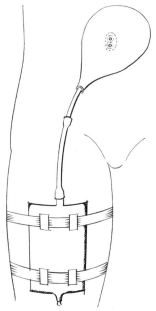

If applied properly, the balloon will remain in place a week or longer. The balloon is held in place with a piece of sponge rubber and ace bandage as shown:

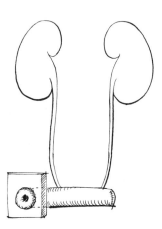

Ureteroileal Transplant

In this procedure the ureters are sutured to an isolated section of ileum connected to an opening in the skin as shown:

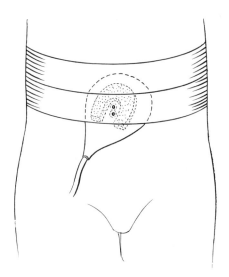

This procedure is believed by its advocates to be more satisfactory than the cutaneous ureterostomy because the ileal stoma will not atrophy as will the ureteral stoma. No drainage tubes are inserted after this operation. A temporary transparent plastic ileostomy bag (see p. 171) is cemented in place in the operating room. The bag is connected to a drainage tube and bottle when the patient returns to his room. The temporary bag is replaced as needed until the wound is healed (7 to 12 days). After this the patient is fitted with a permanent ileostomy bag.

TIDAL DRAINAGE

Tidal drainage is a system in which the bladder is periodically gradually filled and emptied. The system fills by gravity flow and empties by siphonage. Tidal drainage is used to prevent the overstretching of a hypotonic bladder, to prevent the shrinkage of a hypertonic bladder and to restore the muscular function of an atonic bladder. The simplest setup for tidal drainage functions as shown:

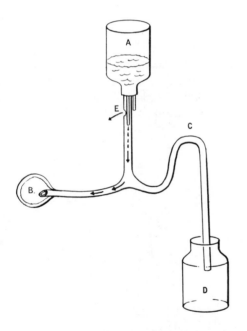

The solution (A) drips into the bladder (B) at a rate of 40 to 60 drops per minute. As the bladder becomes full, it pushes air out through the vent (E). The pressure within the full bladder causes the fluid to rise to the level of the loop (C). As the fluid overflows the loop, a siphonage action is started that drains the bladder into the collection bottle (D). At the end of the siphonage, air enters the vent (E) and stops the siphonage action. The cap-

acity of the bladder is regulated by the height of the loop (C).

One can see from this simple drawing that the relationship of the level of the bladder to the height of the loop is important. The nurse should realize then that if the patient's body is elevated or lowered, it will alter the amount of fluid collected within the bladder. The physician adjusts the apparatus and prescribes the rate of flow for the solution. It is the nurse's responsibility to make certain that the system is functioning properly. The circumstances usually causing malfunction of the apparatus are those involving some obstruction in the tubing. The catheter may be obstructed, the tubing may be kinked, or the patient may be lying on the tubing. Improper placement of the tubing in the drainage bottle may also be the cause as shown:

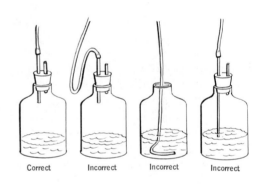

Correct Incorrect Incorrect Incorrect

If the solution is flowing out the air vent or if the patient's bed is wet, the apparatus is not working.

There is a variety of tidal drainage devices and setups. Several are shown here:

A-sterile solution
B-bladder
C-cycle-regulating loop
D-collection bottle
E-air vent.

The Lindsey and McKenna apparatuses are made of glass tubing. The air vents in these are actually the size of a pinhole. The McKenna tube is about 7 inches long, the Lindsey about 12 inches long.

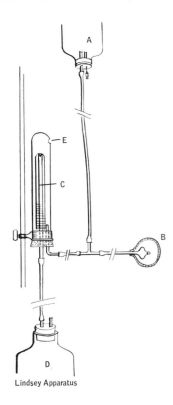

Lindsey Apparatus

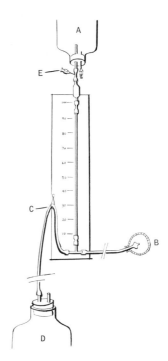

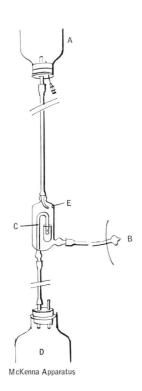

McKenna Apparatus

Points to Remember

1. The tidal drainage stand is set at the level of the symphysis pubis. Keep it at this level. If a Hi-Low bed is used, do not raise or lower the bed.
2. The initial setting of the siphon loop must be set one notch above the marker; otherwise, the set will function as a Y-irrigation.
3. The siphon loop is usually elevated one notch every other day as tolerated by the patient (follow doctor's orders). If the patient cannot tolerate the increased capacity, the loop is lowered to the previous level.
4. Chart output accurately.
5. Make sure there is irrigating solution in the reservoir bottle at all times and that it is dripping at the rate prescribed.
6. Plan nursing care to avoid interrupting the siphonage.
7. The frequency of the bladder's emptying depends upon the rate of flow of the irrigating fluid and the patient's intake. The faster the fluid drips, the more often the bladder empties.

IRRIGATIONS

BLADDER IRRIGATIONS

These are done either with a syringe or an irrigating flask. The syringe used is chosen from the following:

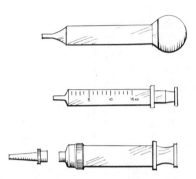

The method with the irrigating flask is the one recommended when irrigations are done several times daily. The irrigating solution is connected to a closed drainage system. With this setup there is less danger of contamination during the procedure. The setup is as shown:

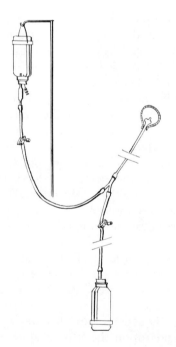

This setup is left in place until the treatment is discontinued. To give the irrigation, the drainage tube leading in to the connection bottle is clamped and the tube leading from the irrigating solution is unclamped.

Sterile normal saline solution is used most frequently for bladder irrigations. Unless otherwise indicated by the physician, enough solution is allowed to flow into the empty bladder until the patient expresses a feeling of fullness. The flow of the irrigating solution is then stopped and the bladder is allowed to drain by opening the clamp to the drainage bottle.

IRRIGATION OF THE KIDNEY PELVIS

Frequently the physician will desire to irrigate a tube placed in the kidney pelvis in order to prevent the tube from becoming clogged. As a rule the physician will perform this procedure; however, in some institutions it is a nursing responsibility. One should keep in mind that the kidney pelvis only has a capacity of between 4 and 5 cc.

When an irrigation is given through an indwelling ureteral catheter, a 2-cc. syringe attached to a No. 18 or 19 needle (depending on the size catheter) is used to inject the fluid as shown:

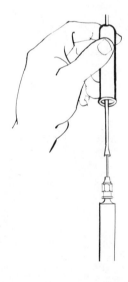

Notice how the catheter is disconnected from the connection tube (see p. 269) and held during the irrigation to prevent contamination to the opening. The fluid is injected slowly and gently. Not more than 2 cc. of solution is used. After all the solution has been injected, it is slowly and gently withdrawn through the syringe. Less than 2 cc. will be withdrawn because some of the solution will run down the ureter.

Never exert any force in injecting or withdrawing the fluid. If the catheter appears to be clogged, notify the physician.

Irrigations of a nephrostomy tube are seldom necessary. A large daily intake of fluid (about 3000 cc.) is usually a good assurance against clogging of the tube. In the event that it becomes necessary to irrigate the nephrostomy tube, the physician usually performs this procedure because of its delicacy. A 5-cc. syringe is used. Some physicians insert a ureteral catheter (No. 6) inside the nephrostomy tube and irrigate through this. If this is not done, a special adaptor must be placed on the syringe so that it will fit tightly in the end of the tube. Large piston syringes and bulb syringes are never used for this procedure because they exert too much force on the renal pelvis.

DRESSINGS AND BINDERS

After most urologic surgical procedures, dressings must be reinforced or changed frequently. This is one area in which the nurse can apply ingenuity in providing the ultimate in patient comfort. There is no excuse for the patient to lie in wet dressings.

After renal surgery, a Penrose drain is left in place to catch the serous material. The original dressings are left in place until changed by the physician. Because there is a profuse bloody drainage for 24 to 48 hours postoperatively, it will be necessary for the nurse to reinforce the dressing frequently. When inspecting the dressings, the nurse should remember that the drainage usually collects at the back and not on the anterior dressings. The reinforcements may be held in place with Montgomery tapes.

After ureteral surgery there may be profuse drainage of urine through the incision. These dressings are also reinforced by the nurse.

After any operation involving a suprapubic cystotomy, the dressings are usually changed by the nurse. In order to prevent skin irritations, the nurse should change the dressings frequently enough to keep them from becoming saturated. The skin around the cystotomy opening should be cleansed with a sterile soap and water solution and dried thoroughly. Special ointments may be prescribed. A plastic film cemented to the skin as illustrated for the colostomy dressing in Chapter 11 also makes a satisfactory dressing for the cystostomy wound.

These dressings are also held in place with Montgomery tapes.

When dressings are placed around drainage tubes, the tube should be anchored to the tapes as shown on page 267.

After a perineal prostatectomy, the perineal drainage is similar to that after the suprapubic cystotomy. In addition, the perineal dressings must be removed when the patient has a bowel movement. The fecal material is cleansed from the perineum with an antiseptic solution poured over the area, as for the obstetric patient.

Perineal dressings are held in place with a T binder. The dressings should be placed in such a way that they support the scrotum, as shown:

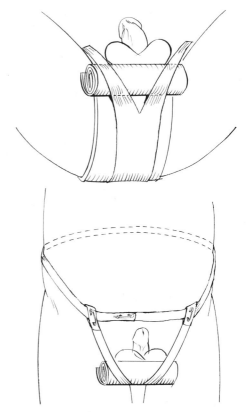

Note the proper placement of the T binder to obtain the ultimate in firmness.

Following the operation for hydrocele and varicocele, an adhesive dressing which gives scrotal support is used as shown:

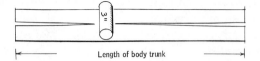

Length of body trunk

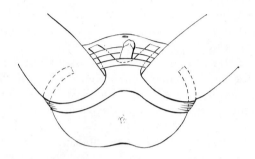

METHODS OF DIALYSIS

The function of the kidney is to filter impurities from the blood by the principle of dialysis. In cases of renal failure, the various waste products resulting from the catabolism of proteins (urea, uric acid, creatinine and creatin) are not excreted. As a result, these waste products accumulate in the blood and cause uremia. Two methods currently used to remove these toxic substances from the body are peritoneal dialysis and the artificial kidney. Both methods depend on the principles of osmosis and diffusion. Dialysis is defined as the separation of solute by differential diffusion through a porous membrane placed between two solutions. Any substance that can pass through a semipermeable membrane will diffuse from the side with the higher concentration until equilibrium is achieved. Any substance whose molecules are too large to pass through the pores of the membrane will, of course, be retained on the original side of the membrane.

The semipermeable membrane used in peritoneal dialysis is the living peritoneal membrane surrounding the abdominal cavity; in the artificial kidney it is cellophane.

Peritoneal Dialysis

In this procedure 2 liters of solution containing concentrations of electrolyte is infused into the abdominal cavity. Peritoneal dialysis solutions containing variable amounts of sodium, chloride, calcium, bicarbonate and dextrose are commercially available (see p. 282). The solution remains in the peritoneal cavity for 60 to 90 minutes, during which time osmosis and diffusion take place across the peritoneal lining. The solution containing the toxic substances is then drained from the cavity, and the entire procedure is repeated as often as necessary. The physician starts the procedure and observes the first infusion. The nurse usually conducts the remaining infusions. The dialysis may be continued for 12 to 36 hours.

During the procedure the nurse is expected to fulfill the following responsibilities:

1. Set up equipment (peritoneal dialysis administration sets commercially available, paracentesis equipment, intravenous tray, infusion stand and medications such as heparin, intravenous tetracycline, parenteral potassium chloride, 2% procaine hydrochloride, and whole blood).
2. Catheterize patient before procedure and place indwelling bladder catheter.
3. Check blood pressure and pulse.
4. Restrain patient's arm if necessary.
5. Add prescribed medications such as tetracycline and heparin to either bottle of dialysis solution, then warm both bottles of solution to body temperature (each bottle contains a different solution).
6. Assist physician with paracentesis.
7. Attach infusion setup to indwelling peritoneal catheter as shown:

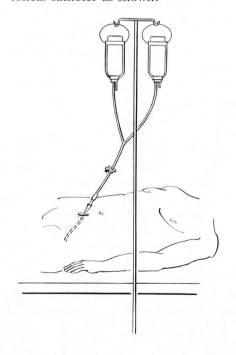

The fluid level should be marked on both bottles.

8. Unclamp tubing and permit solution to run in as rapidly as possible (no longer than 6 to 10 minutes).

9. Clamp tubing when bottles are empty but when there is still solution in tubing, so that siphonage effect can be obtained for drainage.

10. Remove bottles from stand and place on floor on side of bed. Tape tubing to side of bed.

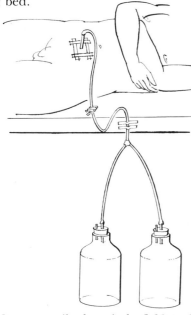

11. After prescribed period of 60 to 90 minutes, remove clamp and allow drainage to begin. Fluids drain out in two steady streams in about 15 minutes. As each bottle fills to the previously marked level, the tubing leading to it should be clamped. Excess fluid is drained in another calibrated container. If steady drainage stops or slows to a drip before most of the fluid has been recovered, the catheter may be obstructed. To correct this, apply brief pressure to lower abdomen as shown:

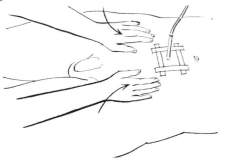

Slightly changing the patient's position from side to side or elevating the head of the bed to 45° may also help. If these measures fail, notify the physician.

Valuable time should not be wasted in waiting for the last 100 to 200 cc. of solution to drain. If 20 minutes have elapsed and the drainage flow becomes a slow drip, start the next exchange.

12. The physician removes the catheter at the termination of treatment. Sterile dressings are placed over the abdominal wound.

Additional nursing care during the procedure includes the following:

Blood pressure and pulse are taken and recorded every 15 minutes during the first exchange and every 60 minutes thereafter if stable. When hypertonic solutions (7 per cent dextrose) are given, blood pressure and pulse are taken every 15 minutes throughout the entire procedure.

An exact record of the amount of solution given and length of time taken for both infusion and drainage is kept. Any excess or deficit greater than 500 cc. is immediately brought to the physician's attention. All other fluid intake and output is also recorded.

During the first few exchanges, the drainage will show evidence of blood. Any later appearance of blood should be reported to the physician.

Abdominal pain may be experienced toward the end of each drainage. An analgesic, sedative or an injection of 5 cc. 2 per cent procaine directly into the peritoneal catheter may be prescribed.

During a period when fluid has been drained from the cavity, the new infusion may be delayed for a short period of time while really necessary nursing measures are completed.

THE ARTIFICIAL KIDNEY

The artificial kidney is a machine designed to perform the work of the kidneys for a short period of time. The basic principle of the machine is the semipermeable membrane comparable to the capillary wall of the glomerular tuft of the human kidney. The membranes used are simple sheets or tubes of cellophane produced commercially for sausage casings. The long cellophane tube is wound spirally on a drum immersed in a tank of rinsing liquid referred to as the bath, dialysing fluid or dialysate. As the blood runs slowly through the long tube on the drum, the impurities and salts diffuse through the membrane into the bath, going from a higher to a lower concentration. The larger protein molecules cannot pass through the membrane. The dialyzing liquid is maintained at about 0.6 per cent sodium chloride, 0.2 per cent sodium bicarbonate, 0.04 per cent potassium chloride and 1.5 per cent glucose. The composition of the bath may be altered to suit the individual need. The bath solution is changed every 2 hours during the procedure.

The average length of dialysis is usually 6 hours. During this time the blood electrolyte levels are usually reduced to one third of the predialysis level.

Approximately 1200 cc. fresh whole blood is used to prime the artificial kidney before use, and the same amount remains in the machine at the end of the procedure.

Heparin is added to this blood to prevent clotting. The patient's blood is drawn from the radial artery through a polyvinyl cannula. From there it goes to the dialyzer and then is pumped through a container that removes air bubbles and clots. Finally it is returned to the patient through a vein (usually the brachial).

There are several types of artificial kidneys currently on the market. In one type the drum containing the blood-filled cellophane rotates in the bath (Kolf). In another type the bath circulates around a stationary drum (Alwall and Skeggs and Leonards). Still another is the Kolf twin-coil kidney, which has a disposable cellophane coil drum. The artificial kidney is used for acute renal insufficiency due to a variety of causes.

The preparation of the patient for dialysis (also called hemodialysis) with the artificial kidney is as follows:

1. In some hospitals an operative permit is signed by the patient.
2. The patient is weighed on a stretcher immediately before and after the procedure with the weight of the stretcher deducted. The average weight loss during the procedure is 4 lbs.
3. The patient is taken to the dialysis unit in his own bed.
4. A sample of arterial blood is taken before the procedure for blood chemistry tests. The tests are also done every 2 hours during the procedure at the time of bath changes.

The team of individuals who conduct the treatment usually consists of several doctors, a nurse and a laboratory technician. The nurse's duties may include the following:

1. Preparation of heparin solutions in two strengths: (1) a concentrated solution of 10 mg. heparin to 1 cc. normal saline for use in the priming blood; (2) a weaker solution of 10 mg. heparin to 50 cc. normal saline for use in intravenous and intra-arterial cannulas.
2. Assisting physician with venesections. A dry dressing and pressure bandage are applied after the cannulas are in place. Local anesthesia is used if the patient is conscious. An arm board is used to immobilize the arm.
3. Placement of blood pressure cuff on the patient's arm and securing the stethoscope in place with tape. After the artificial kidney is turned on, the nurse takes the blood pressure continuously and as rapidly as possible, calling the readings out clearly without waiting to be asked. The doctors rely upon the blood pressures to regulate the flow rate of the blood. The blood pressure drops sharply when blood flows more rapidly into the machine than it is returned into the vein. If the blood pressure stabilizes during the first hour, it may be taken every 15 minutes.
4. Keeping complete records of vital signs, state of consciousness, and return of reflexes in the comatose patient on a special dialysis record sheet.
5. Giving ice chips orally during the procedure.
6. Raising or lowering the head of the bed slightly, if the blood pressure is satisfactory, to relieve the long periods of immobilization.

7. Giving prescribed sedatives for restlessness.
8. Giving drugs such as Sparene for nausea.
9. Changing linen for an incontinent patient.

At the completion of the procedure, protamine sulfate is administered, the cannulas are removed from the arm, the incisions are sutured, and a pressure dressing is applied. The patient is weighed and returned to his room.

Complications that may occur during the procedure include:
1. Bleeding from cannulation site or other tubes in place, such as a nasal tube. This usually occurs after the first 2 hours and may necessitate a change of dressing and bandage.
2. Chills from transfusion reaction.
3. Cardiac arrest (see p. 241).

Care following the procedure includes:
1. Frequent checking of vital signs.
2. Close observation for internal bleeding.
3. Record of intake and output.

Kidney function may be restored after one hemodialysis, or it may require several treatments spaced at intervals of several days apart.

PROCEDURES TO REVIEW

Use of radioactive isotopes for diagnosis (see Chap. 3).
Care of patient receiving radiation therapy as for carcinoma of bladder (see Chap. 3).
Application of hot water bottles and hot baths for renal colic.
Straining urine for calculi.
Catheterization of male and female patients.
Care of comatose patient in event of uremia.
Use of gastrointestinal suction in postoperative care especially after renal and ureteral surgery.
Perineal irrigation for postoperative perineal prostatectomy.
Skin care.
Isolation techniques used in cases of tuberculosis and venereal diseases.
Application of hot or cold compresses for orchitis.
Assisting with rectal examinations used frequently in diagnosis.

Accurate recording of intake and output.
Special mouth care.
Care of geriatric patient.

DIETS TO REVIEW

Low calcium for renal calculi.
Low phosphorus for renal calculi.
Liquid to full consistency following surgery.
High caloric for carcinoma and chronic renal insufficiency.
High protein for chronic renal insufficiency.
Low protein for acute renal insufficiency.

MEDICATIONS TO REVIEW

Inorganic Acids (Acidify Urine). Ammonium chloride, calcium chloride, diluted phosphoric acid and sodium phosphate.

Inorganic Acids (Counteract Acidosis). Potassium citrate, potassium acetate and potassium bitartrate.

Antiseptics (Urinary). Ethoxazene (Serenium) (causes orange-colored urine); hexylresorcinol (Caprokol); mandelamines (Azomandelamine, Mandelamine, Sulamine Plus, Uro-Phosphate tablets), menthenamine (Urotropin, Hexamine, Cystamin, Cystogen); methylene blue (causes greenish urine); nitrofurantoin (Furadantin); pyridium (Sulfid B−A, Azo-Gantrisin, Thiosulfil−A Forte, Urobiotic); phenyl salicylate (Urised).

Anticholinergics. Banthine, Donnatal, Levamine, Mesopin PB, Pro-Banthine, Sedasor and Trolar Elixir.

Cholinergic. Urecholine Chloride.

Anti-infectives (Systemic). Sulfonamides (Gantrisin, Lipo Gantrisin, Madribon, Sulamine Plus); sulfonamide and erythromycin (Ilotycin-Sulfa); sulfonamide and penicillin (Pentid-Sulfas, Gantricillin, V-Cillin Sulfa); sulfonamide and oxytetracycline; Urobiotic; novobiocin sodium preparations (Albamycin, Panalba and Alba-Penicillin); Kanamycin sulfate (Kan trex); tetracycline preparations (Achromycin, Tetracyn, Panmycin, Mysteclin-F); chlortetracycline hydrochloride (Aureomycin); oxytetracycline (Terramycin); penicillin and streptomycin.

Peritoneal Dialysis Solutions. Dianeal and Inpersol.

Bladder Irrigation Solutions. Sterile water, normal saline, silver nitrate 1:8000, protein silver (Protargol) 1:10,000, potassium permanganate 1:5000 to 1:30,000, acriflavine 1:6000, bichloride of mercury 1:10,000.

BIBLIOGRAPHY

Ansell, J. S.: Nephrectomy and Nephrostomy. Am. J. Nurs., *58*:1394, 1958.

Beeson, P. B., and McDermott, W.: Cecil-Loeb Textbook of Medicine. 12th ed. Philadelphia, W. B. Saunders Co., 1967.

Brown, A.: Medical and Surgical Nursing II. Philadelphia, W. B. Saunders Co., 1959.

Brunner, L. S., et al.: Textbook of Medical-Surgical Nursing. Philadelphia, J. B. Lippincott Co., 1964.

Davidsohn, I., and Henry, J. B.: Todd-Sanford Clinical Diagnosis by Laboratory Methods. 14th ed. Philadelphia, W. B. Saunders Co., 1969.

Davis, L.: Christopher's Textbook of Surgery. 9th ed. Philadelphia, W. B. Saunders Co., 1968.

Falconer, M., Patterson, H., and Gustafson, E.: Current Drug Handbook. Philadelphia, W. B. Saunders Co., 1968.

Flitter, H. H.: An Introduction of Physics in Nursing. 5th ed. St. Louis, C. V. Mosby Co., 1967.

Gibson, T. E.: Catheter for Rectal Drainage. J. Urol., *86*:855, 1961.

Goodale, R.: Clinical interpretation of Laboratory Tests. 5th ed. Philadelphia, F. A. Davis Co., 1964.

Goldner, F.: The Artificial Kidney. Southern Med. J., *50(2)*:1301, 1957.

Harmer, B., and Henderson, V.: Textbook of Principles and Practices of Nursing. 5th ed. New York, The Macmillan Co., 1958.

Hodges, C., Lehman, T. H., Moore, R. J., and Loomis, R.: Use of Ileal Segments in Urology. J. Urol., *85*:573, 1961.

Krause, M.: Food, Nutrition, and Diet Therapy. 4th ed. Philadelphia, W. B. Saunders Co., 1966.

McClean, M. M., Creighton, H., and Berman, L. B.: Hemodialysis and the Artificial Kidney. Am. J. Nurs., *58*:1672, 1958.

O'Neill, M.: Peritoneal Dialysis. Nurs. Clin. North America, *1*:309, 1966.

Sadove, M., and Cross, J.: The Recovery Room. Philadelphia, W. B. Saunders Co., 1956.

Taufic, M. P.: Nursing the Patient after Nephrectomy. Am. J. Nurs., *58*:1397, 1958.

Twiss, M. R., and Morton, M. H.: Peritoneal Dialysis. Am. J. Nurs., *59*:1560, 1959.

nursing techniques in the care of Skin Diseases

DIAGNOSTIC PROCEDURES

SPECIAL TESTS

The nurse may be called upon to assist with the following special examinations commonly used in recognizing many dermatoses.

Patch Tests

The identity of the causative agent in contact dermatitis may be elicited by means of the patch tests. The skin is cleaned, and a diluted allergen is applied to the unbroken skin at a site remote from eruptions. The allergen is applied on a piece of cloth about 1 cm. square. This is covered with a piece of plastic about 1½ inches square, held in place with ½-inch adhesive or scotch tape.

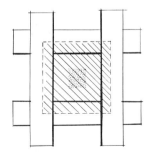

The flexor surface of the forearm or back may be used. The patch is kept in place 24 hours. If the reaction is negative at the end of this period, it should be observed daily for 4 days and periodically for 2 weeks because some agents cause a delayed reaction.

A positive reaction consists of a red area with tiny vesicles.

Scratch Tests

These tests are used in detecting the causative agents in allergies. The patient is stripped to the waist and asked to lie face down. The back is cleansed with soap and water and thoroughly dried. Then numbers corresponding to the number of tests to be done are written on the skin with washable ink. These numbered test areas are placed about 2 inches apart in every direction.

A separate needle is used for each scratch made about ⅜ inch long. The object is not to penetrate the skin but merely tear the surface layer open so that the antigen solution may bathe the cells of the deeper layers. A drop of solution is placed on each scratch. If the test material is sealed in small capillary tubes, it is applied directly from the tube. If the extract is in a bottle, it is applied with a toothpick. A different toothpick is used for each solution. After about 20 to 30 minutes, the extracts are wiped off and the readings are made. The presence of a wheal suggests a positive reading. Positive readings are designated slight, moderate and marked, or +1, +2 and +3.

The scratch tests are checked in 24 hours for delayed reactions.

Scratch test kits containing 44 units are commercially available for basic testing.

Intradermal Tests

These tests are usually done on the arm in groups of 12 or less at a time. The skin is first cleansed and sterilized, then the solution is injected with a small gauge needle (#26). The needle is inserted, bevel side up, until the lumen is barely concealed by the skin.

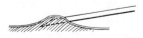

About 0.01 cc. of solution is usually sufficient.

The reaction is checked in 30 minutes. Reactions to bacteria and fungi are usually delayed 24 to 48 hours.

The solutions for intradermal tests are about one hundred times more reactive than scratch tests. For this reason the tests are made on the arm where a tourniquet may be applied proximal to the test site if a reaction occurs.

Specific antigens considered useful in dermatology include the Frei antigen for lymphopathia venereum and various tests employing histamine, tuberculin and trichophytin. Useful fungus antigens include sporotrichin, blastomycin and coccidioidin.

Biopsy. Small sections of skin may be removed for biopsy purposes without much inconvenience to the patient. This is usually accomplished by use of a dermal punch. The dermal punch is an electrically power driven machine which is drilled through the skin to the desired depth. The separated specimen is then lifted from its site and cut off at the base with a scalpel or scissors.

The cutaneous punches vary in diameter from 2 mm. to 6 mm., and the resulting wound seldom needs suturing. A small disc of Gelfoam is placed on the wound and covered with sterile dressings. This procedure is relatively painless and may not require local anesthesia.

Deeper biopsies are removed with a scalpel, and the resulting wound is sutured.

Smears and Cultures. The examination of material from a suspected lesion is helpful in diagnosis of superficial and deep fungus infection such as blastomycosis.

Diascopy. Pressure applied on a lesion with a transparent object such as a microscopic slide reveals the appearance of the lesion after the blood has been driven out of the capillaries. This procedure is used especially in lupus vulgaris.

Microscopy. Hand microscopes which give up to 200 power magnification are sometimes used in the diagnosis of nevi.

Wood's Light Test. A filter is placed over a source of ultraviolet rays to concentrate the rays. All fungi fluoresce when examined in this light. This test is used to diagnose tinea capitis.

Probe Test. A toothpick or similar object is pressed gently against a lesion. In certain tuberculids the point of the probe will painlessly penetrate the lesion and remain fixed when the examiner's hand is removed.

Curette Test. When the scale of a psoriatic lesion is removed with a curette, fine capillary bleeding points are visible.

Capillary Fragility Test. This test is used in diagnosing the purpuras. A blood pressure cuff is placed around the arm for 5 to 7 minutes at a pressure just above diastolic, and the purpuric spots in a square inch are counted. In a positive test the tiny hemorrhages develop within a few minutes.

Dermographia or Artificial Urticaria. The skin is vigorously stroked with a blunt probe. In some individuals this produces whealing. This reaction is frequent in patients with urticaria.

Nikolsky's Sign. The examiner presses his finger gently against the skin and applies traction. The skin separates at the junction of the epidermis and cutis, leaving a raw exuding area. This test is always positive in pemphigus and sometimes in erythema multiforme bullosum and dermatitis herpetiformis.

Transillumination. A small light is held directly against the skin adjacent to a lesion. In nevi that are spreading locally can be seen fine strands of dark pigment invisible on direct examination.

Other Tests. The R. A. test (see p. 177) is used to determine whether arthritis is rheumatoid or caused by lupus erythematosus. The presence of the L.E. cell in bone marrow (see p. 236) is a diagnostic sign of lupus erythematosus. Urinalysis, blood count, blood chemistry, basal metabolism test, blood serologic tests and search for ova in stools are all used in dermatology.

THERAPEUTIC AND REHABILITATIVE PROCEDURES

Many of the therapeutic nursing procedures in dermatology involve the topical application of medications. Numerous improvements in this field simplify these procedures and provide a greater scope of therapy. Solutions used in the application of wet dressings and baths are easily and accurately prepared with the newly available individual packets and tablets. Medications such as tars, topical steroids, antibiotics and fungicides are now dispensed in aerosol form for simplified application. Improvements in a combination of cleansing and healing agents include the newer soaps, i.e., superfatted soaps, soap substitutes and medicated soaps. New shampoo preparations greatly facilitate the treatment of seborrhea capitis. Improvements in the therapy of acne include the new cleansing agents, cosmetic lotions and preparations with which the patient himself can carry out a graded abrasion. There are new preparations of suntan lotions that are helpful in the management of vitiligo. Nonadherent dressings, plastic bases and tapes all make dressings easier to apply and more attractive.

In addition there are several new systemic drugs that have changed the whole concept of therapy for some of the dermatological disorders.

All of these advancements are discussed in detail in this context under the appropriate headings. While the nurse may not encounter some of these newer products in the hospital, she should be aware of their availability in order to provide total patient care.

TOPICAL MEDICATIONS

WET DRESSINGS

Wet dressings are used in the treatment of exudative or highly inflamed lesions.

A wet dressing permits the application of medications to the skin and at the same time provides for drainage of exudate. Wet dressings may also be utilized for the application of heat or cold. The wet dressings may be open or closed. The open wet dressing is not covered. The closed wet dressing is covered with an airtight covering of plastic or wax paper. Since closed dressings applied for prolonged periods cause maceration of the skin, these are seldom used in dermatological nursing.

The physician's orders for wet dressings usually do not specify "open" or "closed"; therefore, the nurse can correctly assume that the open method is to be used in the treatment of skin disorders.

Materials such as broadcloth, percale and soft muslin are preferable to the use of gauze because they absorb and retain more moisture. Absorbent cotton is never used because the fibers adhere to open lesions and are difficult, if not impossible, to remove.

The solutions used in wet dressings include the soothing agents as follows:

Normal Saline Solution. Nonmedicated and hypoallergenic. Used when drainage and heat are desired.

Burow's Solution (¹⁄₂₀) (aluminum acetate solution). Similar to boric acid but less bacteriostatic and more drying. Bur-Veen, Domeboro and Soy-Boro are new products commercially available. Bur-Veen is supplied in packets. One packet of powder added to one pint of water makes an equivalent of a 1:20 Burow's solution in a medium of Aveeno colloidal oatmeal (see colloid bath).

Domeboro is supplied in tablets, powder packets and concentrated solution and can be mixed to produce a 1:10 or 1:20 Burow's solution.

One packet of Soy-Boro dissolved in a pint of water makes a 1:20 Burow's solution reinforced with colloidal soybean.

Milk and Lime Water (4:1). Used cold as a soothing application around eyes or genitalia.

Hypertonic Magnesium Sulfate Solution (25%). Reduces edema and inflammation and provides drainage.

The bacteriostatic and fungistatic solutions are:

Boric Acid Solution (2%). Boric acid may be prescribed in water or in normal saline solution. Used in inflammatory superficial infections.

Potassium Permanganate Solution (1:10,000-1:50,000). Used in the same way as boric acid solution. Leaves a brown stain on the skin. Dalidome may be used instead of potassium permanganate. This is a nonstaining preparation available in powder packets.

Silver Nitrate Solution (0.25-0.5%). Has an astringent effect in addition to being bacteriostatic and fungistatic.

Vleminckx's Solution. A sulfurated lime solution. Available in commercially prepared powder packets under the name Vlem-Dome.

BATHS

Baths are given for the same reasons as wet dressings and are used when the dermatosis is extensive. Baths are used frequently for their antipruritic effect. Baths are given in a regular bathtub (25 gallons of water), as sitz baths for perineal dermatosis (5 to 10 gallons of water) and as foot or arm baths in basins or specially designed tubs.

The medicated baths are as follows:

1. *Colloid Bath.* Starch, Aveeno and Soyaloid are the substances used. Aveeno is a commercial preparation of concentrated colloidal oatmeal made especially for therapeutic purposes. Another preparation, Aveeno Oilated, is composed of colloidal oatmeal impregnated with emollient oils (liquid petrolatum and lanolin) and is used in dry chronic dermatoses such as senile pruritis. Aveeno is supplied in 18-ounce and 4-pound boxes and one cupful is added to a tub (about 25 gallons) of warm water. Aveeno Oilated is supplied in 10-ounce cans and 3 to 4 tablespoonfuls of it is added to a tub of warm water.

Soyaloid is a concentrated colloidal soybean powder with effects similar to those of oatmeal. One packet of powder is dissolved in a tub of water.

Starch is used in a concentration of one cup to a tub of warm water.

The colloid bath is soothing, antipruritic and the least drying of the baths. Warn the patient to beware of slipping when getting in and out of the bathtub.

2. *Potassium Permanganate Bath.* Twenty-five to 50 grains of potassium permanganate are added to 25 gallons of water. The potassium permanganate crystals or tablets should be thoroughly dissolved in water in a basin, then poured into the tub of water to prevent staining of the tub. Undissolved particles of potassium permanganate also cause burns on contact with the skin.

Dalidome may be substituted for potassium permanganate soaks.

3. *Tar Bath.* One-half to 1 ounce of solution of coal tar, N.F. or Alma Tar* is added to the bath water. The tar bath is used in psoriasis, seborrheic dermatitis and chronic eczema.

AEROSOLS

Aerosols are particularly effective on moist lesions. They reduce the likelihood of introducing additional irritants to an involved area, trauma from rubbing and the chance of contamination and infection. Some of the corticosteroid and antibiotic-steroid combinations include Diloderm,* Neo-Diloderm,* Meti-Derm with neomycin, and Tarcortin.* Betadine is a nonstinging, nonstaining iodine spray and, unlike tincture of iodine, can be bandaged. Anesthetic sprays include Americaine and Tronothane Hydrochloride. Desenex is an antifungal spray. Aristoderm foam is a new steroid (triamcinolone) spray. Neo-Aristoderm foam is the steroid preparation containing neomycin.

Aerosols are usually applied several times daily. Shake the container before use; then, with the can upright, spray the area from a distance of 3 to 6 inches. A 2- to 3-second spray is sufficient. Longer spraying wastes medication.

Foams are applied by holding the can inverted next to the skin.

SOAPS AND SOAP SUBSTITUTES

Oilatum soap is a neutral soap containing peanut oil and is used when regular soaps produce excessive dryness and irritation. Fostex cake, Lava soap and Acne-Aid detergent soap are used for oily skins. Medicated soaps include Gamophen and Mycoderm.

When soap is too irritating, soap substitutes are used for cleansing. The soap substitutes include Lowilacake, Acidolate, pHisoderm and pHisoHex (see p. 101).

ABRASIVES

Brasivol is a cleanser containing a graded nonsilicon abrasive plus hexachlorophene in a

---

*Also available in spray foams.

special base of soap and synthetic detergent. This product is available in a fine, medium and rough base and is used in the treatment of acne. It may also be used to remove scales in lesions such as in psoriasis in cleansing the skin prior to the application of an ointment.

SHAMPOOS

Antiseborrheic shampoos include Capsebon, Sebulex, Betadine, Domerine, Ar-Ex Tar, Fostex Cream, and Alvinine, Kwell is a shampoo used to treat pediculosis capitis, phthirius and their nits. The feature of all these shampoos is that no other cleansing or rinsing agents are necessary. After wetting the hair with warm water, apply the shampoo as in any other cleansing shampoo, and allow the lather to remain on the scalp for at least 5 minutes. These shampoos have a pleasant odor and leave the hair soft. The antiseborrheic shampoos are used several times weekly as recommended by the physician.

Only one application of Kwell is necessary in the treatment of pediculosis and phthirius.

OINTMENTS

Ointment is the most widely used type of topical medication. The type of ointment base may be greasy, nongreasy or penetrating. The type of base is chosen to suit the nature of the lesion to be treated as well as to provide the best medium for the drug to be applied. Two ointment bases include Verigerm and Cebum. Both preparations closely approximate the natural lipids and constituents of human sebum. Other ointment bases include petrolatum, lanolin, carbowax, hydrophilic ointment and aquaphor.

Any one of a number of drugs may be combined with an ointment base to form a medicated ointment. The two most commonly used antibiotics applied topically are bacitracin and neomycin. Topical antibiotic therapy is effective only in superficial infections such as impetigo and ecthyma. The topical use of antihistamines is rarely necessary. Topical steroid preparations are now the most widely used group of topical therapeutic agents in dermatologic conditions. All commercially available glucosteroid compounds except cortisone have anti-inflammatory effects when topically applied to the skin. Hydrocortisone and prednisone have been used the most frequently and are the least expensive. Almost all of the newer steroids that have been introduced for systemic administration are also available in preparations for topical application (see "Internal Medication"). Topical steroid therapy is employed in many of the dermatoses such as contact dermatitis, seborrheic dermatitis, neurodermatitis, atopic dermatitis, chronic otitis externa, anal and vulvar pruritis, macerated lesions of psoriasis, some forms of eczema, and herpes simplex.

The steroids are also administered topically in lotions and sprays (Aristoderm foam).

The topical benefits from ointments are increased if interfering scales and crusts are wholly or partially removed before the applications are made. This may be done by having the patient soak in a bath to soften the scales before applying the topical agent.

The steroid preparations should be rubbed in well. When prior removal of scales is not feasible for lesions such as psoriasis, the steroid of choice may be rubbed in with a soft toothbrush, a pumice stone or a tongue blade (clothespins may be used at home), covered with cotton sheeting. In all cases one must of course avoid any degree of damage that might aggravate the lesions. Any change in the lesion and surrounding skin must be noted.

For many chronic lesions dressings are used to cover ointments. The dressings of choice for the steroids and for some of the other ointments currently are thin plastic films. A detailed discussion of the uses of plastic film is included under the heading "Dressings and Bandages" later in this chapter.

INTRALESIONAL INJECTIONS

The treatment of some of the dermatoses by means of local intralesional injections of corticosteroids has been found to be beneficial. Hydrocortisone acetate, prednisolone acetate, and triamcinolone diacetate suspensions are currently used in this manner to treat conditions such as alopecia areata, psoriasis, granuloma annulare, lichen simplex chronicus, hypertrophic lichen planus, and chronic discoid lupus erythematosus.

The frequency of injections varies with the disease. Ordinarily a single injection is sufficient. Not more than three or four injections given several weeks apart are required. In alopecia areata, hair regrowth usually occurs after one injection.

The steroid suspensions may be injected with a tuberculin syringe attached to an ordinary No. 26 to No. 21 gauge needle, which is introduced just under and parallel to the skin surface. Another method is to insert the needle perpendicularly at multiple sites approximately ¼ inch apart. A device consisting of a specially designed syringe to which a vial of solution is attached is used with short-beaded needles. An adjustment on the device regulates the amount of solution given each time the plunger is pushed. The needles used are beaded to control the depth of injection.

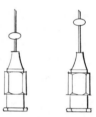

A complication of intralesional steroid therapy is temporary depression of the skin. This usually becomes indiscernible within about one year.

INTERNAL MEDICATIONS

A number of systemic medications are used in treating the dermatoses. A complete list of these medications is given at the end of this chapter. Several medications that have revolutionized dermatological therapy are mentioned here.

GRISEOFULVIN

Until a decade ago the specific therapy of many varieties of superficial and deep mycoses was completely lacking. The introduction late in 1958 of the drug griseofulvin (Fulvicin, Grifulvin) has proved to be what amounts to a revolutionary advance in the management of certain of the superficial fungus infections. Griseofulvin is obtained from a penicillin strain and is the first antifungal antibiotic effective in the treatment of fungal dermatoses. The drug has found its greatest usefulness in the treatment of tinea capitis, tinea corporis, tinea barbae, tinea cruris, tinea pedis, tinea manum and onychomycosis.

Griseofulvin is administered orally in doses of 250 mg. 4 times daily or 500 mg. twice daily. Tests show that the drug may also have some usefulness in topical application.

The administration of the drug to this date has been remarkably free of adverse effects.

HORMONES

The advancements in hormone therapy in dermatology have been centered on the uses of the synthetic adrenocorticotropic hormones. In medical literature this group of hormones is referred to as adrenocorticals, corticosteroids, glucosteroids or steroids. (A review of anatomy and physiology may help the nurse more clearly understand the basis for this variety of terms.) This group of drugs is most likely used more frequently than any other group in dermatologic therapy and can be used in treating more conditions than can any other. The steroids actually cure nothing; yet therapy is much more effective because of their use in relief of symptoms. They are used in many of the dermatoses, including psoriasis, lupus erythematosus and drug allergies. In addition to their usefulness in topical therapy, the steroids are also administered orally, intravenously and intramuscularly. The systemic therapy is sometimes combined with topical therapy. The two steroids used most frequently are hydrocortisone and prednisolone. A number of additional synthetics are also currently in use. A complete list of these and their trade names are listed at the end of this chapter.

One of the reasons for the increase in the number of new synthetic steroids is that an effort is continuously being made to formulate a steroid that has fewer or no undesirable side effects. The undesirable effects are seen especially when prolonged use of the steroids is necessary. The potassium secretion and sodium retention common in the use of cortisone and hydrocortisone have been nearly eliminated in the newer prednisone, prednisolone, triamcinolone, methyl prednisolone and dexamethasone.

Undesirable effects of current steroids are their ability to mask infection, interference with the formation of fibroblasts, producing an osteoporosis that can result in fracture, and redistribution of fat causing moon face and buffalo hump. Habituation to these hormones is also common.

Symptoms the nurse may look for include
1. hypertension
2. gastric distress (milk may be given with the oral dose to eliminate gastric distress)
3. insomnia (usually disappears 1 to 2 weeks after initiation of therapy)
4. weight gain
5. edema
6. purpura
7. vertigo
8. headache
9. abnormal growth of hair
10. emotional disturbances.

Upon reading this list of undesirable side effects, one may wonder why these drugs are even considered remarkable; however, for every one who suffers an ill effect from a corticosteroid, there are 20 others who can obtain relief that no other medication available today can give them.

Intermittent intravenous therapy rather than continuous oral therapy is known to reduce the undesirable effects from the corticosteroids.

ANTIMALARIALS

Drugs such as Atabrine, Aralen, and Plaquenil which have a history in the treatment of malaria, now have uses in the treatment of skin diseases. They are remarkably effective in the treatment of chronic discoid lupus erythematosus. They are also used in conditions such as dermatomyositis, polymorphous light sensitivity reactions, sunburn, poison ivy, verruca plana, acne, and rosacea.

DRESSINGS AND BANDAGES

DRY DRESSINGS

Dressings are used on the diseased skin to cover medications, to provide a covering that prevents touching, picking and scratching, and to protect the skin from general hazards.

The best dressing materials for a covering over greasy preparations are soft, closely woven cotton cloths like broadcloth, muslin, percale or poplin.

Tubular cotton materials like stockinette, Surgitube and Tubegauz are most suitable for holding the dressings in place. Circular gauze bandages are cumbersome, constricting, more time-consuming to place, and generally less satisfactory than tubular forms.

Adhesive tape is sometimes required to hold the entire dressing in place. When adhesive is used in the treatment of skin diseases, it should not be placed next to the skin because of the possibility of sensitivity.

Some practical ways of holding dressings in place on different portions of the skin are as follows:

The use of tubular gauze on the fingers and 2- to 3-inch stockinette on the remainder of the hand holds a cotton dressing in place on the fingers, palm and dorsa, as shown.

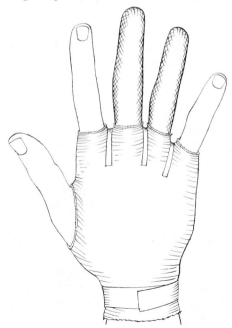

When the heel does not have to be covered, stockinette may be placed over foot dressings as shown:

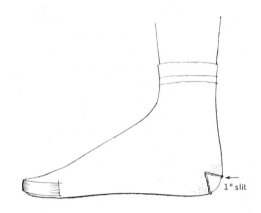

Adhesive tape may also be placed on either side of the slit at the heel if necessary.

Socks (preferably two) may be used to hold dressings in place on the foot. Gloves are not useful on the hands because they move too much.

A sling dressing may be used for the axilla.

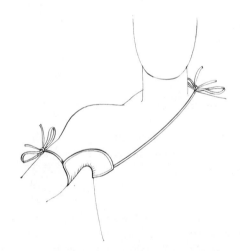

The face, ears and neck and scalp are rarely covered for psychologic reasons.

The trunk is seldom covered. When eruptions are this generalized, the patient is placed on bed rest and medication is carried out on a relatively naked, sheet-covered body.

Stockinette is used for the limbs and should be cut so that it extends well above and below the underdressing.

The secret in getting the stockinette in place over underdressings merely lying in place is in rolling the stockinette before application. The roll is slipped over the limb to the place where the dressing is to begin, then unrolled over the underdressing as shown:

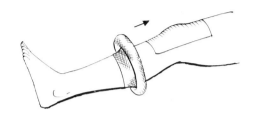

Adjustments in the underdressing are made as the stockinette is unrolled.

UNNA'S PASTE DRESSINGS

Unna's paste (see p. 245) is sometimes used in the treatment of neurodermatitis and stasis dermatitis. The commercial preparation (Medicopaste or Cruricast) of this dressing is usually used.

PLASTIC FILM DRESSINGS

Preliminary experience with several topical agents, especially the steroids, suggests that their therapeutic effectiveness is enhanced when applied under plastic films. Saran Wrap, available at the food market, is the plastic film most frequently employed.

The ointment of choice is applied to the skin, then covered with the plastic. Saran Wrap may be used to cover the arms and legs, including the feet, but not the hands. The plastic is held in place with scotch tape. The tape need not touch the skin. In some cases this is all that is necessary to hold the dressings in place. In other cases the plastic must be covered with gauze bandage or preferably with the knitted tubular cotton dressings. Stockings or socks may be used for the legs and feet. Thin plastic gloves are used to cover the hands and do not require a covering dressing. The plastic film may be used in the genital area in females and held in place with a sanitary belt and pad, over which tight panties are worn. On ambulatory patients disposable diapers (Chux) may be placed on the areas on the back and buttocks. The plastic is worn against the skin. On the torso may be used plastic garment bags used in dry cleaning. The necessary holes are cut for the head and arms, and the bag is slipped on over the head and held in place with tight-fitting underclothes.

Hospitalized patients are usually treated in this manner around the clock for 24 hours. The dressings may be changed once or twice daily. Ambulatory patients are usually treated only during the night.

When the dressings are removed, little or no ointment remains on the skin, and as a rule no special cleansing is necessary to remove the ointment.

In a small percentage of cases, skin irritations may follow the use of plastic film dressings. These usually disappear when the dressings are eliminated for several days.

WET DRESSINGS

The uses of wet dressings have been included in the discussion on "Topical Medications."

PHYSICAL THERAPY

LIGHT THERAPY

Since the newer drugs have come on the market, the use of ultraviolet rays is no longer necessary for many of the dermatoses.

RADIOTHERAPY

Roentgen rays, radium and radioactive isotopes are effectively used in dermatological therapy for conditions such as malignancies and benign new growths and granulomas. Radiation is used to inhibit the activity of sebaceous glands (in acne, seborrhea, etc.), to inhibit the activity of sweat glands, and for their antipruritic and depilatory effect.

For a complete discussion on the uses of radiotherapy and care of the patient receiving this treatment, see Chapter 3.

REFRIGERATION

Liquid nitrogen and solid carbon dioxide are used in removing unsightly scars and growths such as warts, particularly on the hands and fingers, x-ray keratoses on the hands and fingers, senile and seborrheic keratoses, Bowen's disease, small recent hypertrophic scars, granuloma annulare, pigmented nevi, and synovial cysts at finger joints.

The temperature of liquid nitrogen is

$-320.5°$ F. $(-195.8°$ C.); the temperature of solid carbon dioxide is $-110°$ F. $(-78.5°$ C.).

Liquid nitrogen is applied with a cotton-tipped applicator of appropriate size. The cotton tip, soaked with liquid nitrogen, is held on the lesion until all the liquid has evaporated; then it is replaced with a freshly soaked one. This procedure is repeated until the lesion is frozen (about 30 seconds to 3 minutes). Severe stinging occurs as the lesion first starts to freeze and again when thawing takes place. The treated area is uncomfortable for an hour or two thereafter. A blister containing clear or bloody fluid forms under and around the lesion in 3 to 6 hours. The blister is drained with a sterile needle each time it fills, usually several times in the first 48 hours after the treatment. Patients are warned against removing the vesicle roof for 2 to 3 weeks, when healing occurs. The site of the lesion does not have to be bandaged or protected from water. One treatment is usually sufficient to remove a lesion. The lesion disappears several months following the treatment.

PSYCHOTHERAPY

The psychosomatic approach to certain dermatologic problems is becoming more and more helpful. In some instances, the dermatologic disorders are symptoms of an underlying emotional disorder; in others the emotional impact resulting from the dermatologic problem may be important.

The nurse can help by being a sympathetic, understanding listener and by overcoming any reluctance to look upon or touch the patient's skin.

SURGERY

DERMABRASION

Extensive pitting facial scars resulting from some dermatologic lesions, especially in acne, may be removed by dermabrasion. This is a surgical procedure in which the skin is planed with small, high speed abrasive brushes of various types. This is carried out on skin which is first hardened (frozen) by the local appli-

cation of a refrigerant spray. For several years after the initial use of this procedure, it was highly publicized by the laity as a quick, simple, and painless operation for the complete removal of scars. This unfortunately is far from the truth. The enthusiasm for dermabrasion has diminished.

The nurse should be aware, however, that although dermabrasion is not a procedure which miraculously transforms a bizarre skin to a "peaches and cream" complexion, it does produce some improvement in every case. The degree of improvement varies with each case. Keeping this in mind, the nurse should refrain from making any statements to the patient that may give him false hopes.

Since general anesthesia is not needed for this procedure, it may be done in the doctor's office. In the event that this procedure is carried out in the hospital, the nurse should understand several factors about the post-dermabrasive patient, as follows:

1. Sterile dressings are applied rather firmly. Some surgeons use ointments such as sterile petroleum jelly or antibiotics.
2. Dressings that become blood-tinged are removed 24 hours after surgery. No further dressings are required.
3. A burning sensation—as from brush burns —is experienced by some patients for the first few days.
4. When the dressings are removed, the skin is red, markedly swollen—enough to shut the eyes in some cases—and covered with dried blood and scabs as though the face had been badly burned.
5. The scabs drop off in 7 to 10 days. The redness usually continues for 3 or 4 weeks.
6. The optimum in improvement is experienced in 6 months.

PLASTIC SURGERY

Nursing techniques encountered in plastic surgery of the skin include the following:
1. The area to be grafted is rendered free of infection prior to grafting with antibacterial skin cleansers. Dressings may be placed over the area.
2. The donor area of skin is prepared as for any other general surgery.

3. After surgery dressings are rarely used on the face. Dressings elsewhere are changed in 3 to 5 days by the physician.
4. The slight oozing of blood from an uncovered incision on the face must be wiped away with an alcohol sponge so that clot formation does not occur. An infection may occur under the clot and spoil the cosmetic effect.
5. When flaps are used as the corrective technique, the flaps must be observed for circulation. Warm wet dressings are sometimes used to improve the circulation in flaps. Care must be used to keep this procedure aseptically sterile.

PROCEDURES TO REVIEW

The application of heat and cold to the body
Uses of various new dressing materials (Chapter 8)
Intravenous and intramuscular injections (Chapter 6)
Radiotherapy (Chapter 3)
Isolation techniques (Chapter 7)
Catheterization of patient
Use of the indwelling catheter used for the patient with severe burns (see p. 266)
Use of Stryker frame for patient with burns and extensive dermatoses (see p. 198)
Prevention and treatment of shock in patient with burns
Emergency treatment of burns and drug reactions
Giving a shampoo
Use of heated and unheated bed cradles
Supervising and assisting with the tub bath
Use of devices to prevent decubitus ulcers
Methods for maintaining good body alignment for the patient
Lifting and moving the patient
Special mouth care as necessary when lesions are also present in the mouth
Eye irrigations given when dermatoses affect the eyes
Maintenance of an allergen-free environment
Application of lotions and powders
Care of the aging skin
Exercises to prevent contractures in healing burns

Recording intake and output
Use of deodorants for foul-smelling dressings

DIETS TO REVIEW

Liquid to soft consistencies for patients with lesions of mouth
Elimination diet for allergy
Diabetic diet for patients with skin inflammations resulting from diabetes mellitus
High caloric and high protein diet used in burns and other debilitating conditions
Low carbohydrate and fat in acne
High protein diet used with administration of some steroids.

MEDICATIONS TO REVIEW

The following is a list of systemic medications used in dermatology. The commonly used topical medicaments have been discussed in the context of this chapter. Many of the systemic medications listed here are also available in topical forms.

Antihistamines. Antistine, Dimetane, Clistin, Tagathen, Chlor-Trimeton, Allercur, Benadryl, Hispril, Decapryn, Neohetramine, Thenfadil, Pyribenzamine, Histadyl, Neo-Antergan, Thephorin, Temaril, Perazil, Phenergan.

Antibiotics. Sulfonamides (Madribon, Medicil, Kynex); penicillins; tetracycline; erythromycin; novobiocin; isoniazid (for tuberculosis of skin).

Antimalarials. Aralen, Atabrine, Plaquenil, Camoquin, Triquin.

Tranquilizers. Thorazine, Serpasil, meprobamate (Miltown, Equanil).

Vitamins. Vitamin A (Aquasol A and Aquasynth A); vitamin B complex; vitamin D_2(Calciferol); and vitamin E.

Adrenocorticosteroids. Hydrocortisone acetate (Cortef Acetate); hydrocortisone (Cortef, Terra-Cortril, Hydrocortone Acetate, Compound F); prednisone (Meticorten); prednisolone acetate (Delta-Cortef); methylprednisolone (Medrol); deoxycorticosterone acetate (Doca, Cortate); dexamethasone (Decadron, Deronil, Gammacorten); triamcinolone (Kenacort); fluorohydrocortisone acetate (Florinef).

BIBLIOGRAPHY

Beeson, P. B., and McDermott, W.: Cecil-Loeb Textbook of Medicine. 12th ed. Philadelphia, W. B. Saunders Co., 1967.

Berger, Robert A.: An Improved Technique for the Intracutaneous Injection of Steroid Suspensions. Arch. Dermatol. *82*:271, 1960.

Brown, A.: Medical and Surgical Nursing II. Philadelphia, W. B. Saunders Co., 1959.

Brunner, L. S., et al.: Textbook of Medical-Surgical Nursing. Philadelphia, J. B. Lippincott Co., 1964.

Burrill, B. B.: Recent Advances in Dermatology. J. Med. Soc. N.J., *57(11)*:623, 1960.

Davidsohn I., and Henry, J. B.: Todd-Sanford Clinical Diagnosis by Laboratory Methods. 14th ed. Philadelphia, W. B. Saunders Co., 1969.

Davis, L.: Christopher's Textbook of Surgery. 9th ed. Philadelphia, W. B. Saunders Co., 1968.

Falconer, M., Patterson, H., and Gustafson, E.: Current Drug Handbook. 1968-1970. Philadelphia, W. B. Saunders Co., 1968.

Goodale, R.: Clinical Interpretation of Laboratory Tests. 5th ed. Philadelphia, F. A. Davis Co., 1965.

Hall, F. A.: Advantages and Limitations of Liquid Nitrogen in the Therapy of Skin Lesions. Arch. Dermatol., *82*:9, 1960.

Harmer, B., and Henderson, V.: Textbook of Principles and Practices of Nursing. 5th ed. New York, The Macmillan Co., 1958.

Krause, M.: Food, Nutrition, and Diet Therapy. 4th ed. Philadelphia, W. B. Saunders Co., 1966.

Lewis, G. M., and Wheeler, C. E., Jr.: Practical Dermatology. 3rd ed. Philadelphia, W. B. Saunders Co., 1967.

Montag, M., and Swenson, R.: Fundamentals in Nursing Care. 3rd ed. Philadelphia, W. B. Saunders Co., 1959.

Pillsbury, D. M., Shelley, W. B., and Kligman, A. M.: A Manual of Cutaneous Medicine. Philadelphia, W. B. Saunders Co., 1961.

Price, A.: The Art, Science and Spirit of Nursing. 3rd ed. Philadelphia, W. B. Saunders Co., 1965.

Sulzberger, M. B., and Whitten, V. H.: Thin Pliable Plastic Films in Topical Dermatologic Therapy. Arch. Dermatol., *84*:1027, 1961.

Williamson, P.: Office Procedures. 2nd ed. Philadelphia, W. B. Saunders Co., 1962.

Witten, V. H., and Sulzberger, M. B.: Newer Dermatologic Methods for Using Corticosteroids More Efficaciously. Med. Clin. North America, *45*:857, 1961.

nursing techniques in the care of
Diseases of the
Nervous System

DIAGNOSTIC PROCEDURES

NEUROLOGICAL EXAMINATION

The clinical examination of the human nervous system differs considerably from that of other areas of the body. From the neurological examination the physician attempts to gather data that will aid in localizing a disease process. In addition to noting the general physical and mental status of the patient, the neurological examination includes the following:

1. Speech and language functions
2. Head and neck
3. Motor system
4. Station and gait
5. Coordination
6. Cranial nerves
7. Reflexes
8. Sensibility
9. Other special tests
10. Spinal column

The nurse should have some understanding of what the physician hopes to determine through the examination so that she can assist efficiently.

SPEECH AND LANGUAGE FUNCTIONS

The testing of these functions may include:
1. Observation of patient's spontaneous speech
2. Recognition and naming of objects such as pencil, key, penny, matches and scissors
3. Repetition of words, phrases and short sentences
4. Understanding of a series of commands such as "Protrude tongue," "Close eyes," or "Raise hand"
5. Tests for ability to read
6. Ability to write name and address or short sentences, or copy a paragraph.

HEAD AND NECK

Examination of the head includes observation of shape and size, palpation for depressions and ridges, percussion to detect tenderness or to detect abnormal sounds and auscultation to detect abnormal circulatory murmurs.

MOTOR SYSTEM

Muscle status is determined by palpation, observation and by comparing measurements of the two sides of the body.

The examiner may discover alterations in the muscle tone of the extremities by passively and slowly moving the relaxed extremity in all possible directions. He discovers extensor hypertonus of the leg by lifting the thigh just above the popliteal fossa. When the patient is instructed to relax the leg at the knee, the foot normally drops to the bed. If extensor hypertonus is present, the foot will drop slightly, then kick upward.

The tone of specific muscles is determined with a percussion hammer.

Decreased muscle tone is determined by hyperflexion and hyperextension of the limbs. If the examiner stands behind the patient and swings the patient's relaxed arms back and forth across the chest, floppiness or hypotonia of the hands can be seen.

Muscle power is determined by flexion of various parts of the body against resistance.

Abnormal movements such as tremors are noted during rest or action.

STATION AND GAIT

The examiner detects gait disturbances by asking the patient to walk forward, backward and sideways, turn quickly, run and stand or walk with eyes closed.

COORDINATION

Tests to determine incoordination include touching the tip of the nose with the index fingers with eyes open and closed, touching the tips of the index fingers; pouring water from one glass to another; and placing the heel of one foot on the knee of the opposite leg and sliding the heel down the anterior border of the tibia with eyes open and shut.

CRANIAL NERVES

Disturbances of the cranial nerves are determined as follows:

I. Olfactory
Substances with characteristic odors such as coffee, tobacco, soap, oil of cloves and oil of peppermint are placed beneath each nostril separately with the other nostril occluded to test the sense of smell.

II. Optic
Visual acuity (see p. 333) is tested with specially designed cards. The patient's corrective glasses should be worn.

Color vision is tested with various colored yarns or cards.

The examiner tests the visual field by asking the patient to sit and gaze at the examiner's eyes. Covering one of the patient's eyes, the examiner moves a finger or small object in an arc from behind the patient toward his visual field. The patient indicates when he first sees the object (see p. 334).

An ophthalmoscopic examination is carried out to determine the size of vessels and observe the optic disc. A complete examination requires the instillation of a mydriatic.

III, IV and VI. Oculomotor Trochlear and Abducens
The third, fourth and sixth cranial nerves are examined together, since they are all

concerned with movements of the eyeballs.

The size and shape of pupils are observed in a semidarkened room. A light is flashed into the eye to determine reaction to light.

To test ocular movements the examiner asks the patient to hold the head still and follow the movement of a moving object or finger.

V. Trigeminal

The fifth cranial nerve supplies all superficial sensation to the face and mucous membranes of the eye and buccal cavity. Sensations are tested with cotton, pinprick, heat and cold. The corneal reflex is elicited by touching the corneoscleral junction with a wisp of cotton. The response is a sudden wink. To test the muscles of mastication the examiner has the patient open the jaw, move the jaw from side to side, and bite firmly. The jaw reflex is obtained by tapping the chin horizontally with the mouth half open.

VII. Facial

Taste is tested by placing sour, salt, sweet and bitter stimuli on the protruding tongue with a cotton applicator. Voluntary and involuntary facial movements are observed while the patient smiles, whistles, wrinkles his forehead, closes his eyelids and holds his eyelid closed against resistance.

VIII. Acoustic

Hearing tests with a pocket watch and tuning fork are used to test cochlear function. (See also page 347.)

Labyrinthine functions are examined with the caloric and rotation tests. The caloric test consists of stimulating the semicircular canals and recording the responses. Normally when the right ear is stimulated, there is nystagmus to the left and pass pointing to the right. To determine pass pointing, the examiner asks the patient, with arm out-stretched, to point to the examiner's finger. Following right ear stimulation, the normal patient will consistently pass point the finger to the right. The semicircular canals are stimulated by an irrigation of the ear (see p. 350) for about 40 seconds with water at 12° F. above and 12° F. below body temperature. About 2 quarts of solution is needed for each irrigation. During the irrigation the patient lies on a table with the head elevated about 20° above the horizontal, thus bringing the horizontal canal into its maximum position for caloric excitation.

For the rotation test the patient is placed on a revolving chair and rotated ten times in 20 seconds. The rotation is stopped, and the patient is tested for nystagmus and pass pointing.

The caloric test and the rotating test cause vertigo, nausea and sometimes vomiting.

IX and X. Glossopharyngeal and Vagus

These two nerves are tested together. The glossopharyngeal enervates the taste buds on the posterior tongue and is rarely tested. To test the vagus nerve, concerned with the muscles of the larynx, pharynx, and soft palate, the examiner produces the gag reflex with a cotton-tipped applicator and observes the movement of the palatal dome as the patient says "Ah." Nasal speech, regurgitation of fluids through the nose, difficulty in swallowing and a hoarse voice also indicate paralysis of the vagus nerve.

XI. Spinal Accessory

The nerve is tested by means of movements of the sternocleidomastoid muscle by asking the patient to rotate his head and shrug his shoulders.

XII. Hypoglossal

The examiner tests the movements of the tongue by having the patient protrude the tongue, push it against the inside of each cheek, and rapidly move the tongue in and out of the mouth.

REFLEXES

The commonly tested reflexes, the methods of testing, and the normal effects are listed in the table on page 298.

SENSIBILITY

Superficial and deep sensations and the methods of testing are listed in the table on page 298.

REFLEX	METHOD	EFFECT
Jaw	Light blow on center of slightly opened jaw	Closure of jaw
Biceps	Blow on examiner's thumb placed over biceps tendon	Flexion of elbow
Brachioradialis	Styloid process of radius is tapped while fore-arm is in semiflexion and semipronation	Flexion of elbow
Triceps	Blow on triceps tendon just above olecranon	Extension of elbow
Finger flexion	Examiner taps his index finger placed across volar surfaces of phalanges of patient's four fingers	Flexion of fingers and distal portion of thumb
Patellar	Blow on patellar tendon	Leg extends
Achilles	Blow on Achilles tendon	Plantar flexion of foot
Abdominal	Stroke skin of upper, middle and lower abdomen	Contraction of abdominal wall
Cremasteric	Stroke medial surface of upper thigh	Elevation of scrotum and testicle
Anal	Stroke perineal region	Contraction of external anal sphincter
Plantar	Stroke sole of foot	Flexion of toes

SENSE	METHOD
Touch	A wisp of cotton or hair is touched to the skin.
Superficial pain	Sharp point of straight pin or needle is touched to skin.
Temperature	Test tubes containing cracked ice and warm (110° F) water are placed on the skin.
Position	With eyes closed, patient indicates which finger or toe is being grasped. With eyes closed, patient uses one index finger to find that of opposite hand, which is being moved away from searching finger.
Vibratory	A vibrating tuning fork is placed over various bony prominences.
Pressure	A blunt object is used to apply pressure.
Deep pain	Digital compression of increasing intensity is applied.
Two-point discrimination	Two pins, a compass or small pair of calipers are used to determine the minimal distance at which the patient can discriminate between one and two points.
Graphesthesia (traced-figure identification)	Figures are traced slowly on the palm with a pencil or head of a pin.
Stereognosis	The blindfolded patient is asked to identify objects such as a key, pencil, coins and a paper clip by handling them.
Tactile localization	The blindfolded patient is requested to identify with his finger the point where his skin was touched by the examiner.

OTHER SPECIAL TESTS

Special methods used frequently to discover signs of meningeal irritation are as follows.

Nuchal Rigidity. Passive lateral movements of the head are possible, but when the chin is brought forward on the chest, there is limitation of motion and extreme pain.

Brudzinski's Sign. Passive flexion of the head on the chest is followed by flexion of both thighs and both legs.

Kernig's Sign. One leg is flexed at a right angle at the thigh, then an attempt is made to extend the leg at the knee as shown in the opposite column.

When pain and resistance due to spasm of the hamstrung muscles prevent complete extension of the knee, it is known as a positive Kernig's sign.

Lasègue's Test. An attempt is made to flex the thigh at the hip with full extension maintained at the knee. Lasègue's sign is positive when a full 90° angle cannot be formed at the hip joint.

These signs are also present in diseases other than meningitis. Nuchal rigidity is present in

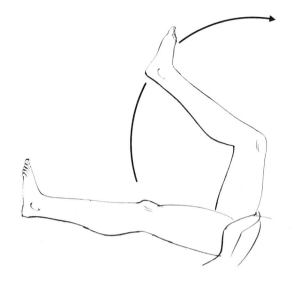

or radiation irritation due to neoplasm in the sacral region.

Examination of the vertebral column includes inspection, palpation, percussion and traction and compression of the neck.

SUPPLEMENTARY EXAMINATIONS

Additional procedures that may be used in diagnosing neurological disorders include an examination of cerebrospinal fluid, x-rays, electroencephalography, electrical testing of muscles, psychological testing and laboratory tests.

EXAMINATION OF CEREBROSPINAL FLUID

neck trauma, cervical arthritis and myositis. The Kernig and Lasègue signs are positive in disorders such as herniated intravertebral disc

The cerebrospinal fluid is obtained for examination by means of a lumbar puncture

CHARACTERISTICS	NORMAL	ABNORMAL INDICATIONS
Pressure	100-200 mm. of water with patient lying on side	Increased in certain brain tumors, hydrocephalus, meningitis, intracranial hemorrhage, brain abscess, cerebral thrombosis, decompensation, uremia, erythremia, edema of brain and sometimes in anterior poliomyelitis and encephalitis. Decreased in a block of the subarachnoid space of the spinal cord and in shock, fainting, dehydration and obstructive hydrocephalus.
Color	Clear and colorless	Bloody in hemorrhage due to trauma or central nervous system pathosis. Yellow (xanthochromic) in fluids removed from below obstructing tumors of spinal cord or vertebrae. Cloudy in meningitis. A fine web (pellicle) forms on top of the specimen when left standing at room temperature in tuberculous meningitis, intra-spinal tumor, anterior poliomyelitis, general paresis and occasionally epidemic encephalitis.
Cell count (lymphocytes)	0-10 per cu. mm.	Increased in all types of pyogenic meningitis, brain abscess impinging on surface of brain, anterior poliomyelitis, some brain and spinal cord tumors, syphilis of central nervous system and sometimes in multiple sclerosis.
pH range	7.35 to 7.40	Fresh fluid less alkaline in pyogenic meningitis.
Total protein*	15-40 mg. per 100 cc.	Increased in conditions due to infection such as meningitis and brain abscess impinging on meninges or ventricular wall; in hemorrhage, cerebral, traumatic, or from brain tumor; in thrombosis; in virus diseases such as poliomyelitis and encephalitis; and after convulsion, in chronic alcoholism or in paralysis agitans.
Glucose	50-80 mg. per 100 cc.	Increased in epidemic encephalitis and anterior poliomyelitis. Decreased in meningitis and metastatic carcinoma in meninges.
Chlorides	720-750 mg. per 100 cc.	Decreased in tuberculous and pyogenic meningitis.

*Pandy's test and Ross-Jones test are sometimes requested for the determination of total globulin.

and a cisternal puncture. The cisternal puncture is used less frequently than the lumbar puncture and is used only when a spinal puncture cannot be performed at the lumbar site.

The equipment is the same for both the lumbar and cisternal puncture.

For the cisternal puncture the patient's neck is shaved as high as the external occipital protuberance. During the procedure the patient lies on his side with his head flexed maximally on the chest.

The specimen of cerebrospinal fluid should be sent to the laboratory as soon as it is obtained because the cell count and sugar values decrease on standing.

The normal characteristics and composition of adult spinal fluid and the abnormal indications are listed in the table on page 299.

Various tests conducted with cerebrospinal fluid include the following:

Colloidal-Gold Reaction. This test is based upon the fact that in certain diseases the sodium chloride content of cerebrospinal fluid precipitates colloidal gold with characteristic color changes. In normal cerebrospinal fluids, the color does not change from the deep red of the gold chloride reagent. Various dilutions of spinal fluid are poured into ten specimen tubes, which are divided into three groups of zones (Zone I, II and III). The color changes are numbered from 0 to 5. The normal deep red is number 0, and a clear color is designated 5. The normal reading for the colloidal gold reaction is 0000000000. A Zone I reaction, read 5555432000, is suggestive of general paresis, taboparesis and multiple sclerosis. A Zone II reaction such as 1123210000 is seen in tabes dorsalis and meningovascular syphilis. A Zone III reaction, 0001234530, is seen in meningitis.

Colloidal-Mastic Test. The principle of this test is the same as that of the colloidal gold test. A gum-mastic reagent is used instead of gold chloride, and the results are read in the same manner as in the colloidal gold test.

Levinson Test. This test is based upon the reaction of an alkaloidal and metallic precipitate. In tuberculous meningitis the precipitate in the metallic dilution is three times greater than the precipitation from the alkaloid dilution. In pyogenic meningitis the ratio is reversed.

Serum Test for Meningococcic Meningitis. A positive reaction is indicative of meningitis.

Bacteriological Studies. Normal cerebrospinal fluid is sterile. A culture is carried out to determine the causative organism in purulent meningitis. Causative organisms may be meningococci, *Hemophilus influenzae*, pneumococci, hemolytic streptococci, staphylococci and occasionally *Escherichia coli*, *Eberthella typhosa* and *Mycobacterium tuberculosis*.

Queckenstedt's Test. This test is done during the spinal puncture when a spinal block is suspected. With the pressure manometer attached to the inserted lumbar puncture needle, pressure is applied to the jugular veins for 6 to 8 seconds. This normally causes a rise in the column of fluid in the manometer. The pressure normally drops upon the release of the jugular compression. When a spinal block is present, the pressure will either rise and fall more slowly on jugular compression and release or will not rise at all.

X-RAYS

Plain Views

The skull, vertebrae and other bones are frequently examined by x-ray. Intracranial calcifications are encountered in chronic subdural hematomas, arteriosclerosis of the larger vessels of the circle of Willis, toxoplasmic encephalitis, tuberous sclerosis, gliomas and other neoplasms.

Because of the importance of diseases of the chest in the production of neurological manifestations, x-rays of the chest are also of value in the neurological investigation.

Contrast Studies

These studies include the ventriculogram, pneumoencephalogram, cerebral angiogram and myelogram.

Ventriculogram. A ventriculogram is done on those patients in whom there is reason to suspect a space-occupying lesion and in whom a localizing diagnosis is difficult. Patients with known or suspected cerebral neoplasms are not subjected to this procedure. In this procedure gas is introduced directly into the cerebral ventricles for the purpose of x-ray visualization. Ventriculography is considered a surgical procedure because two small holes must be made in the skull for the introduction of the needle. Preoperative preparation includes shaving the posterior half of the crown and withholding foods as for general or local anesthesia.

Postoperatively the vital signs are checked frequently (see p. 304). Any evidence of intracranial pressure is reported immediately. The patient is kept in bed with the head elevated 12 to 18 inches for 24 to 48 hours. Sterile brain cannulae are kept at the bedside in case the ventricle must be tapped to relieve increased pressure:

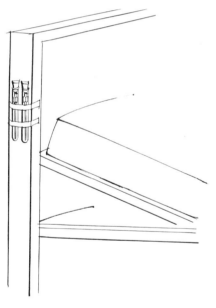

Headaches, nausea and vomiting may occur postoperatively. Ice bags and medications such as caffeine with sodium benzoate and codeine may be used to relieve the headaches that persist until the air or gas is absorbed (2 to 3 days).

Pneumoencephalogram.   Pneumoencephalography is a procedure in which air or other gas such as helium is injected into the cerebrospinal fluid spaces in and around the brain and spinal cord by means of a lumbar

puncture. The patient is seated upright for the procedure, which is carried out in the x-ray department. The patient receives heavy sedation prior to the procedure. General anesthesia is seldom used.

Pneumoencephalography is used more frequently than ventriculography; however, it is not a substitute for ventriculography. Whereas the ventriculogram is useful in intracranial space lesions, the pneumoencephalogram is contraindicated in such cases. Pneumoencephalography is used in cases where an atrophic or degenerative process is suspected.

Food is withheld several hours prior to the studies because of the danger of vomiting.

After following the procedure the vital signs are checked frequently, with special alertness for any signs of intracranial pressure. The degree of nausea, vomiting and headache varies with each patient. Measures to relieve these discomforts include the administration of sedatives and analgesics and the application of an ice bag to the head. The patient is kept in bed with his head slightly elevated for 12 to 24 hours after the pneumoencephalogram.

Cerebral Angiogram.   This method includes the injection of a radiopaque substance (Diodrast or Hypaque) into the blood vessels (see p. 230) for the purpose of visualizing the major vessels of the brain by x-ray. Tumors are thus located by the vessels they displace. Vascular anomalies such as aneurysms are also demonstrated by cerebral angiography. The vertebral and carotid arteries are used to make the injection, the carotid being used more frequently. Injections in both the carotid and vertebral arteries are usually made through the skin. Most surgeons use local anesthesia, but a few give general anesthesia.

After the procedure the patient should be observed for hypotension and shock-like symptoms resulting from hypersensitivity to the iodide contrast media. Other complications to watch for are cerebral swelling and bleeding in the neck.

Myelogram.   To obtain this study, Pantopaque is introduced into the lumbar subarachnoid space, and the dye is observed fluoroscopically in its course along the sub-arachnoid space as the patient lies on a tilting table. This procedure is used to locate intraspinal lesions and other obstructing conditions.

After this procedure the patient is observed for symptoms of meningeal irritation.

Electroencephalography. The electroencephalograph records the electrical activity of the brain and is used most frequently in the diagnosis and classification of the epilepsies and allied disorders. The electroencephalogram is also useful in the localization of brain tumors.

ELECTRICAL TESTING OF MUSCLES

Several methods are used to measure muscle activity. One such test involves the electrical stimulation of a muscle. If the muscle fails to contract when stimulated, *reaction of degeneration* is said to be present. Reaction of degeneration indicates a lesion of the lower motor neuron.

A more exacting test is the strength-duration test. The test reveals the length of time (duration) it takes for a muscle to react to electrical currents of varying intensity (strength). The results of the test are read according to curves. The curve from a degenerated nerve is steep; from a normal nerve it is flat.

Electromyography is used in measuring the activity of the skeletal muscles. Electrode needles are inserted directly into the muscle. The electrical activity of the deep muscle is then recorded as sound and on film. This test is used in the study of lesions of the lower motor neuron. Several weeks after muscle is denervated, spontaneous irregular contractions of individual muscle fibers begin. This is called fibrillation and is not visible to the eye. On the electromyograph, fibrillation produces a clicking when converted to sound. This test is helpful in the differential diagnosis of muscular dystrophy, myositis and neurogenic atrophy.

LABORATORY TESTS

Laboratory tests used in studying the neurological manifestations of metabolic disorders include the benzodioxane test, ferric chloride test, neostigmine test, porphobilinogen urine test, regitine test, and the Thorn test. All of these are discussed in detail in Chapter 20.

Tests for the diagnosis of syphilis include the Wassermann, Kolmer, Kline and VDRL tests. More recently the TPI (treponemal immobilization) test and the TPIA (treponema pallidum immune adherence) test are specific for syphilis, yaws, pinta and bejel but do not differentiate among these disorders.

PSYCHOLOGICAL TESTING

Psychological testing is used to estimate the general intellectual functioning, to recognize special disturbances of brain function and to evaluate the effects of the neurological disorder upon personality behavior.

It is not within the scope of this text to describe in detail all of the tests that can be employed. However, some of the tests in common usage are reviewed in order to correlate their neurological significance.

The Wechsler-Bellevue Intelligence Scales

All of the Wechsler-Bellevue Intelligence Scales are built upon the same model and comprise eleven tests—six are verbal and five are performance. The parts, a brief description, and their significance are listed on the opposite page.

In organic disease the similarities test, block design and digit symbol tests are performed poorly while the information, comprehension and vocabulary tests are less impaired.

Memory Tests

The Wechsler Memory Scale and the Revised Visual Retention Test are two such tests. In these tests the patient is requested to repeat numbers and words and draw designs from a card displayed for a brief period. In cerebral disease the performance of either copying designs or reproducing them from memory is generally inadequate.

WECHSLER-BELLEVUE TESTS

PART	DESCRIPTION	SIGNIFICANCE
Information test	25 questions covering knowledge of every-day subjects common to everyone	Estimates alertness of patient to environment
Comprehension test	10 items in which a hypothetical situation is given with a selection of one of several action responses	
Memory to digits	Numbers are given verbally in forward and reverse order and subject is asked to repeat them	Concerned with attention, maintenance of concentration and memory
Arithmetic test	10 problems to be solved without pencil and paper	
Similarities test	12 items requiring the patient to state in which way certain objects are alike and how they differ	Tests thinking processes in area of verbal concept formation. Concept formation is common to all thinking processes and is thus vulnerable to both maladjustment and disease
Vocabulary test	42 words to be defined	A good single test of intelligence
Picture arrangement	6 sets of cartoon drawings, each with a set of pictures that, when arranged in proper sequence, tell a story	Includes elements of planning, anticipation, and problem solving
Picture completion tests	15 cards upon which are printed a picture with a single part missing. The subject states which part is absent.	Measures basic perceptual and conceptual abilities
Object assembly test	3 jigsaw problems	Tests visual-motor coordination, perception and visual organization
Block design test	Colored blocks to be assembled into a design drawn on cards	Tests spatial organization process in visual-motor coordination
Digit symbol test	An encoding test involving numbers and symbols	Visual and motor activities as well as learning process

Specific Tests of Brain Disease

Some of the specific tests are the Babcock-Levy Mental Deterioration Test, the Hunt-Minnesota Test for Organic Brain Damage and the Shipley-Hartford Retreat Scale for measuring intellectual impairment and deterioration. These tests employ factors such as psychomotor speed, memory reasoning and various performance tests. Most of them use a vocabulary test as a measure of original capacity for comparison. This is a questionable technique.

OTHER TESTS

Several other tests used in diagnosing neurological disorders include the following.

Sweating Pattern Tests. Loss of sweating on a skin area corresponds closely to the sensory loss which accompanies peripheral nerve injuries. Sweating pattern tests are carried out following the induction of perspiration by giving the patient aspirin and hot tea and placing him in a warm room or by giving pilocarpine hydrochloride.

In the starch-iodine test, also called Minor's test, the area is painted with an aqueous iodine solution, then dusted with powdered starch. Where sweating occurs, a blue-black color appears, while the dry areas remain white.

In the cobalt chloride test the area is painted with a saturated cobalt chloride solution in 95 per cent alcohol, and the perspiring area turns from blue to red.

For the quinizarin dye test the area is powdered with the reddish-gray dye, and the sweating changes the color to a deep purple.

Several tests used in diagnosing myasthenia gravis may include the following:

Neostigmine Test. Neostigmine methylsulfate (1.0 to 2.0 mg.) is administered intramuscularly. If the patient has myasthenia gravis, a definite increase in muscle strength is seen in 30 minutes. When larger doses of neostigmine are used (1.5 to 2.0 mg.), 0.6 mg. atropine sulfate is usually given shortly before the neostigmine to prevent abdominal cramps.

Tensilon Test. This is a more rapid test in which 2 mg. Tensilon is administered intravenously. Increased strength occurs within one minute.

Curare Test. A small dose of curare is administered intravenously. If myasthenia gravis exists, the patient will suddenly feel weaker. This test has hazards and is carried out only when equipment and personnel are on hand for intratracheal intubation and resuscitative methods.

Cystometry as discussed on page 261 is used in evaluating bladder function.

THERAPEUTIC AND REHABILITATIVE PROCEDURES

Because of the multiphasic character of many of the neurological disorders, the format of this chapter is altered somewhat from that of the remaining chapters. Here nursing techniques are discussed in their relationship to specific problems commonly encountered in neurological nursing.

OBSERVING THE STATE OF CONSCIOUSNESS

One of the most important observations of the neurological patient is that of the state of consciousness. This observation is essential following any interference in the brain and spinal column whether it be through disease, trauma or surgical procedures.

Unconsciousness may be slight, moderate or profound. It is described in the milder instance as a feeling of being dazed or as being able to hear but not understand what occurs in the environment. In more severe cases it varies from loss of contact with the surroundings with awareness but not identification of happenings to stupor and coma.

When frequent observations of the state of consciousness are important as after cranial surgery or cranial trauma, the state of unconsciousness can best be determined by noting the degree of disorientation at frequent intervals. The degree of disorientation can be determined by addressing the patient by name. If he responds, he can be asked what day of the week it is and the time of the day as morning, afternoon or evening. If the patient does not respond to questions, he should be commanded to move a part of his body, as open

the mouth or stick out the tongue. If he does not respond to a command, observe his reaction to a painful stimulus such as a pinch.

A continued record of these observations is important for comparison of progress. If the patient's response is reduced or slower than before, the resident should be called immediately.

OBSERVATION OF VITAL SIGNS

Next to the degree and duration of unconsciousness, marked changes in body temperature and respiratory rate are the best index of the severity of brain trauma. Changes in pulse rate and blood pressure may also be significant. Actually, no specific change in any of the vital signs can be singled out as being indicative of cerebral trauma. For example, the temperature may be abnormally elevated or lowered, the respirations may be rapid and irregular or slow and irregular, the pulse may be rapid and weak or slow and full, and the blood pressure may be elevated or lowered. For this reason any marked change in vital signs should be reported immediately.

CARE OF THE EYES

Frequently an eye may become edematous after intracranial trauma (as after a craniotomy, cerebrovascular accident, or injury resulting from an accident). When conjunctival edema occurs, the treatment includes normal saline eye irrigations and compresses to keep the exposed edematous eye moist and clean. Antibiotic solutions may be used to prevent infection. Periocular edema is reduced by the application of ice. Ice is best applied in a small plastic bag held in place with scotch tape.

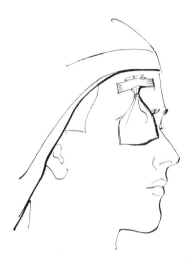

A rubber glove may be used if a plastic bag is not available.

A complication of facial nerve paralysis is corneal drying because the patient cannot close his eyelid. To protect the eye from drying, scarring and ulceration, a transparent protective shield is placed over the eye and sealed to the face around the edges. Moisture condenses on the inside of the shield, thus preventing dryness. The method of making this protective shield (Buller shield) is described and illustrated in detail on page 339. Note that when using a shield for this purpose the shield is sealed around the entire edge rather than left open at the outer edge as mentioned on page 339. Some physicians prescribe an eye instillation of mineral oil or castor oil and the application of eye dressings instead of the Buller shield. The techniques for the eye instillation and dressings are discussed in Chapter 18.

RESTLESSNESS

When the patient is extremely restless and apprehensive, side rails are put on the bed. Restraints are seldom used because tugging and straining at restraints causes the arterial

blood pressure to rise. Such a rise in blood pressure may precipitate intracranial bleeding after a cerebrovascular accident or after brain surgery. Sedation and narcotics are used with caution because they mask the signs of intracranial pressure. Aspirin is usually given for headache after intracranial trauma and surgery. Paraldehyde and chloral hydrate may be given for restlessness. The nurse should realize that restlessness may be due to another factor such as a distended bladder. When there is danger that the restless patient will remove dressings or tubes, the hands can be mittened with cotton stockinette as shown:

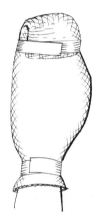

CONVULSIONS

Convulsions may occur after craniotomy, cerebrovascular accident, and head injury in patients who have no previous history of seizures. For this reason padded tongue blades are kept at the bedside of such a patient for insertion between the teeth in the event of a convulsive seizure.

SEEPAGE OF CEREBROSPINAL FLUID

Occasionally, after head injury and craniotomy, cerebrospinal fluid drains from the nose and ear. This drainage should be encouraged. If possible place the draining area lowermost. The nose and ear should not be plugged with cotton or gauze. The patient should be instructed not to sniff back the drainage, blow his nose or smoke.

Cerebrospinal fluid drainage may be seen

on dressings as a clear wet area surrounding a bloody stain.

RESPIRATORY PROBLEMS

Maintenance of an adequate airway is of particular importance for comatose patients, convulsive patients, and patients with cervical lesions of the spinal cord.

Methods of maintaining an adequate airway and preventing pulmonary complications are as follows:

1. The comatose patient is placed flat in bed, preferably on his side to aid drainage of tracheobronchial secretions. The pharynx and trachea are suctioned as often as necessary (see p. 220).
2. In patients with bulbar paralysis, a tracheotomy may be necessary (see p. 353).
3. Oxygen by mask or tent (see Chap. 4) is administered to comatose patients and to patients with pulmonary complications. Carbogen (95 per cent oxygen, 5 per cent carbon dioxide) may be administered by mask in preference to oxygen.
4. Pulmonary complications are frequent in cerebrovascular accidents and in cervical cord lesions; therefore, particular attention is given to turning these patients frequently and to carrying out measures to evoke coughing (see p. 219). Quadriplegic patients have weak abdominal muscles and consequently find it difficult to cough. An abdominal binder is sometimes prescribed to give the patient abdominal support.
5. The artificial respirator may be needed in cases of cord lesion (see Chap. 5).
6. Drugs such as morphine are avoided because of their medullary depressant action.
7. Special mouth care (see p. 159) is a prophylactic against pulmonary complications.

THE NEUROGENIC BLADDER

A bladder disorder due to neurologic disease is called neurogenic bladder.

Bladder dysfunction is the rule in numerous neurological disorders. In order to have a better comprehension of this consequence in neurologic disorders, the reader should review the anatomy and physiology of the vegetative nervous system. The five types of neurogenic bladder are summarized in the following outline.

I. Sensory atonic bladder
  A. Lesions
    1. Acute shock stage of spinal injury
    2. Tabes dorsalis
    3. Diabetic radiculitis
    4. Subacute combined sclerosis
  B. Bladder sensation—none
  C. Capacity—greatly increased
  D. Residual urine—present in large volumes
  E. Early signs—incomplete emptying
  F. Late signs—overflow incontinence, dribbling
  G. Comments
    1. This type merges into reflex bladder as shock subsides unless overdistention causes loss of muscle control
    2. Danger of infection is great. Infection may prevent improvement.
II. Motor atonic bladder
  A. Lesions
    1. May be part of result of spinal shock
    2. Poliomyelitis
  B. Bladder sensation—present
  C. Capacity—greatly increased
  D. Residual urine—present in large volumes
  E. Early signs—incomplete emptying, sensation of distention
  F. Late signs—overflow incontinence, dribbling
  G. Comments—Infection is common. It delays and may prevent restoration of muscle control.
III. Autonomous bladder
  A. Lesions
    1. Traumatic lesions of sacral cord or conus
    2. Spina bifida
    3. Traumatic lesions of nervi erigentes
  B. Bladder sensation—none
  C. Capacity—variable, usually under 600 cc.
  D. Residual urine—small amount
  E. Early signs—inability to void, distended bladder

F. Late signs—straining or dribbling

G. Comments—Infection is likely but not as pronounced as with atonic types. Patient may be able to express some urine by straining or manual compression.

IV. Reflex bladder

A. Lesions

1. Traumatic lesions above sacral level after period of shock
2. Spinal cord tumor
3. Multiple sclerosis

B. Bladder sensation—vague sense of fullness

C. Capacity—slightly increased or reduced

D. Residual urine—present in variable amounts

E. Early signs—inability to void, large volume of residual urine

F. Late signs—voiding sudden and uncontrollable

G. Comments—Infection a danger. Patient may discover "trigger areas" for induction of micturition such as friction on thighs or pressure on lower abdomen.

V. Uninhibited bladder

A. Lesions

1. Cerebral arteriosclerosis
2. Brain tumor
3. Brain injury
4. Incomplete lesions of spinal cord

B. Bladder sensation—normal

C. Capacity—decreases

D. Residual urine—none

E. Signs—urgency incontinence, frequency of urination

F. Comments—Function is regained more rapidly than in other forms.

Incontinence due to neurogenic causes may be managed in several ways. An indwelling catheter may be inserted into the bladder. If there is hope that bladder function can be restored, the catheter may be clamped and opened for drainage at 2- to 4-hour intervals. A bladder that is drained continuously will lose its muscle tone and its normal capacity. Sometimes tidal drainage apparatus is used to provide automatic filling and emptying of the bladder (see p. 274).

As a rule, an indwelling catheter is not used for long periods of time because of the danger of infection. As a foreign body it causes irritation of the mucous lining of the bladder and in turn predisposes to cystitis. In the male patient prolonged use of an indwelling catheter predisposes to epididymitis.

When the patient has an indwelling catheter all measures used for the maintenance and function as discussed in Chapter 15 are also applicable here.

Drugs such as Banthine and atropine are used in controlling bladder function. Infection is kept at a minimum with the aid of drugs such as calcium mandelate and Gantrisin.

Urological care is important especially in the rehabilitation of the quadriplegic and paraplegic patient both during hospitalization and following discharge. The restoration of bladder function for this group of patients is directed toward training the bladder to empty on a schedule. In the hospital a routine should be set up so that the patient attempts to void at regular intervals. Hourly intervals are sufficient for a beginning. When this is achieved, the interval is gradually lengthened. The schedule should be maintained for 24 hours. The patient is taught manual expression of urine. When possible, the sitting position should be maintained between voidings, as this helps the patient to retain urine. A long-term regimen during and after hospitalization includes an adequate daily intake of fluids, observation of urine for cloudiness, frequent urinalysis and acid-alkaline tests, periodic flat plate of kidneys, report of a persistent temperature elevation and maintenance of good health through diet, exercise and rest.

Until a schedule for emptying the bladder is achieved by the patient, there will be continual dribbling of urine. Urinals or other external collection devices are usually used for the collection of urine. A number of male and female urinals are currently designed for use.

The male urinals are designed for both ambulatory (through wheelchair, etc.) and bedridden patients. Most are made with shields of soft rubber that fit snugly over the penis. A urinal for an ambulatory patient is shown here.

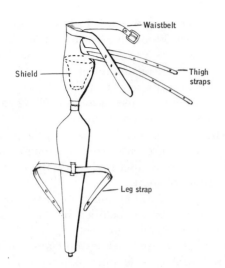

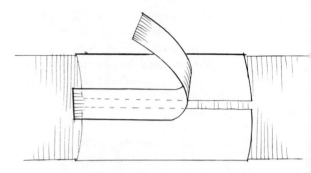

The lined strip may then be pinned to a sanitary belt as shown:

A urinal can also be made by taping a piece of Penrose drain to a rubber drainage tube as shown:

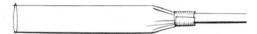

To apply this device, the penis is first cleansed and dried. Tincture of benzoin can be applied to the skin. The foreskin is pulled back over the glans and the Penrose drain, rolled back, is then rolled over the penis. Thin adhesive or elastoplast tape may be used to prevent the Penrose drain from sliding off the penis. The drain should fit snugly but should not be constricting.

When these devices are being used, the penis should be checked frequently for areas of excoriation.

The female patient usually finds urinals unsatisfactory and prefers the use of pads. A sanitary belt with two pads may be worn under rubber-lined panties. A number of styles of plastic panties with inner pockets for disposable absorbent pads are also currently available at surgical supply stores; with a little ingenuity the nurse can design protective briefs for the hospitalized female patient. The design of the brief should suit the patient's pelvic structure and should be made to accommodate the patient's needs.

A strip of muslin or old sheeting about 5 inches wide may be lined with plastic. The plastic can be fastened to the outside of the material with masking tape as shown.

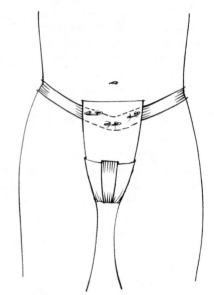

The patient can loosen and fasten this arrangement herself.

A more satisfactory arrangement for the patient who is unable to help herself can be made with two triangles lined with plastic fastened to the inside with tape.

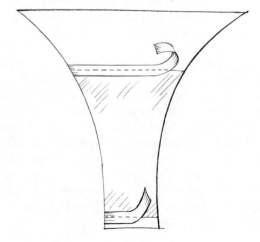

The triangles are pinned at the waist and overlapped and pinned at the perineum as shown.

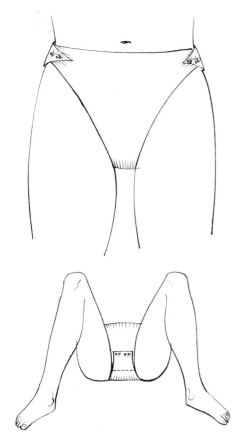

This arrangement enables the nurse to open the bottom and change absorbent pads without removing the entire garment. This protective garment fits snugly and will hold several surgical absorbent pads in place.

Any protective covering the nurse may design for the female patient should be as brief as possible and should not be bulky. Anything large, square and bulky looks too much like a diaper and has a negative psychological impact on the patient. Even though the patient may not express such feelings, she cannot help being embarrassed.

GASTROINTESTINAL PROBLEMS

Nursing procedures related to the gastrointestinal system include special feeding methods and methods to maintain or restore bowel function.

Feeding may be a problem in a number of neurological disorders. Tube feedings (see p. 161) are given when oral feeding is not possible within several days after a cerebrovascular accident. In high lesions of the spinal cord, such as those resulting in quadriplegia, peristalsis may be absent for a week or longer. During this time gastrointestinal suction (see p. 158) and rectal tubes (see p. 310) are used to relieve distention. When peristalsis returns, oral feeding is begun. In the paraplegic, oral feedings are usually tolerated from the start. The hemiplegic, paraplegic and quadriplegic usually have poor appetites and are fed small amounts at frequent intervals.

When facial paralysis is present as after a cerebral accident or a craniotomy, it is easier for the patient to eat if he lies on the unaffected side. A facial sling on the affected side as shown may give support to the drooping mouth and lessen excessive drooling.

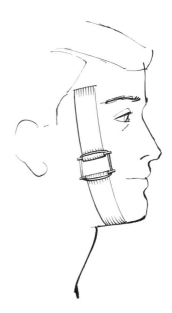

When facial paralysis is present, it may be also helpful at first to give liquids with a rubber-tipped Asepto syringe.

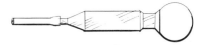

Frequent enemas are necessary to prevent a fecal impaction and, in some cases, to aid in restoring bowel function. When the condition of the bowel is such that retention of the enema solution is impossible, special techniques must be employed in order for the enema to be effective.

One method of helping the patient retain the enema solution is to hold the buttocks together during the administration as shown:

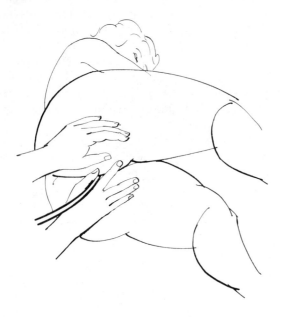

It may be necessary to leave the tube in place and hold the buttocks in this manner for 10 or 15 minutes after the total amount of enema solution has been given.

The Virden-Bardex enema tube is also a useful device. This tube has a 30 cc. inflatable balloon which helps the patient to retain the solution. The balloon is inflated with a compression bulb as shown.

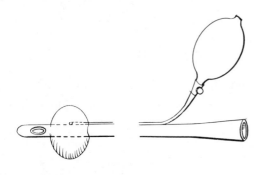

The inflatable enema tube is inserted about 4 to 5 inches, then the balloon is inflated by compressing the bulb 3 to 4 times. The metal

screw is then tightened so that the air remains in the balloon. The inflated tube is left in place for 10 to 15 minutes after the solution is administered, then the airflow valve is released and the tube removed.

When the establishment of automatic bowel control is attempted, the patient should be placed on the bedpan at the same time daily. When daily enemas are part of the bowel control program, the enema should be given at the same time daily. While the patient is on the bedpan, his abdomen should be gently kneaded as shown to aid evacuation.

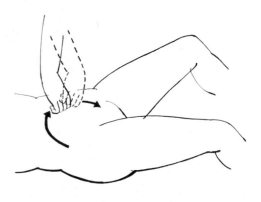

The patient may be taught to do this himself.

Applying pressure to the abdomen with the palms of the hands while the patient blows air through tightened lips will further aid evacuation. When reflexes become more active, pinching the abdomen or scratching the thigh may be of help.

With a program such as this, the bowel can be trained to evacuate regularly and completely at the established time daily or every other day.

Until the bowel is trained, it may be necessary for the patient to wear a protective garment of some sort. Here again the nurse is left to devise some type of protection that best suits the patient's particular needs. Unlike the brief garments illustrated for urinary incontinence, the protective garment for fecal incontinence must cover the buttocks and fit snugly around the upper thighs. In spite of this, the protective covering need not be large and bulky.

A large square of old sheeting folded and fastened like this seems to be the best suited to the contours of the adult pelvis.

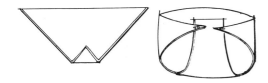

This design fits snugly, is neat in appearance, and comfortable to the patient. The fact that the pins are not fastened at the area over the bony prominences of the pelvis is also helpful in preventing skin excoriations.

The best inner lining for the protective panty is a disposable diaper with a plastic backing. The side with the plastic is placed away from the patient's skin. By all means, do not get the disposable diaper confused with the disposable bed pads, which have a stiff paper backing. Believe it or not, we have seen disposable bed pads used for this purpose!

In addition to all of the techniques just mentioned as being part of the bowel rehabilitation program, the patient's diet also plays an important role. The diet must contain enough bulk to prevent constipation and must eliminate foods that cause liquid stools. The dietary requirements for bowel regulation will be different for each patient.

SKIN PROBLEMS

The nurse is well aware of the ever-present possibility of the decubitus ulcer on the bedridden patient. This possibility is even greater in the paralyzed patient. For this reason the use of soap and water, heat lamps, doughnuts, air rings, bed cradles, foam mattresses and alternating pressure pads should be emphasized here. Frequent back rubs and turns in bed are also important. Vigilance in the prevention of decubitus ulcers cannot be dismissed after the patient is allowed out of bed. Even then, excoriations may develop on the paralyzed part from bumping it against the wheelchair or from dragging it across the sheets.

The unconscious patient should be bathed daily and the skin should be dried briskly to stimulate circulation. If the skin is dry it should be lubricated with lanolin or cold cream. The nails of an unconscious patient should be kept short. Many patients scratch themselves as the depth of consciousness becomes more shallow.

ORTHOPEDIC PROBLEMS

The rehabilitation of the paralyzed patient may be hindered by the development of muscle and joint deformities. Many of these deformities can be prevented by the application of a few simple nursing techniques employed in the daily care of the patient. For some reason nurses seem to associate the principles of good body mechanics only with the normal moving body and forget that the same principles also apply to the paralyzed body. It is erroneous to assume that the responsibility for muscular rehabilitation of the paralyzed patient rests entirely upon the physiotherapy department. The patient may not be referred to the physiotherapy department for several weeks or more after the initial onset of paralysis. In this length of time numerous deformities will develop if measures are not incorporated in the nursing plan to prevent them.

When joints are not exercised in their full range of motion daily, the muscles supplying the motion gradually shrink, forming what is known as a contracture. When a contracture is allowed to develop, the contracture must first be corrected before the patient can begin learning how to use the part. For example, if a paraplegic patient develops foot drop, the foot drop must be corrected before retraining can be begun to teach the patient to walk. It may require several weeks or months to correct the contracture.

Certain contractions are common in the hemiplegic, paraplegic and quadriplegic. Measures to prevent these should be incorporated immediately in the daily care of the patient.

PREVENTIVE MEASURES FOR THE HEMIPLEGIC

The usual position of the affected side in the hemiplegic is as shown:

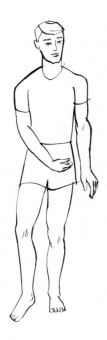

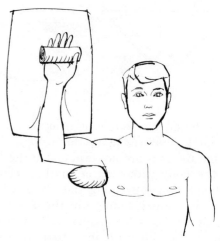

Notice sandbag under axilla, pillow elevating arm, elbow in slight flexion, wrist in extension and fingers in extension.

With the patient in the sitting position the arm is as shown:

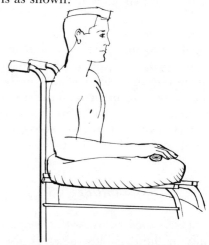

Notice the dropped shoulder, the flexed wrist and hand, the outward rotation of the leg and the extended foot. Keeping this in mind, one can visualize the areas of the body that need attention in positioning the patient.

Alternate resting positions for the arm when the patient is lying on his back are as shown:

The resting position for the leg should include the use of sandbags to prevent outward rotation and a foot board to prevent foot drop as shown.

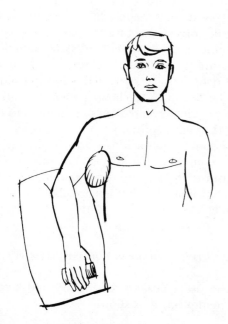

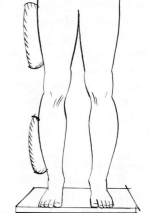

In spastic paralysis, splints are useful for the prevention of wrist drop and foot drop.

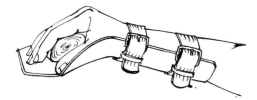

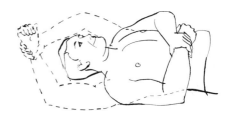

The affected hand must be bandaged to the pulley hand bar to hold it in place.

An exercise for the elbow is as shown. Notice the three positions of motion of the hand.

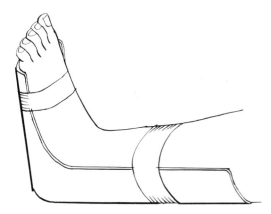

Passive exercises that should be incorporated in daily care include full joint motion of all joints. This need not be a laborious, time-consuming ritual. Five or six motions per joint each day would be helpful. These motions may be done at the time of the daily bath. As soon as the patient's condition permits, he may be taught how to move the affected arm with the unaffected arm. The shoulder is exercised either with or without the use of pulleys as shown.

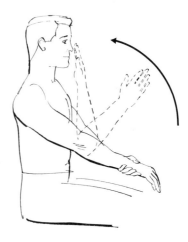

As a hand exercise the patient should be asked to try to flatten his hand on a tabletop. When he can do this, he should extend each finger and the wrist with the unaffected hand.

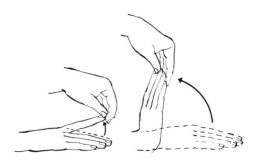

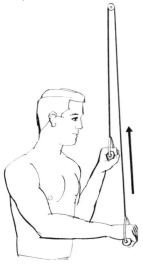

The affected leg may also be moved with the use of the unaffected arm and pulleys and ropes attached to the knee and foot.

A leg exercise known as quadriceps setting should be begun immediately. The popliteal space is pushed downward while an attempt is made to lift the heel.

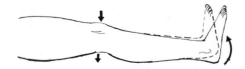

PREVENTIVE MEASURES FOR THE PARAPLEGIC AND QUADRIPLEGIC

The common areas of contracture in the paraplegic are the knee and hip. A complete range of passive motion of these joints should be performed twice daily. For extension of the thigh, the patient must be turned on his abdomen.

Quadriplegia may be caused by trauma' or disease. Traumatic quadriplegia is seen more frequently, and the greatest number have lesions of the sixth or seventh vertebra. A typical patient with a lesion of the sixth or seventh vertebra retains certain movements of the shoulder. In addition, the extensors of the hand may be only partially enervated, so that the patient retains enough grasp to hold large objects in his hand. When the traumatic quadriplegic is first admitted to the hospital, he will be placed in traction (see p. 190) for periods up to 6 weeks. During this time the patient's extremities should be carried through a complete range of motion of all joints twice daily. Finger motion may be maintained by squeezing a rubber ball.

The resting position of the limbs of the paraplegic and quadriplegic should be changed frequently, with specific attention directed toward the prevention of wrist drop and foot drop.

The position of all paralyzed patients must be changed at least every two hours. The hemiplegic should not be turned on the affected side because of circulatory complications. The paraplegic and quadriplegic are placed on special frames discussed in detail in Chapter 12.

AIMING TOWARD SELF-CARE

The ultimate aim, of course, in any rehabilitative program is to gradually retrain the patient to the point where he can achieve the optimum in function. In many neurological disorders the retraining program directed toward self-care begins in the hospital with the nurse playing an important role.

Since the approach toward self-care varies somewhat with various disabilities, each will be considered separately.

APHASIA

Most aphasic patients are those who demonstrate aphasia with accompanying hemiplegia after a cerebrovascular accident. These aphasic patients range from those completely unable to communicate to those who have some command of the language with only minor deficiencies.

At best, aphasia rehabilitation is a slow process. If there is a speech therapy department in the hospital, the aphasic patient is started on a speech rehabilitation program at about the same time an attempt to reestablish balance is begun (see p. 317). Whether or not a trained speech therapist is available, there are several things the nurse can do to help.

1. Talk to the patient as much as possible and then some more. Auditory stimulation through repetitive listening is an important part of the rehabilitation process, since perceiving usually precedes language production.

2. By all means, find some way for the patient to communicate. Unfortunately, there is no standard sign language or code in common use among nurses for use with an aphasic patient. Some institutions have a hand talking chart that contains a few basics in sign language. In some instances it may be difficult for the patient to learn a sign language. Here is a simple device every nurse can make herself that requires no additional learning (i.e. memorizing a sign language) on the part of the persons who are in contact with the patient. Take a piece of cardboard about the size of a sheet of typewriter paper and print a few basic words on it with a heavy crayon or marking pen like this:

YES	SIT	RADIO
NO	LIE	HUNGRY
REPEAT	READ	THIRSTY
COLD	NURSE	PAIN
WARM	DOCTOR	LIGHT
BEDPAN	FAMILY	SMOKE
MOVE	DOOR	WINDOW

0 1 2 3 4 5 6 7 8 9

A B C D E F G H I J K L M

N O P Q R S T U V W X Y Z

The patient expresses himself by pointing to words, numbers or letters. The cardboard ("talking card") can be hung on the head of the bed with a hook made from a large paper clip. Thus it is plainly visible to anyone who approaches the patient for conversation. A second talking card for use in discussing dietary likes and dislikes may be made by using different words or possibly pictures pasted on a piece of cardboard.

3. Encourage the patient to move his tongue from side to side as rapidly as possible and to try to whistle. This helps in regaining control of the muscles of speech.

4. When the patient begins to make sounds, repeat a letter of the alphabet to him while at the same time encouraging him to speak the same letter.

Persons working around an aphasic patient should be cautioned not to treat the patient like a child. Even though the tasks he must learn are those taught to children, he is not a child and does not think like one.

HEMIPLEGIA

In the absence of any medical contraindications, self-care and other nonwalking daily activities are taught as soon as the patient is conscious enough to assist in rolling over in bed, in feeding himself and in sitting up. In retraining for these activities, emphasis is placed on the use of the unaffected limbs. If there is sufficient sensory and motor function in the affected limbs, they may be used as well.

The first three activities, then, that the nurse should begin teaching simultaneously to the hemiplegic patient are rolling over in bed, feeding himself and sitting. Perhaps it might be well to mention at this point that it most certainly is much easier and less time-consuming for the nurse to do all of these things for the patient than for her to teach him to do them for himself. It is also difficult for the nurse to stand by and watch the patient struggle in his attempt at self-care. The nurse should realize, however, that by encouraging the patient to do things for himself, she is really suggesting that he will be able to learn these activities. This creates and maintains a hopeful atmosphere. It is a known fact that once the patient feels hopeless, his chances for rehabilitation are reduced. For this reason also, the importance of initiating the self-care program as soon as the patient is conscious is emphasized. The longer the self-care program is delayed, the more hopeless the patient becomes.

Teaching the Hemiplegic to Roll Over

1. A firm mattress with a bed board makes all bed activities easier.

2. Teach the patient to assist himself in moving by grasping an overhead trapeze bar (see p. 183) or the side rails on the bed.

3. Put the bedside table on the affected side so that he can turn over and reach for articles he needs.

Teaching the Hemiplegic to Sit

The objectives in teaching the hemiplegic patient to sit are twofold:

1. He must learn to pull himself to a sitting position.

2. He must learn to balance himself in the sitting position. A heavy rope tied at the bottom of the bed as shown

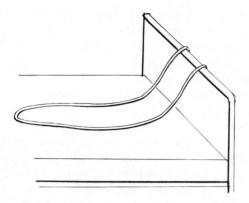

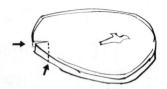

If the meat is hard to cut, a sharp knife is a necessity.

3. He can break bread or rolls like this:

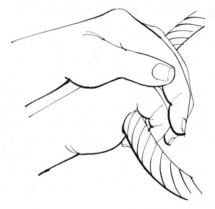

seems to be the most suitable device for assisting the patient. The patient places his affected hand over the rope and holds it in place with his good hand as shown.

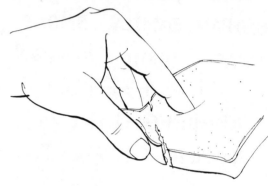

In this manner he can pull himself to a sitting position and steady himself while he is sitting.

With hard rolls, first crush the roll in the fist before breaking it. Bread or rolls can be buttered by merely pressing down fairly hard on the butter knife as the butter is drawn across it. This pressure keeps the bread from sliding.

Teaching the Hemiplegic to Eat

1. Allow him to practice first with soft foods such as mashed potatoes, puddings, etc.
2. Teach him how to cut his own meat. Meat can be cut with one hand by holding the knife like this and cutting away from him.

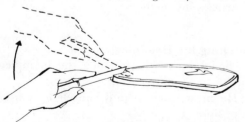

A small cut is made like this. To make a larger cut, simply remove the knife and start afresh. Remove a bite at a time like this:

Teaching the Hemiplegic to Stand

Shortly after the patient has begun to learn to roll over, eat and sit, he learns to stand. The patient need not learn to sit by himself, etc., before he begins standing. If the patient is able to stand with assistance, he should be placed between two chairs placed about 2 feet apart as shown:

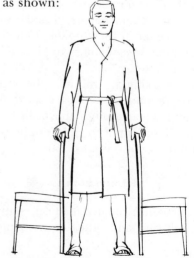

The paralyzed hand is held on one chair by an attendant. The patient is asked to put weight first on one foot, then the other. This maneuver helps to regain standing balance. As soon as this is mastered, ambulation training should be started.

Sitting and standing balance may develop slowly, especially in elderly hemiplegic patients. It is advisable to have such patients rise slowly and pause following a change from supine to sitting position and from sitting to standing position. Quick head turning should also be avoided when the patient is in the erect position because he may lose his balance.

The Tiltboard

When the patient is unable to stand with assistance, it is often helpful to start training in standing balance with a tiltboard. Actually the tiltboard has a number of worthwhile effects. It improves circulation and metabolism and helps to prevent decubitus ulcers. It helps in regaining bladder control and in the prevention of urinary infection. The patient's morale as well is improved by being in the upright position for several hours daily.

There are a number of tiltboards (also called tilt-tables) currently on the market with designs similar to this:

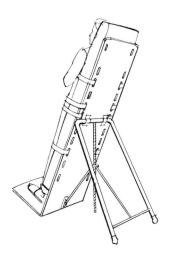

There are also several designs of tilting hospital beds currently being used. One such design is similar to this:

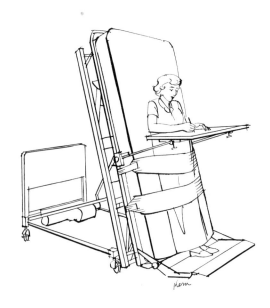

When a tilt-table or bed is not available, an ordinary board 24 inches wide, padded with foam rubber, may be used for short periods of standing like this:

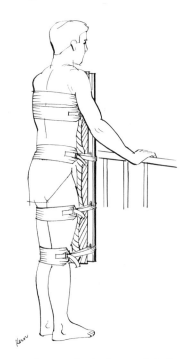

This type is particularly useful for patients who have severe decubitus ulcers.

A board with a footrest is initially better tolerated by the patient because the degree of tilt may be adjusted at various angles.

The board is placed on one side of the bed as shown:

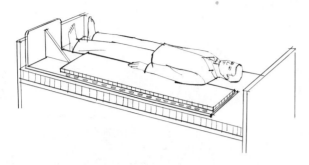

The patient is then placed on the board, and the padded straps are secured in place. By means of the straps, the board is lifted over the bottom of the bed.

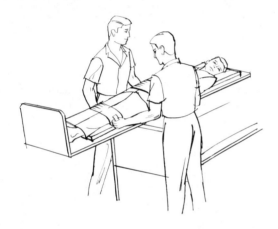

A "homemade" tiltboard may be propped against the foot of the bed like this:

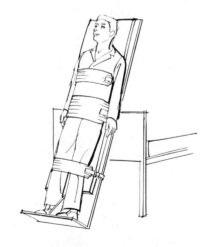

Notice the position of the padded straps—one directly over the knees, one over the pelvic region, and one over the chest. To prevent sliding, the bed wheels are in the locked position. Also the bottom edge of the

tiltboard is covered with protective rubber.

The degree of tilt and the length of time the patient is to remain in this position are prescribed by the physician. While the patient is on the tiltboard, the feet and legs should be kept in good body alignment. A small pillow is placed under the head for support, and a bedside table is placed in front of the patient.

Teaching the Hemiplegic to Walk

As soon as the patient can stand unsupported at a rail or chair, ambulation training is begun. In most institutions ambulation training is directed by a trained physical therapist.

The first step in teaching the patient to walk is gait training. The patient learns this by standing between parallel bars or two chairs (as illustrated previously). He stands on the paralyzed leg and tries to take a step forward with the good leg. Keeping the bad leg in one place, he practices this forward step with the good leg until he is able to achieve a functional step. After he accomplishes a step with the good leg, he tries the same procedure for the paralyzed leg.

A good bed exercise that prepares the patient for the reciprocal gait motion needed in walking may be carried out with a rope and pulleys as shown:

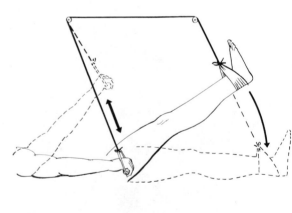

The patient is instructed to pull the arm up by pushing the leg down and vice versa.

Rehabilitative exercises to teach coordination of the upper and lower limbs may be done as follows. The patient lies flat in bed with the bedclothes removed and his head elevated on pillows high enough so that he can see his feet. Three of four sandbags are placed across the foot of the bed, and the patient is instructed to lift a leg and place the heel in the center of each bag. To improve coordination of the arms this exercise is helpful. Place the patient's arms at the side and have him attempt to touch the fingers together. Both exercises are shown here:

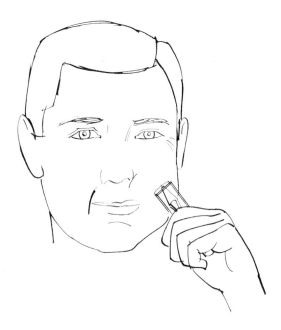

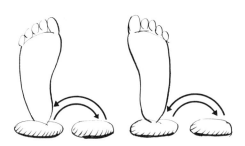

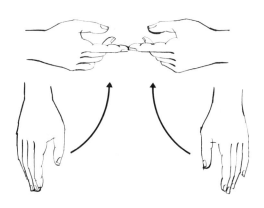

Dressing. Pajama tops, shirts and blouses are put on by first slipping the paralyzed arm into the sleeve, then slipping the good arm in the other sleeve. Outer garments should open in front and have large buttons or snaps. Undergarments which have wide straps and open in front are fairly easily managed. Shoes without laces are more practical. A long-handled shoe horn is sometimes helpful. Buttoned shirt sleeves should be buttoned before putting the shirt on. To unbutton the sleeve before taking off, grasp the outer corner with the teeth as shown and pull open.

Other Activities

Depending upon the extent of the hemiplegic patient's disability, the nurse may be called upon to suggest self-help methods for use both in the hospital and in the home. The nurse should be reminded that, if the patient shows some signs of being able to use his affected arm, he should be encouraged to use it rather than become completely dependent on the unaffected arm.

Shaving. Two-handed people pull on the skin with one hand to tighten the skin while shaving with the other. The same effect is achieved by blowing up the cheek.

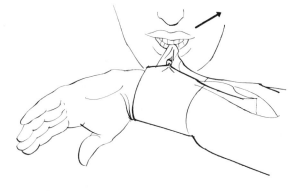

Neckties, both the bow tie and the four-in-hand knot type, are now available in clip-on styles.

Getting a glove in place with one hand is

possible by sewing a loop to the cuff. Hook the loop over a nail or coat button and then slip the fingers in position.

Bathing. Brushes with suction cups attached allow the patient to wash the uninvolved hand and fingers. These brushes look like the surgical scrub brush the nurse uses for handwashing. Two suction cups are fastened on the brush. The brush can be fastened to the washbowl.

A stall shower with side handgrasps is advisable. If a bathtub must be used, the patient can use a portable rubber shower head while he sits on a board which rests on both sides of the tub or on a portable chair in the tub.

Bathroom Needs. Incontinence usually disappears after the patient begins standing. As soon as the patient learns to get in and out of bed without assistance, the bedside commode may be preferable to having the patient walk to the bathroom in the dark. A rail fastened adjacent to the toilet on the unaffected side helps the patient achieve independence in toilet activities.

Housekeeping Activities. Every woman who does her own work knows that a great portion of her time is spent in the kitchen. The nurse can assure the female hemiplegic patient that there are hundreds of other women with her same condition who have learned to function very well in the kitchen. Here are a few suggestions which can be given to the patient for help in kitchen activities.

A board with thin nails protruding holds food items in place for scraping, peeling, slicing and dicing.

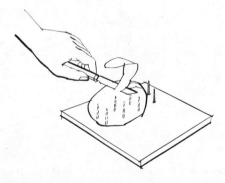

Linens are opened by unfolding rather than shaking.

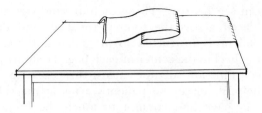

Eggs can be broken with one hand and a mixing bowl can be held in place with a specially designed suction cup, as shown, available at houseware stores:

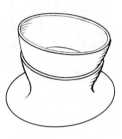

It saves steps to carry articles on a movable cart or a wheelchair tray.

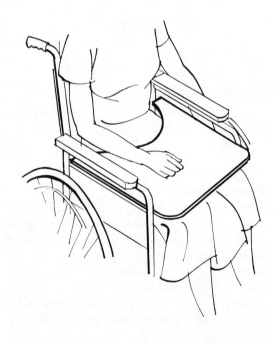

The wheelchair tray also provides work space.

Social Activities. An unawkward handshake is accomplished with the left hand by offering the hand with the palm outward like this:

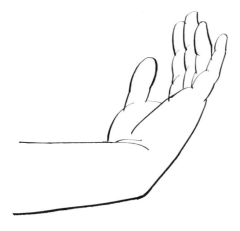

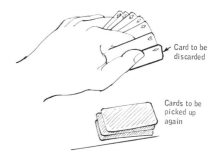

Cards can be shuffled and dealt with one hand like this:

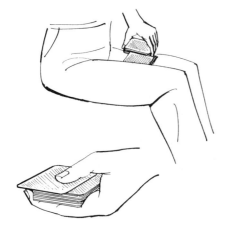

Cards may be fanned out in the hand with the thumb and forefinger like this:

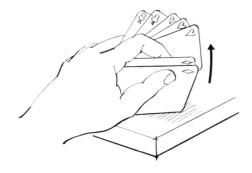

To discard a card or to rearrange the hand, the cards preceding the desired card are placed on the table, then the desired card is pushed out of the hand by holding the next two cards between the hand like this:

Naturally this takes practice. If only two people are playing cards, the patient can place the arranged cards face up on a book held on his lap. Gathering and straightening cards at the end of a game is fairly easy with one hand providing about one third of the cards are straightened at a time.

Wheelchair Activities. If the hemiplegic patient is confined to a wheelchair, he can propel and steer the chair with his good arm and foot as shown:

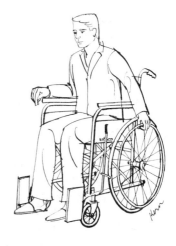

Notice the type of wheelchair that must be used, i.e., one with large wheels in the back, 8-inch wheels in the front and a hand brake. This type of chair is more practical for continued use than one equipped with a one-arm drive because the operation of such a chair requires too much coordination for most hemiplegic patients who require a wheelchair.

The patient should be taught to move from the bed to the wheelchair as shown:

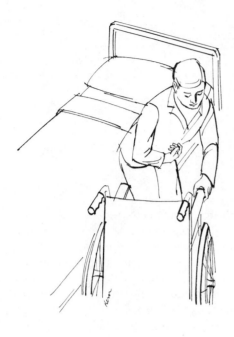

possible, since they discourage independence and rob the patient of a natural form of exercise beneficial for him.

Bed Activities. As soon as the patient is able he should be encouraged to participate in any bed activity which exercises the shoulder depressors, triceps and the latissimus dorsi. Push-up exercises are the most important bed exercises and can be done in these various ways.

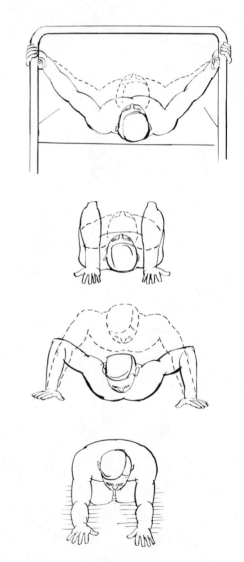

PARAPLEGIA

When the paraplegic patient is first admitted to the hospital, he is placed on an ordinary hospital bed with a foam mattress and bed board or on a Stryker frame (see p. 198). Special nursing care during the early weeks of hospitalization is directed toward skin care (p. 311) and posture (p. 314). Shortly after hospitalization a laminectomy may be done to determine the exact condition of the cord. As soon as the condition of the cord is determined, a rehabilitation program is begun. If there is some hope of return of muscle function, a more conservative approach is usually used. These patients must be protected orthopedically as outlined on page 311 as long as necessary. Those patients whose spinal cord has been irreparably damaged, as determined by an early laminectomy, usually are approached more directly.

The paraplegic must depend solely on the arms and shoulder girdle for locomotive power. He must learn to move in bed, dress and undress himself and put on braces. To do these things, he must learn to sit, change position in bed and roll from side to side. For these operations, it may be necessary at first to use an overhead trapeze and pull-up rope as illustrated on page 183. These devices, however, should be eliminated as soon as

After the patient regains arm and shoulder strength, he should be encouraged to help himself in sliding from one side of the bed to the other, rolling over, pushing himself from the supine to the sitting position and manipulating the bedpan as shown:

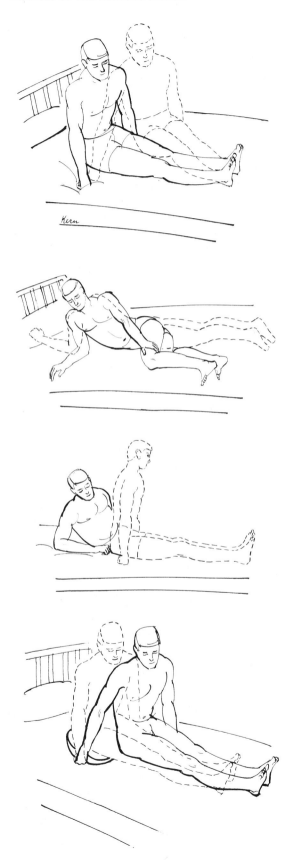

After the patient can sit up by himself, he can begin practicing moving his legs with one arm while leaning on one elbow as shown:

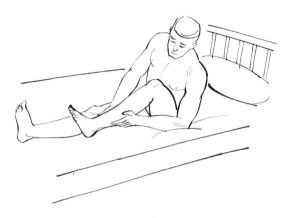

When he is able to do this, he will be able to dress himself and put on braces.

Early Standing. It is important that the paraplegic patient be put in a standing position as soon as possible. Long before many of the bed activities just mentioned are begun, the patient is placed in the erect position on a tiltboard (see p. 317). The initial angle of tilt is usually 20 to 30 degrees. The patient should be watched closely for signs of insufficient cerebral circulation—pallor, sweating, and tachycardia. The angle of tilt and the length of time that the patient can stand are gradually increased.

Other Activities. After the patient is allowed out of bed, he is taught how to move from bed to wheelchair (see p. 325), and other wheelchair activities. During some phase of the retraining program, the patient is fitted for braces. He is then taught crutch walking and the ways in which many activities of daily living are conducted with the aid of crutches. The care and uses of braces are discussed in Chapter 12.

QUADRIPLEGIA

This group of patients will always need some help. Usually they are unable to get from bed to wheelchair without assistance.

A quadriplegic patient with a lesion of the sixth or seventh cervical vertebra should be able to propel his wheelchair if knobs are added to the hand rims so that he can use his biceps rather than triceps muscles. This will enable him to move about in his home, but he will need help outside of his home. With lesions above the sixth cervical vertebra, a patient will be able to do less for himself.

The retraining program for the quadriplegic usually begins with re-education for the muscles that can be used. In the meantime he is placed on the tiltboard starting with a narrow angle and gradually increasing the angle until the erect position is tolerated.

With the aid of self-help devices, many quadriplegic patients can live productive lives. Some of these devices will be discussed here.

Devices to Aid or Support Arm Motions. The selection of a self-help device naturally depends upon the specific needs of the patient. Devices to aid shoulder and elbow motion include the overhead slings and a ball-bearing arm support:

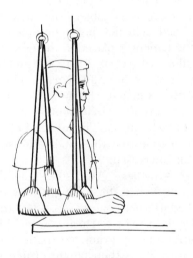

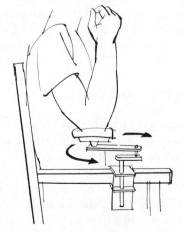

A number of arm splints and braces are also available to aid and support a part or the whole arm.

Eating Devices. Special eating equipment may include suction cup dishes, long straws, nonspillable training cups as used for infants, and knives, forks and spoons with altered handles. Handles fixed onto ordinary items are shown here:

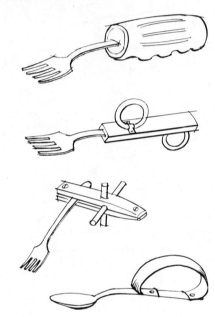

The wooden peg handle assists a weak grasp. The leather strap handle is used when there is complete loss of grasp. The finger rings encourage holding (with thumb and little finger) while using a minimal amount of grasp, and the bicycle grip over glued-on plastic is used when there is limited grasping power.

Dressing Aids. A stick with a closet hook on one end may be useful in removing a garment from the shoulders.

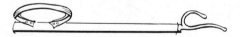

Vertical rather than horizontal buttonholes are helpful.

For men, tapes secured to the shirttail and sock tops help to keep the shirt tucked in. Short-sleeved shirts or blouses with action back pleats are most suitable.

Devices Helpful for Other Activities. A large cork with a hole burned or drilled in it or a clothespin make a pencil-holder.

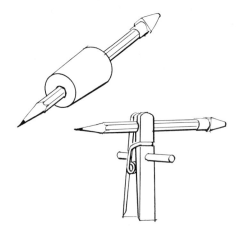

A small piece of plastic (available in sheet or bar form at a hobby shop) glued to a radio knob with plastic cement makes it possible to turn on a radio.

A toothbrush can be made useful by taping it to two tongue depressors.

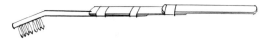

Large plastic curtain rings taped to various articles give added grip. Here rings are used on an electric shaver and cigarette holder.

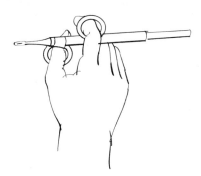

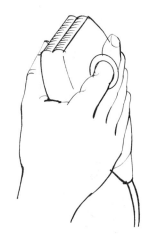

A box will make a card rack as shown:

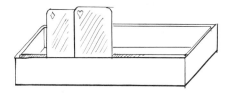

Many additional self-help devices are currently manufactured for the quadriplegic. These include items such as book holders, page turners, telephone holders and a portable mechanical lift to assist the patient in and out of the car.

Suggestions for Assistance. Several suggestions for assisting the quadriplegic patient in moving from one place to another are worth mentioning here.

One person can slide the patient from a wheelchair to a bed like this:

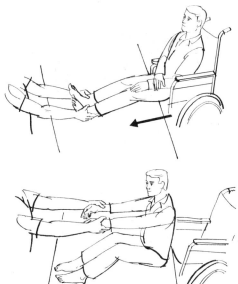

In order for this to be accomplished, the bed (high-low bed) must be level with the chair, the chair must be close to the bed, and the chair must be locked in place. To get the patient out of bed, grasp the arms like this, and stand first on the side of the chair, then step to the back of the chair.

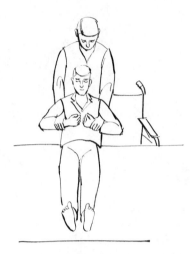

The same method can be used in sliding the patient in and out of a car with a board between the car seat and the wheelchair. When the patient is being moved from the chair to the car, one end of the board is placed under the wheelchair cushion, and the other end is placed on top of the car seat.

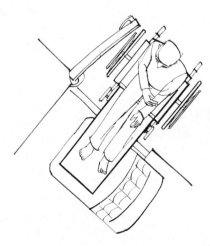

When moving the patient from the car to the chair, place the board on top of the wheelchair cushion.

When constant irritation and discomfort

are caused by the quadriplegic's spastic knees drawing together, something must be placed between the knees to keep them separated. A medium-sized plastic beach ball (inflated by blowing air into it) is a practical device for this purpose. The ball can be inflated with as much or as little air as needed. In addition, it is lightweight, easily cleaned, and inexpensive.

NEUROSURGICAL NURSING TECHNIQUES

BRAIN SURGERY

After brain surgery all the neurological nursing problems discussed previously in this section will be applicable. Immediately after surgery the patient is transferred from the operating room table directly to his own bed in order to eliminate unnecessary moving. The patient's head is placed at the foot of the bed to permit easier access for treatments. The patient is kept quiet and flat in bed. When prescribed, the head of the bed may be elevated about 25° by placing the legs of the bed on shock blocks. The immediate problems include maintenance of an open airway (p. 65), attention toward urinary output and the indwelling catheter (see p. 266), checking the vital signs (p. 304) and state of consciousness (p. 304), watching for convulsions (p. 305) and relieving restlessness (p. 305). The nurse should be aware that hypotensive drugs are administered during brain surgery; hence the blood pressure may be lowered during the immediate postoperative period.

Profound hypothermia (see p. 10) is also used by some brain surgeons. In this event the patient may or may not have a thoracotomy. Recently, profound hypothermia through extracorporeal circulation has been accomplished without a thoracotomy by inserting cannulas through the jugular vein and into the right atrium, and from the femoral vein into the inferior vena cava, and returning the oxygenated blood into the femoral artery. When hypothermia is used, the patient is cared for as outlined on page 15.

The continued care of the patient includes

eye care (p. 304), skin care (p. 311), nutrition (p. 309), bowel care (p. 309), attention toward orthopedic problems (p. 311), and aiming toward self-care (p. 314) in the event of paralysis.

Head dressings are initially changed by the resident and reinforced by the nurse when necessary.

SPINAL CORD SURGERY

The reader is referred to Chapter 12 and to topics earlier in this chapter which pertain to the subject.

PROCEDURES TO REVIEW

Administration of oxygen (Chap. 4)
Radiotherapy used for brain tumors (Chap. 3)
Radioactive isotopes used in scanning for brain tumor (Chap. 3)
Use of respirators (Chap. 5)
Isolation techniques (Chap. 7)
Preoperative and postoperative procedures (Chaps. 9 and 10)
Gastric gavage (p. 161)
Use of orthopedic devices (Chap. 12)
Nasopharyngeal suction (p. 158)
Care of tracheotomy (p. 353)
Special mouth care for comatose patient (p. 159)
Application of heat by means of hot water bottle, heat lamp, etc., for pain of neuralgia and neuritis
Application of cold to reduce edema and relieve headache
Lumbar puncture
Care and observation during a convulsive seizure
Cautious administration of enema with small amounts of fluid to prevent strain
Use of hypothermia apparatus to regulate temperature when heat-regulating mechanism of body is affected (p. 11)
Use of special bedpans for spinal injuries and following lumbar surgery

DIETS TO REVIEW

Liquid to solid consistencies
High thiamine in neuritis due to thiamine deficiency
High caloric, high vitamin, high protein for spinal cord lesions
High protein, between-meal nourishment for patients who cannot eat large amounts at mealtime
Ketogenic for convulsive seizures

MEDICATIONS TO REVIEW

Skeletal Muscle Relaxants. Carisoprodal (Soma, Rela), chlormethazanone (Trancopal), chlorzoxazone (Paraflex), curare (Tubocurarine Chloride, Intocostrin), biperiden (Akineton), diethyl propanediol (Prenderol), mephenesin (Lissephen, Oranixon, Dioloxol, Tolulexin, Tolserol, Sinan, Tolyspaz), methocarbamol (Robaxin), orphenadrine (Disipal, Norflex), phenyramidol HCl (Analexin), styramate (Sinaxar), zoxazolamine (Flexin).

Anticonvulsants. Amino-glutethimide (Elipten), diphenylhydantoin (Dilantin), ethotoin (Peganone), meprobamate (Equanil, Miltown), methsuximide (Celontin), methylphenylethylhydantoin (Mesantoin, Nirvanol), paramethadione (Paradione), phenacemide (Phenurone), promoxolane (Dimethylane), trimethadione (Tridione), primidone (Mysoline).

Tranquilizers. Acetylpromazine (Plegicil), amphenidone (Dornwal), azacyclonol hydrochloride (Frenquel), captodiamine hydrochloride (Suvren), hydroxyzine hydrochloride (Atarax), mepazine (Pacatal), methaminodiazepoxide hydrochloride (Librium), methoxypromazine maleate (Tentone), oxanamide (Quiactin), perphenazine (Trilafon), phenaglycodal (Ultran), prochlorperazine (Compazine), prothipendyl (Timovan), thiopropazate dihydrochloride (Dartal), thioridiazine (Mellaril), triflupromazine hydrochloride (Vesprin).

Parasympathetic Stimulants (for Myasthenia Gravis). Ambenonium (Mytelase, Mysuran), isoflurophate (D.F.P., Floropryl), neostigmine (Prostigmin), pyridostigmine bromide (Mestinon).

Parasympathetic Depressants (for Parkinson's Disease). Belladonna—atropine, hyoscine, hyoscyamine and stramonium—benztropine methane sulfonate (Cogentin), trihexyphenidyl hydrochloride (Artane), cycrimine hydrochloride (Pagitane), ethopropazine

hydrochloride (Parsidol), caramiphen hydrochloride (Panparnit), procyclidine hydrochloride (Kemadrin).

BIBLIOGRAPHY

Alpers, B. J.: Clinical Neurology. 5th ed. Philadelphia,
F. A. Davis Co., 1963.

Beeson, P. B., and McDermott, W.: Cecil-Loeb Textbook
of Medicine. 12th ed. Philadelphia, W. B. Saunders
Co., 1967.

Brown, A.: Medical and Surgical Nursing II. Philadelphia,
W. B. Saunders Co., 1959.

Brunner, L. S., et al.: Textbook of Medical-Surgical
Nursing. Philadelphia, J. B. Lippincott Co., 1964.

Davidsohn, I., and Henry, J. B.: Todd-Sanford Clinical
Diagnosis by Laboratory Methods. 14 ed. Philadelphia, W. B. Saunders Co., 1969.

Davis, L.: Christopher's Textbook of Surgery. 8th ed.
Philadelphia, W. B. Saunders Co., 1968.

DeGutierrez-Mahoney, C. G., and Carini, E.: Neurological
and Neurosurgical Nursing. 4th ed. St. Louis, C. V.
Mosby Co., 1965.

Falconer, M., Patterson, H., and Gustafson, E.: Current
Drug Handbook. 1968-1970. Philadelphia, W. B.
Saunders Co., 1968.

Frost, R. and A.: Handbook for Paraplegics and Quad-
riplegics. New York, Robert Frost, 1951.

Gardiner, M. A. M.: Responsiveness as a Measure of
Consciousness. Am. J. Nurs., *68*:1034, 1968.

Goodale, R.: Clinical Interpretation of Laboratory Tests.
5th ed. Philadelphia, F. A. Davis Co., 1964.

Harmer, B., and Henderson, V.: Textbook of Principles
and Practices of Nursing. 5th ed. New York, The
Macmillan Co., 1958.

Krause, M.: Food, Nutrition, and Diet Therapy. 4th ed.
Philadelphia, W. B. Saunders Co., 1966.

Olsen, E. V.: Hazards of Immobility. Am. J. Nurs., *67*:
779, 1967.

Price, A.: The Art, Science and Spirit of Nursing. 3rd ed.
Philadelphia, W. B. Saunders Co., 1965.

Rothberg, J. S. (ed.): Symposium on Chronic Disease and
Rehabilitation. Nurs. Clin. N. America, *1*:352-532,
1966.

Rusk, H. A.: Rehabilitation Medicine. 2nd ed. St. Louis,
C. V. Mosby Co., 1964.

Sadove, M., and Cross, J.: The Recovery Room. Philadelphia, W. B. Saunders Co., 1956.

Sorensen, K. M., and Amis, D. B.: Understanding the
World of the Chronically Ill. Am. J. Nurs., *67*:811,
1967.

Wohl, M. V.: Long-Term Illness. Philadelphia, W. B.
Saunders Co., 1959.

18

nursing techniques in the care of
Diseases of the Eye

DIAGNOSTIC PROCEDURES

An examination of the eye consists of an external examination, examination by ophthalmoscope and other objective methods, and an examination of the functions of the eye.

EXTERNAL EXAMINATION

The anterior segments of the eyes and their appendages are examined in the most part without the use of special apparatus. The physician notes the general appearance of the eyelids, lashes and eyebrows and lacrimal apparatus. While the patient looks in various directions, the position and motility of the eyeballs are noted. To inspect the conjunctival surface of the upper lid, the physician must evert the lid. The nurse uses the same method when called upon to look for a foreign body. Face the patient when his head is supported by a headrest. When the patient

is sitting in an ordinary chair, it is better for the nurse to stand behind the patient, with the patient's head resting against her body.

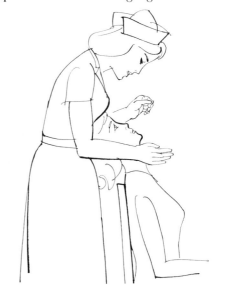

The patient is asked to look down but to keep both eyes OPEN. This is a most important part of the procedure, for in this way the sensitive cornea is kept away from the surface of the lid as it is being turned. Also normal blinking carries with it an upward turning of the eyeball. Grasp the upper lid by the eyelashes and pull down and out.

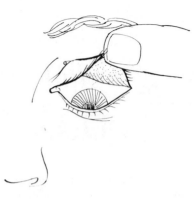

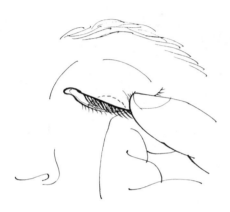

The stick can be removed and the lid held everted with one hand, leaving the other free for further examination.
The lower lid is everted like this:

An applicator, cotton-covered toothpick or pencil is placed on the lid at a spot above the tarsal cartilage, which is firm and cannot be bent. The location of the stick and tarsal cartilage is shown here.

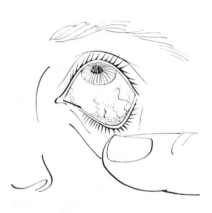

When it is necessary to use a lid retractor, the physician may wish to use a paper clip bent like this:

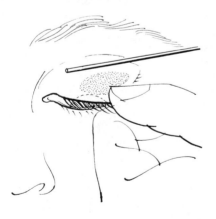

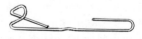

Before a retractor is used, the eye is anesthetized with a few drops of 0.5 per cent Pontocaine, then allowed to rest 5 to 10 minutes.

The physician examines the cornea with a condensing lens, an electric light and magnifying glasses like this:

Press gently backward and downward with the stick, and at the same time pull up on the lashes.

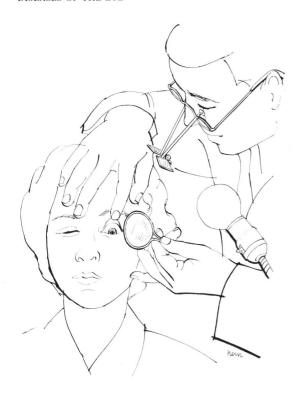

EXAMINATION BY OPHTHALMOSCOPE

By looking through the milled disk of the ophthalmoscope, which carries various lenses, the physician can see various structures of the eye. An ophthalmoscopic examination is best done in a darkened room. See the table below.

EXAMINATION BY OTHER OBJECTIVE METHODS

The Slit Lamp

The slit lamp, an instrument second to the ophthalmoscope in diagnostic importance, is used to examine the anterior segment of the eye. With the slit lamp a brilliant beam of light is focused in such a way that the anterior segments (cornea, lens, and aqueous humor) are seen in layers. This instrument is of value in detecting early cataractous changes.

Transillumination

This method is often necessary in diagnosing intraocular tumors. The value of this procedure lies in the fact that light thrown through the sclera will illuminate the interior of the eye so that a red reflex is seen in the pupil. Any abnormal solid mass of tissue blocks the red reflex. For transillumination a local anesthetic is placed in the eye, and the room is completely dark. The transilluminator is placed against the eye as shown:

The condensing lens is held in such a way that the light is focused on the cornea. Abrasions of the cornea may be detected by instilling one or two drops of 2 per cent aqueous solution of sodium fluorescein. After a few seconds the excess dye is washed out with normal saline solution. The abrasion will show a green coloration. See page 332 for the procedure of a more detailed examination of the cornea.

THE OPHTHALMOSCOPIC EXAMINATION

ANATOMICAL PART	NORMAL	ABNORMAL INDICATIONS
Vitreous body	Transparent	Opacities occur in diseases of the choroid. Patient complains of spots before eye
Optic disk	Vertical oval in shape. Pink in color with a white area where central vessels enter and leave disk. Depression or cupping of disk occurs in temporal area of disk	Disk swollen and margins blurred in optic neuritis as from retinitis, multiple sclerosis, herpes zoster, syphilis, tuberculosis, acute infectious diseases (malaria, measles, pneumonia) and intoxication by poisons such as tobacco and lead. "Choked disk" occurs in brain tumors, brain abscesses, and subarachnoid hemorrhage. Cupping occurs in glaucoma
Retinal arteries and veins	Veins are larger and darker than arteries	The character of the crossing of arteries and veins is important among the first signs of arteriosclerosis

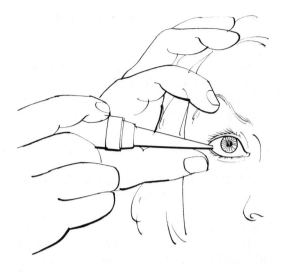

The Tonometer

The tonometer is used to determine the intraocular pressure of the eyeball. The tonometer is an instrument that consists of a footplate curved to fit the average normal cornea. Through the center of the footplate runs a plunger upon which various weights are placed. On top of the plunger rests a lever, the long arm of which is a pointer, the position of which is read against the scale.

The instrument is used like this:

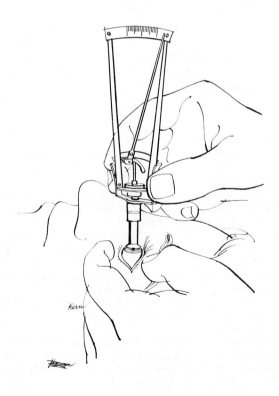

After the eyes have been anesthetized with an instillation of one or two drops of 1 per cent Pontocaine or 0.5 per cent Ophthaine, the patient is placed in a supine position and is asked to look directly upward at some fixed object. The tonometer is placed directly over the cornea and held steady so that the pointer becomes fixed at one of the scale markings.

Normal pressure is from 15 mm. to 30 mm. mercury. A continual increase in intraocular pressure is termed glaucoma. Glaucoma may be primary or secondary; it occurs after iritis, occlusion of the central vein, intraocular tumors, change in position of lens, and trauma. If the eye is painful after the anesthesia wears off, it is very likely that an abrasion has occurred from the use of the tonometer. An antiseptic ointment is used, and the eye is patched (see pp. 336 and 338).

Medications that cause pupillary reactions should never be instilled in the eye when the intraocular pressure is above normal.

Corneal Sensitivity

A wisp of cotton drawn out to a few threads is touched to each cornea to determine corneal sensitivity. The lids are held apart, and the patient is told to tell when he feels the slightest touch. Impairment of corneal sensitivity occurs with an intracranial lesion of the fifth nerve.

Examination of Pupil

The general appearance of the pupils, and their size, shape, situation and equality are noted with the patient facing a diffuse light. Normal pupils are centrally placed, round and in the majority of people, equal in size. Inequality of the pupils, however, is not by itself a sign of disease. About 25 per cent of normal individuals have pupils slightly unequal in size.

Further examination of the pupil is done by testing the pupillary reflexes.

Reaction to Light. The patient is seated in an even light, and a flashlight is brought directly in front of one eye. The opposite eye is kept covered, and the patient is told to maintain his gaze on some fixed object. The pupil

REACTION TO CERTAIN DRUGS

DRUG	NORMAL REACTION	ABNORMAL REACTION
Eserine	Contraction	Ineffective if postganglionic fibers have degenerated
Atropine	Dilation	In neurosyphilis the pupil will not dilate
Mecholyl 2.5%	No change	Constricts pupil in some conditions

normally contracts as a result of direct light. This is called direct reaction. When the exposed pupil contracts, the covered pupil should also contract. This is called consensual reaction.

Near Point Reaction. When the gaze is changed from a distant object to an object close at hand, the pupils contract.

Reaction to Painful Stimuli. Both pupils normally dilate to painful stimuli. This is tested by pulling a few hairs at the nape of the neck.

Abnormal pupils may be classified as follows:

PUPIL	DISEASE	DESCRIPTION
Argyll Robertson pupil	Neurosyphilis (tabes)	Impairment of contraction both directly and consensually. Contraction at near point normal. Pupil is miotic. No response to painful stimuli. Pupils irregular in diameter. No reaction to atropine
Adie's or Tonic pupil	Probably partial degeneration of postganglionic fibers	Direct and consensual light reaction abnormal. Near point reaction abnormal. Reacts to mecholyl 2.5%
Paralysis of pupil	Luetic meningitis, vascular syphilis, diphtheria, encephalitis, botulism and lead poisoning	Fails to react to all stimuli

FUNCTIONAL EXAMINATION OF THE EYE

An examination of the functions of the eye includes testing of visual acuity, testing the focusing power, testing the visual fields and tests for color sense.

TESTING VISUAL ACUITY

Visual testing is done with the Snellen chart or one of its modifications. The test is carried out at a distance of 6 meters (20 feet), since at this distance rays of light from an object are practically parallel and no accommodation is necessary to focus the object. The reading chart contains letters of various sizes. At the side of each line of letters is given the distance at which that letter should be read. If the patient who is seated 6 meters from the chart reads the line of letters labeled 6, his vision is expressed by the fraction 6/6 (or 20/20). Vision is expressed by a fraction, the numerator denoting the distance in meters at which the test is conducted and the denominator denoting the smallest letters read at that distance. If one or more letters are missed in the line, this is recorded as 6/6−1 or 6/6−2, etc.

If the largest letter (150) on the chart cannot be seen at a distance of 6 meters, the patient is brought toward the chart until he can read the letter. The distance at which the letter is read is recorded as 3/150−meaning it was read at a distance of 3 meters. If the patient is unable to see the large 150 letter at a distance of one meter, he is asked whether or not he can see the examiner's hand. If he cannot see the examiner's hand at a distance of one or two meters, a light is thrown into his eye from different directions, and he is asked to tell when the light goes on and off. If he can do this, the notation "light perception present" is made. A person is technically blind when no light perception is present.

The vision of each eye is tested separately both with and without glasses. Since there is only one line of letters representing each fraction of visual acuity on each chart, the chart is changed frequently in order to prevent the subject from memorizing the letters.

TESTING FOCUSING POWER

The focusing power or power of accommodation is determined by placing a line of print close to the eye, then slowly removing it to the point at which the patient is able to read it. The nearest point at which it is readable is the near point of accommodation.

TESTING THE VISUAL FIELDS

Determination of the visual fields is known as perimetry. This includes the range of vision when the eye is fixed on one object.

The simplest method of testing the visual fields is the confrontation method. For this method the doctor and patient are seated facing each other about a meter apart with the light coming from behind the patient. One of the patient's eyes is covered and he is instructed to look steadily at the doctor's eye. The doctor then moves his hand in a circumference midway between himself and the patient and the patient is requested to tell when he sees the doctor's hand come into the field of vision, as shown.

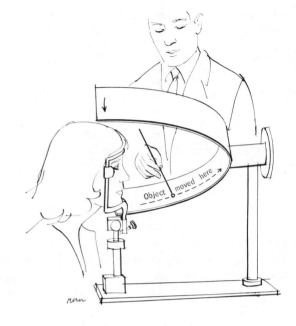

The metal arc is marked in degrees so that an exact recording of the test can be made by the examiner. A normal visual fields recording for the right eye looks similar to this. The unshaded area is the extent of vision.

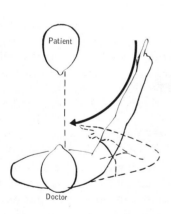

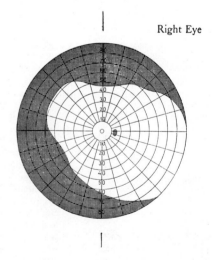

Right Eye

Other more exacting methods of testing the visual fields include the use of the perimeter and tangent screen. The perimeter contains a metal arc that can be revolved 360 degrees. The patient sits with one eye closed and his head supported and tells the examiner when he sees the object moved along the arc, as it is here:

Defects of the central visual field are detected with a tangent screen. The tangent screen is merely a flat black screen with circular markings (as on the recording chart) invisible to the patient. With one eye covered, the patient sits at a distance of 1 to 2 meters away from the screen and tells when he sees an object as it is moved from the periphery to the center of the screen. The points at which the object is seen are marked with small black pins. The recording of the visual fields with the use of the tangent screen looks similar to that of the perimeter.

Testing the visual fields is important in the

diagnosis of glaucoma, brain tumors, optic nerve disease, retinal tumors and detachment and in various other systemic infections. The interpretation of visual fields is not only of importance in making the diagnosis but is also of value in localizing a lesion.

THERAPEUTIC AND REHABILITATIVE PROCEDURES

INSTILLATION OF EYEDROPS

The technique of administering eyedrops would appear to be of such simplicity that it hardly bears mention. There are, however, several factors of considerable importance in making certain that the administered medication will be effective.

The eyedrop is administered into the lower fornix.

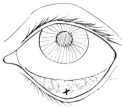

In order to make certain that the eyedrop falls exactly in this small spot, the patient's head must be straight—that is, not turned toward the side—and leaning slightly backward. The patient should be lying flat in bed or sitting on a chair. During the procedure the nurse's hand must be steadied against something so that the movements of the dropper may be controlled in order to prevent the dropper from touching any part of the eye or lid. (If the dropper touches the lid, it is contaminated, and a fresh sterile one must be used.)

If the nurse is right-handed, she should stand on the left side of the patient lying in bed and administer the drops like this:

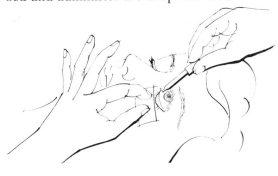

When the patient is sitting in a chair, the nurse should stand in back of the patient and support his head against her body to give the drops. Instruct the patient to look up at the hand holding the dropper during the procedure. This gives him something to think about and helps in holding the eye steady. After the drop has been introduced into the conjunctival fornix, the eyelid should be closed lightly. Squeezing the eyelid tightly shut causes the medication to be completely expressed from the eye. This of course must be explained to the patient before the procedure is begun. In giving poisonous solutions such as atropine, it is important to prevent the solution from being absorbed into the tear duct. To prevent this, the nurse should press the inner angle of the eye like this after the drop is instilled and the patient closes the lid.

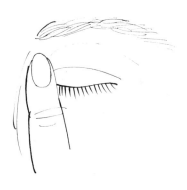

Any excess solution that gathers on the eyelashes is wiped off with cotton or gauze. (The conjunctival sac can retain only 0.1 ml. of fluid.)

One reminder: Different medications may be ordered for each eye: o.d. means right eye, o.s. means left eye, and o.u. means both eyes.

APPLICATION OF OINTMENTS

The position of the patient and the nurse is the same in applying an ointment as in introducing drops. The ointment is applied directly to the fornix from the ointment tube, care being taken not to allow the tip of the tube to touch any part of the eye, thus becoming contaminated. A ribbon of ointment long enough to cover the length of the fornix is expressed. Because the ointment tube is held slightly away from the eyelid, the ribbon must be twisted off before the lower eyelid is filled. Twist the ribbon off at about this point.

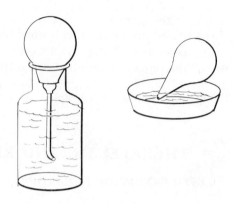

An undine, which looks like this, may also be used.

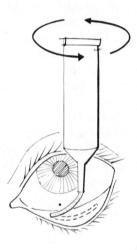

Cold ointment is difficult to manage. It tends to slide along the fornix and is difficult to twist off; therefore, the ointment tube should be held in the hand a few minutes to warm the ointment before use. After the application, instruct the patient to close his eye lightly and roll the eyeball in all directions.

EYE IRRIGATIONS

Eye irrigations should be given in such a manner as to cleanse the entire surface of the globe and all the crevices of the conjunctival sac. The equipment for the irrigation varies with the amount of solution prescribed. As a rule, massive irrigations are no longer used since the advent of antibiotics. For irrigations involving small amounts of fluid, syringes like these are used.

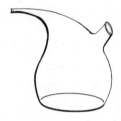

The prescribed solution, at body temperature, is poured over the eye so that it flows from the nasal side toward the outer side. Because it will be impossible for the patient to refrain from closing his eye during the procedure, the nurse should hold the upper eyelid open and ask the patient to look downward. It is easier to have the patient lying flat in bed with his face turned toward one side. If the nurse is right-handed, she should stand to the right of the patient and direct the flow of solution as shown.

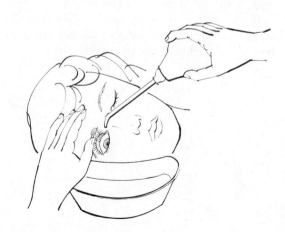

Notice the use of the emesis basin to catch the overflow. The patient can be instructed to hold the emesis basin against his cheek.

WET COMPRESSES

All of the materials used for hot and cold moist compresses on the eyes must be sterile. Ice should be rinsed with cold water before using.

A compress that requires a minimum of handling on the part of the nurse can be made with gauze and wide tongue blades. A 4 × 8 gauze dressing, or preferably a piece of cotton flannel of equal size and thickness, is folded and tied tightly on a wide tongue blade like this.

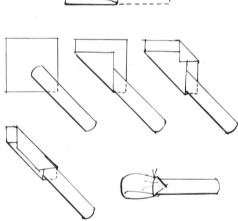

These dressings (we call them lollipops) are made up and sterilized in packets of four. In applying moist heat or cold to the eye, the excess moisture is squeezed from the gauze or flannel by pressing two lollipops together like this.

The desired temperature is maintained on the eye by alternating the dressing every 30 to 60 seconds. The handle must be held in the upright position at all times during use to prevent cross contamination. Do NOT allow this to happen.

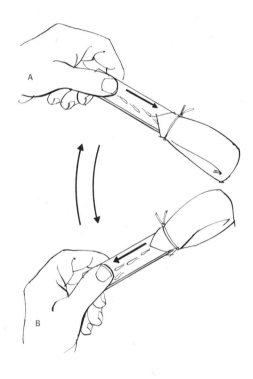

Before applying moist heat or cold to the eye, a protective layer of sterile petroleum jelly is applied to the lid. When compresses are applied to both eyes, separate equipment is used for each eye. Hot moist compresses are given at a temperature as hot as is tolerated by the patient.

MASSAGING THE EYEBALL

Massage to the eyeball is sometimes prescribed to reduce intraocular pressure in glaucoma. Massage is applied by alternating pressure with the two index fingers, as shown. Just enough pressure is applied to indent the globe slightly and to avoid producing pain or

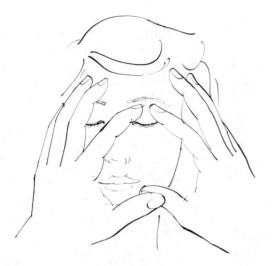

discomfort. As a rule, the massage is carried out from 1 to 5 minutes several times daily. The patient should be instructed to look downward during the entire procedure.

EYE DRESSINGS

Eye dressings are prepared by placing two layers of cotton batting between two layers of gauze roller bandage like this.

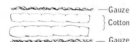

The layers are then cut in an oval shape like this.

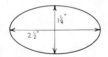

These eye pads are sterilized in packets of two.

When dressing an eye that is deep set, two eye pads should be used on one eye.

Eye dressings are held in place with scotch tape placed in this direction.

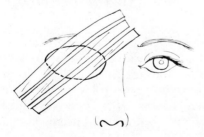

When the normal eye must be bandaged to protect it from an infection present in the opposite eye, a Buller shield is made. The Buller shield is made from a watch glass and adhesive tape or moleskin. To make the shield, place two pieces of adhesive 4 inches square on a flat surface and lightly trace the circumference of the watch glass in the center of each like this:

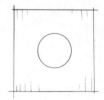

Then cut the center out of each, leaving a margin of about 1/4 inch between the cut mark and the pencil mark like this.

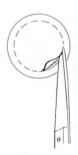

The watch glass is placed in the center of one piece of adhesive, and the adhesive is trimmed in a small circle. The adhesive surface of this circle is placed next to the adhesive surface of the other tape like this:

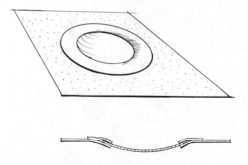

The large adhesive square is then trimmed and placed on the patient like this.

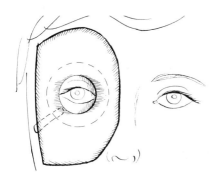

A small piece of gauze is placed at the outer edge for ventilation in order to prevent moisture from forming on the inner surface of the glass.

A circle of transparent x-ray film cut and overlapped to form a cone like this may be used instead of a watch glass.

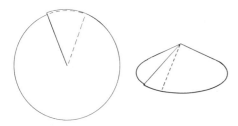

The use of the Buller shield necessitates shaving the eyebrow. The patient can be assured that this will soon grow in and that protection of the good eye is of extreme importance.

Pressure dressings are sometimes used in eye treatments and usually following an enucleation. The pressure dressing consists of several eye dressing pads (enough to fill out the orbital space) held in place with 2-inch elastic bandage like this:

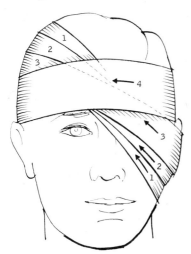

MASKS AND SHIELDS

An eye mask is used when both eyes are covered with dressings. The mask prevents displacement and touching of the dressings by the patient's hands. The diseased eye should always be marked by placing a small piece of adhesive tape on the appropriate side as shown:

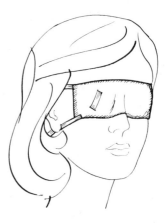

A protective eye shield is made of flexible aluminum that can be bent to fit the contours of the face. A shield like this is held in place over the eye dressing with scotch tape.

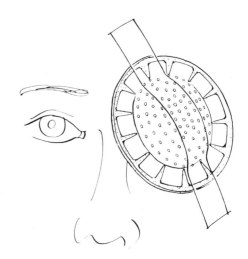

DARK GLASSES

Glasses with dark lenses are worn whenever the sensitive eye is to be protected from light. They are worn in many eye conditions and after dressings are removed following surgery.

Pinhole glasses that look like this are worn before and after corrective surgery for retinal detachment.

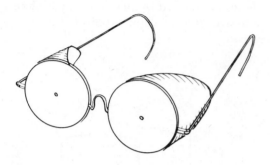

These glasses allow vision only through the tiny hole in the center of each lens.

CLEANSING THE EYELIDS

The eyelids must be cleansed frequently in the care of patients with eye disorders. The eyelids are always cleansed prior to the instillation of any medication and the application of compresses. The eyelids must also be cleansed by the nurse after the dressings are removed following eye surgery.

The eyelids are cleansed with cotton balls moistened in sterile normal saline. Being careful not to exert any pressure on the globe, cleanse the upper lid while the patient looks downward. The upper lid may be held taut like this.

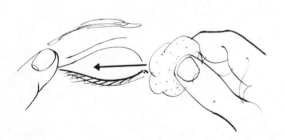

The lower lid is cleansed while the patient looks upward. It is important to clean thoroughly the inner angle of the lids also. A clean cotton sponge is used for each eyelid on each eye.

REMOVING FOREIGN BODIES FROM THE EYE

Nurses are frequently called upon by numerous persons to remove fallen eyelashes or small particles of dirt from the eye. Evert the eyelids as illustrated on page 330 and, after locating the object, remove it with a cotton-tipped applicator moistened with sterile normal saline solution.

Foreign objects other than these are not tampered with by the nurse.

EYE INSTRUMENTS

Several instruments the physician may request for use in areas other than the operating room are identified here.

The Stevens tenotomy scissors—straight

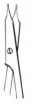

Straight iris scissors—suture

Foreign body spud

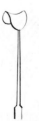

Desmarres lid retractor

Rake retractor

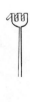

Chalazion forceps

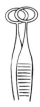

Cilia forceps

To obtain akinesia of the orbicularis, Procaine is injected into the seventh nerve.

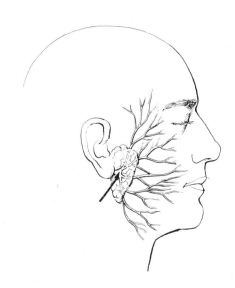

EYE SURGERY

Several recent advances in the techniques of ophthalmic surgery have also revolutionized the nursing care of these patients. The general advancements include the use of local anesthesia which has several advantages over the use of general anesthesia and the development of finer suture material and nontraumatic corneal needles which make it possible to suture the cornea and sclera.

Local Anesthesia

Most eye operations are now done under local anesthesia. Local anesthesia consists of an eye instillation, a retrobulbar injection and an injection into the seventh nerve. The local preparation with the use of eyedrops may be started in the patient's own room, however some surgeons prefer that part or all of the preparation be done in the operating room.

Eyedrops such as Pontocaine, Larocaine, Metycaine, Nupercaine and Butyn are instilled in the eye. Epinephrine hydrochloride 1:1000 is instilled with some of the eye anesthetics. In the operating room Procaine or Xylocaine with hyaluronidase is injected into the retrobulbar area as shown:

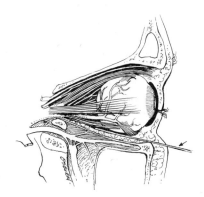

Some of the advantages of local over general anesthesia are: earlier ambulation and oral feeding, less nausea and vomiting, lower incidence of pulmonary and embolic complications, and less danger of aspiration pneumonia.

General anesthesia is still used when the eye operation is extremely lengthy, as in orbital tumors; and for patients who are highly nervous.

Corneoscleral Sutures

Previously intraocular incisions were held together by conjunctival sutures or no sutures at all, and the patient had to lie absolutely quiet so that the surgical wound would properly adhere. Now surgeons have fine suture materials and improved nontraumatic needles at their disposal, which make it possible to suture the cornea and sclera. Because of this the patient need no longer lie flat in bed with the head immobilized between sandbags. Early ambulation is now considered an important part of postoperative eye surgery and is handled in the same manner as after other surgery. The patient is also allowed a full diet as soon as possible, since it is no longer necessary to immobilize the facial muscles.

The two specific aspects of importance in mobility after intraocular surgery now are:
1. The patient should never bend over, causing venous pressure within the head to

rise. The nurse must make certain that the patient does not lean over the side of the bed to vomit or to put on slippers, tie shoes, pick up articles from the floor, etc. The patient is instructed to refrain from these activities during hospitalization and for about 2 to 3 weeks after discharge.
2. The patient should refrain from activities that require sudden jerking movements of the head such as might be encountered when brushing the teeth and combing the hair, for instance.

Additional advancements of specific surgical techniques and the general plan of care for several types of eye surgery are summarized in the following table:

	CATARACT	RETINAL DETACHMENT	CORNEAL TRANSPLANT KERATOPLASTY
Improved surgical technique	Intracapsular method now perfected. Patient can be treated sooner.	Retinal-scleral adhesions created by diathermy or shortening of sclera. Injection of donor vitreous also used; 75% of cases can now be treated because of new methods.	Improvements in care and handling of donor material* and techniques in placement of graft.
Pre-operative management	Admitted 1 to 2 days prior to surgery.	Admitted 3 to 7 days prior to surgery. Both eyes covered with bilateral mask or pinhole goggles. Bed rest and no bending over or sudden movements so that retina will fall back in place for surgery.	Admitted several days before surgery. Cultures of eyeball and lid taken daily. Antibiotic ointments instilled. Attention to cleanliness of face and other eye. Pupil dilated for lamellar graft and constricted for deep (penetrating) graft.
Post-operative management	Bathroom privileges as early as day of surgery. No bending over for about 1 month. One eye bandaged. Dressings changed by physician. Corticosteroid instillation used. Dark glasses worn 1 month. Fitted for cataract glass in one month.† Discharged in 8 to 10 days (diabetic patient longer).	Bathroom privileges in 1 to 2 days. No bending over or jerky movements. Both eyes bandaged for about 1 week. Dressings changed every other day by doctor. Pinhole glasses worn after dressings are removed for about 1 month. Discharged in about 2 weeks after surgery.	Bathroom privileges in 1 to 2 days. Both eyes bandaged for several days. Note: A number of these patients are also deaf; therefore, some system of communication such as the use of letter blocks must be worked out before surgery. Dark glasses worn after dressings removed.

*The donor eye must be enucleated within 24 hours after death and can be kept up to 3 days. Largest eye bank is Eye Bank, Inc., New York, N.Y.

†Quite an adjustment must be made when wearing cataract glasses. When the patient looks directly through the center of the cataract glass, vision is perfect, but any slight deviation from the center of the glass causes objects to look distorted and displaced in their space relationships.

ENUCLEATION

An injured or diseased eye is removed when it is beyond repair. There are several advancements in the technique of enucleation. One is the use of implants.

An implant is a hollow plastic sphere (sometimes covered with fine wire mesh) placed beneath the rectus muscles after removal of the eyeball. The purpose of the implant is to provide movement of the prosthetic eye, to prevent the formation of a deep sulcus in the upper lid and to preserve the normal contour of the lids by volume replacement. Implants are either buried or exposed. The buried implant is covered by the muscle and conjunctiva. Here is a lateral view of a buried implant and prosthetic eye in place:

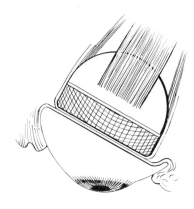

The exposed implant is not completely covered. A portion is left exposed to be fixed to the artificial eye. Here is one type of exposed implant, the Johnson implant:

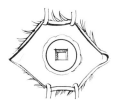

After surgery, a conformer is put in place in the socket for several weeks until the patient receives his artificial eye. The conformer is a clear plastic shell similar in shape to the artificial eye. It looks like this:

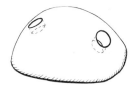

The aftercare of the exposed implant is extremely important because of the danger of infection. For this reason, this type of implant is used only when the physician is certain that the patient is capable of giving meticulous care to the eye socket. Daily continuous care includes:

1. An antibiotic ointment is instilled into the socket every night.
2. The prosthesis is always left in place.
3. The socket is irrigated every morning with a solution such as Zephiran chloride 1:1000. An all-rubber ear syringe is used to flush the eye. The syringe is placed beside the lower edge of the prosthesis in the depth of the socket as shown so that all secretion is flushed from behind the prosthesis:

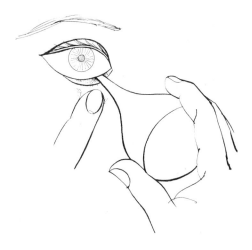

These procedures are carried out as routinely as one brushes one's teeth.

A moderate amount of secretion occurs for the first 2 to 3 weeks after surgery but should not continue thereafter unless there is an infection in the socket. The patient is instructed to carry a small packet of sterile facial tissues with him at all times to blot the lids. The fingers should never touch the lids. The patient is also advised never to allow his socket to get wet during swimming. If this does occur, a large amount of an antibiotic ointment must be put in the socket immediately.

ARTIFICIAL EYES

Artificial eyes are made of plastic and glass. Both types look the same and allow the same degree of movement, but plastic eyes give considerably more service because plastic will not break, crack or shatter.

To Put the Artificial Eye in Place. Wash hands thoroughly and wet the eye. Lift the upper lid and slip the eye under the upper lid as far as possible:

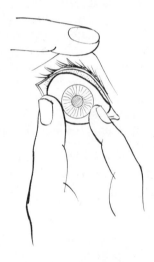

The point of the eye is held toward the nose. Hold the eye in the socket, then pull the lower lid down until it slips over the lower edge of the eye:

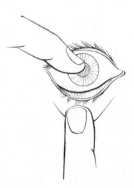

To Remove the Artificial Eye. Pull the lower lid down and press in under the eye and the eye will slip out.

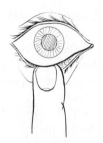

Hold a hand under the eye to catch it when it falls out.

Care of an Artificial Eye
1. Clean with soap and lukewarm water, rubbing it between the thumb and forefinger. Never use extremely hot or cold water.
2. A soft cloth or tissue may be used to polish the eye.
3. Keep the eye in plain water when it is not being worn.
4. Never put a plastic eye in alcohol. Other solutions which damage a plastic eye are Gantrisin, sulfadiazine ointment, carbolic acid, peroxide, phenol solution, Dobell's solution, lighter fluid, and ether.*

PROCEDURES TO REVIEW

All procedures related to the care of the diabetic (see Chap. 20)

Application of bed sides to bed of patient who has both eyes bandaged

Use of elbow splints when there is danger that a restless patient will remove eye dressings

Mouth care without the use of a toothbrush following intraocular surgery

Methods of assisting the blind patient in all activities, including bathing, dressing, ambulation, and eating

Creation of a safe environment for the blind or partially blind patient

Methods for reducing light in the patient's room

All general procedures involved in pre- and postoperative nursing (Chapters 9 and 10)

Use of diversional therapeutic methods to

---

*Personal communication from American Optical Company, Southbridge, Mass.

prevent depression, a common feeling among eye patients

Acquaintance with the addresses of local organizations that help the blind patient

Measures to prevent the spread of infection (Chap. 7)

Care of the patient undergoing radiotherapy (Chap. 3)

Fever therapy

Instructing the patient in the importance of hand washing and other hygienic measures essential to the prevention of eye infections

MEDICATIONS TO REVIEW

Ophthalmic Antibiotic Ointments. Penicillin, crystalline penicillin G, penicillin with dihydrostreptomycin, Sulamyd, Terramycin, Aureomycin, bacitracin, neomycin, Neosporin, Chloromycetin.

Mydriatics and Cycloplegics. Homatropine hydrobromide 2%, atropine sulfate 1%, Neo-Synephrine Hydrochloride 10% viscous sol., Cyclogyl 1% and atropine ointment.

Miotics. Pilocarpine nitrate 0.5 to 4.0%, Eserine salicylate 0.25 to 1.0%.

Carbonic Anhydrase Inhibitors (to Reduce Intraocular Pressure). Diamox, Cardrase, Daranide.

Local Corticosteroids (Ophthalmic Solution and Ointment). Cortisone acetate (Cortone, Cortogen), hydrocortisone (Cortef, Cortril, Hydrocortone), prednisolone (Delta-Cortef, Meticortelone), methylprednisolone (Medrol), triamcinolone (Aristocort, Kenacort), dexamethasone (Decadron).

BIBLIOGRAPHY

Adler, F. H.: Textbook of Ophthalmology. 7th ed. Philadelphia, W. B. Saunders Co., 1962.

Brown, A.: Medical and Surgical Nursing II. Philadelphia, W. B. Saunders Co., 1959.

Brunner, L. S., et al.: Textbook of Medical-Surgical Nursing. Philadelphia, J. B. Lippincott Co., 1964.

Clark, G., and Shaw, C. L.: The Patient with Retinal Detachment. Am. J. Nurs., 57:868, 1957.

Duke-Elder, S.: Parsons' Diseases of the Eye. 13th ed. London, J. and A. Churchill Ltd., 1959.

Duke-Elder, S.: System of Ophthalmology. Vol. VII. The Foundations of Ophthalmology. St. Louis, C. V. Mosby Co., 1963.

Manhattan Eye, Ear and Throat Hospital: Nursing in Diseases of the Eye, Ear, Nose and Throat. 10th ed. Philadelphia, W. B. Saunders Co., 1958.

Rycroft, B.: Keratoplasty. In The Yearbook of Ophthalmology. Chicago, Yearbook Medical Publishers, 1961-1962, pp. 5-28.

Saunders, W. H., et al.: Nursing Care in Eye, Ear, Nose and Throat Disorders. St. Louis, C. V. Mosby Co., 1968.

19

nursing techniques in the care of

Diseases of the Ear, Nose and Throat

DIAGNOSTIC PROCEDURES

EXAMINATION OF THE EAR

An examination of the ear also includes an examination of the nose and throat because an infection in these areas may be a contributing cause of ear disease.

The physician examines the auditory canal by means of an otoscope, head mirror and ear speculum. The patient usually sits in an upright position for the examination. The nurse may be needed to steady the patient's head. During the examination the physician may need swabs and irrigation equipment to cleanse the auditory canal.

Ear swabs are made by twisting a few wisps of cotton from a cotton ball around the end of a toothpick or wire (a wire probe may be used) so that the cotton extends beyond the end of the wire like this.

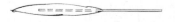

The physician may wish to make the swabs himself.

The equipment needed for an ear irrigation is discussed on page 350.

The patency of the eustachian tube is tested in several ways. The simplest method is done by holding the nose shut and asking the patient to swallow. If both eustachian tubes are open, the patient will experience a clicking sensation in both ears during the swallowing act. If this method is not successful, the Politzer bag is used. The Politzer bag looks like this.

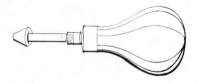

It is inserted in one nostril while the other nostril is held shut with the finger. The pa-

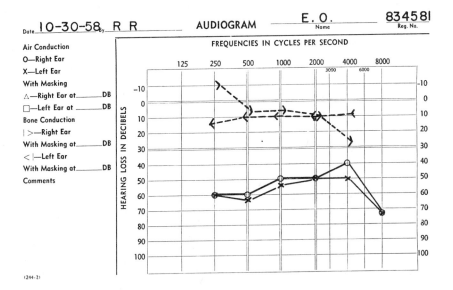

tient is instructed to repeat the letter "K" or the word "kick," or swallow water. At the moment of saying "K" or swallowing, the Politzer bag is forcibly compressed. A clicking sound is experienced in both ears if the eustachian tubes are open.

X-ray studies of the ear are made in cases of chronic middle ear suppuration and in cases of acute otitis media that do not respond to therapy.

HEARING TESTS

The hearing is tested with an instrument called the audiometer. The audiometer is an apparatus that produces sounds of definite frequencies and intensities. There are two general types of audiometers, the step type and the sweep type. The step type has a limited number of specific frequencies while the sweep type has a continuous range of frequencies.

The hearing is often tested at 125, 250, 500, 750, 1000, 2000, 3000, 4000, 6000, 8000 cycles per second. The percentage of loss is shown on a graph like that shown at the top of the page.

The figures at the left of the graph represent the percentage of loss, which is determined by regulating the loudness of the frequency tone. If, for instance, the patient cannot hear a certain frequency at the normal tone, the volume is gradually turned up to a

point at which it can be heard. This of course is a basic screening method of giving the test. For more detailed information a number of other variations in volume (decibels) are used. Methods for bone conduction as well as air conduction are also used. Each ear is tested separately.

For the audiometry test, the patient sits in a soundproof room and listens to the sounds by means of an earphone placed on his head. The patient signals that he hears the sound by raising a finger or by pressing a button. The test is carried out in a special department in the hospital.

Actually the physician can derive all the necessary information concerning the patient's hearing from the audiogram. However, for practical purposes, not every patient who enters the hospital with ear complaints can be immediately scheduled for audiometry.

Thus the physician uses other preliminary methods of testing the hearing. Three such tests making use of the tuning fork are as follows:

Schwabach's Test. This test is performed by placing the tuning fork on the mastoid and timing the duration of sound in seconds. Since sound is transmitted to both ears by bone conduction regardless of where the sound source is applied on the skull, one ear must be masked. This is done by rapidly rubbing a sheet of glazed paper over the ear to eliminate it from the test.

Weber's Test. The tuning fork is placed on the forehead and/or upper teeth, and the patient is asked to state in which ear the sound seems to be louder. In unilateral conduction deafness the tone will be heard best in the diseased ear. In unilateral perception deafness the sound is heard in the good ear. This test obviously is useful only when the hearing in one ear is affected.

Rinne's Test. This test is based upon the principle that the duration of sound by air conduction is about twice that of sound traveling by bone conduction. The tuning fork is placed against the mastoid, and the sound duration is timed. The same is done with the tuning fork held close to the external auditory meatus. In conduction deafness the duration of hearing the sound by bone conduction is longer than by air conduction. In perceptive deafness the air conduction—bone conduction ratio is normal. When the air conduction—bone conduction ratio is normal, the Rinne test is said to be positive. When this ratio is reversed, the test is negative. The ear not being tested is masked in the same manner as for the Schwabach test.

CLASSIFICATION OF HEARING LOSS

In order better to understand the partially deaf patient, the nurse should know something about the variation in hearing losses. Generally speaking, air conduction hearing loss occurs either in high tone or low tones. When the patient with high tone loss is spoken to in normal conversational tones, then, he would be able to hear words said in a low pitch but would not be able to hear the words said in a high pitch. For this reason the nurse erroneously assumes that the patient "hears what he wants to."

In addition, in some types of deafness such as in early Ménière's syndrome, the quality of sounds is distorted, causing loud sounds to be disagreeable and painful. When a patient with this type of deafness is spoken to, he may not hear and ask "What did you say?" Then with repetition only slightly louder, he may say, "Don't shout at me!"

The air conduction tone loss experienced with the various types of deafness are listed here:

Conduction deafness: mild—low or high tone loss. Severe—uniform loss in both tones.

Nerve deafness: high tone loss greater than low.

Deafness due to malfunction of hair cells: low tone loss in Ménière's syndrome. High tone loss in acoustic trauma and labyrinthosis.

OTHER TESTS

Labyrinthine Tests. These tests, useful in the diagnosis of diseases of the inner ear and its pathways to the brain, include the caloric and rotation tests (see p. 297).

Fistula Test. This test is used in cases of chronic suppuration of the middle ear to determine the presence of an erosion through the horizontal semicircular canal. A Politzer bag is used to compress air into the external canal. If vertigo and nystagmus result, fistula is present.

EXAMINATION OF THE NOSE AND THROAT

While examining the nose and throat, the physician wears a head mirror. The anterior portion of the nose is examined with the aid of a nasal speculum.

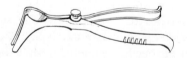

After an initial inspection, a constricting agent such as epinephrine or ephedrine is applied to the nasal membrane by means of an atomizer so that the membrane tightens and enlarges the nasal cavity. The nasal cavity is then inspected again with the speculum. A blunt probe is used for palpation when necessary.

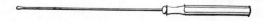

A small amount of anesthetic agent such as cocaine 4 per cent or Pontocaine 1 per cent is applied to the nasal membrane, and an electrically lighted nasopharyngoscope is inserted to examine the posterior part of the nose and nasopharynx.

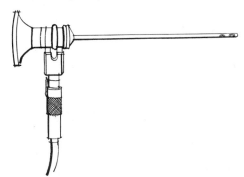

When the nasal mucous membrane is edematous, it is difficult to anesthetize and shrink the membrane. In this event the physician applies the medications by means of a strip of cotton about this size,

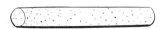

first moistened in the solution, then placed in the nose by means of a bayonet forceps.

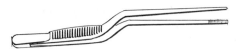

The cotton pledget is left in place several minutes. A mixture of Pontocaine-ephedrine solution may also be used instead of the separate solutions. Next, the tongue is depressed, and a postpharyngeal mirror is inserted through the mouth to the oropharynx to further examine the nasopharynx.

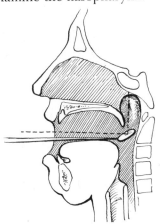

A laryngeal mirror is used to visualize the base of the tongue, the hypopharynx and the larynx.

Before mirrors are inserted, they must be warmed to prevent fogging. This may be done by dipping them in a glass of hot water, then drying.

In the event that a laryngoscope must be used to examine the larynx, the throat is sprayed several times with an anesthetic. The patient's head is then extended over the end of a table and supported by the nurse in this position.

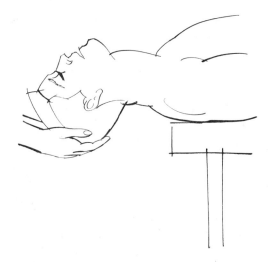

Make certain that dentures are removed before this procedure is begun.

The care of the patient following laryngoscopy is the same as that following bronchoscopy (see p. 211).

EXAMINING THE MOUTH

To examine the mouth, the physician uses the head mirror, tongue blades and retractors. A sterile finger cot or glove should be on hand

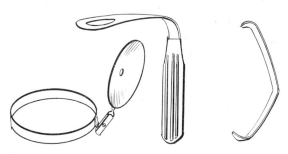

in the event that it is necessary to palpate the salivary ducts with the fingertip. Before a finger is inserted in the patient's mouth, two tongue blades taped together are inserted between the teeth like this.

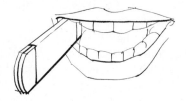

Cotton tipped applicators are needed to wipe away secretions and obtain smears.

Sialography.   This is an x-ray examination of the salivary glands after the injection of Lipiodol Lafay into the salivary ducts. The aftercare of the patient consists of massage of the salivary gland region and instructions to chew gum for a period of 1 to 2 hours 3 to 4 times daily for 2 or 3 days to aid in emptying the Lipiodol from the gland.

THERAPEUTIC AND REHABILITATIVE PROCEDURES

SPECIAL IRRIGATIONS

Irrigating the Ear

The physician may prescribe ear irrigations to cleanse the external auditory canal of purulent discharge or to remove impacted cerumen or foreign bodies. An ear irrigation is never used to remove vegetables such as beans and corn from the ear because the solution makes them swell, thus making them more difficult to remove. (These are usually removed with a knife or hook.) When a hard impacted mass of cerumen is present, hydrogen peroxide is instilled into the ear about 15 minutes before the irrigation. Sometimes it is necessary to instill mineral oil in the ear several days prior to the irrigation to soften cerumen. Bugs are killed prior to irrigation by filling the canal with mineral oil, olive oil or Cresatin.

The type of irrigating syringe used may be one of these three:

the rubber bulb syringe,

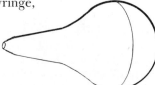

the glass syringe,

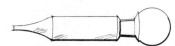

and the metal Pomeroy syringe.

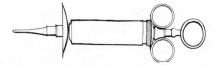

The Pomeroy syringe is the one preferred by most individuals.

Solutions used for the irrigation may be normal saline, water or bicarbonate of soda, depending upon the purpose. The solution should be warmed to around 105°F. Cool solutions are extremely painful to the patient.

When the irrigation is given, the curved auditory canal must be straightened in order for the treatment to be effective. The adult canal is straightened by pulling the auricle upward and backward. It is best to grasp the auricle between the middle and index finger of the left hand. This sounds awkward and impossible but is really quite easy provided the auricle is grasped between the base of the fingers like this

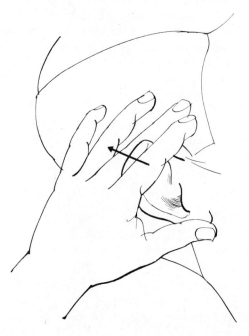

rather than between the tip of the fingers, as one is inclined to do.

The advantage of this method is that the thumb is free to act as a rest for the syringe. This is especially useful when using the Pomeroy syringe because it is rather heavy.

The tip of the syringe should be placed just inside the meatus with the angle of flow directed toward the side of the canal like this:

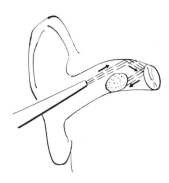

If the solution is directed toward the center of the canal, it will push the plugging substance back against the drum and may cause injury. There is also danger involved if the solution is administered too forcefully. If the nurse has never used a Pomeroy syringe before, she should practice filling and emptying it with water before using it on the patient. This type of syringe is heavy, and it is easy to empty the syringe with too much force.

The best position for the patient for this procedure is sitting on a chair with his head leaning only slightly toward the affected side. The patient is instructed to hold the emesis basin against his face and under the ear to catch the return flow.

Up to 500 cc. of solution is usually a sufficient amount to cleanse the canal.

Nose Irrigation

Nasal irrigations are seldom used, and when they are used, the patient is taught to do the procedure because it is done for a chronic condition, chronic atrophic rhinitis. Nasal irrigations are given at least once daily in this condition to keep the nose free of crusts. Normal saline solution is used unless local applications of estrogenic compounds are part of the therapy. In this event the nose is irrigated with an alkaline solution such as sodium bicarbonate prior to each application.

The irrigation is given with an irrigating can. A nasal irrigating tip is used.

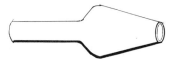

If a nasal irrigating tip is not available, an ordinary glass connection tube serves the purpose just as well. During the procedure the patient should sit with his head held over the lavatory (or a large basin) in this position.

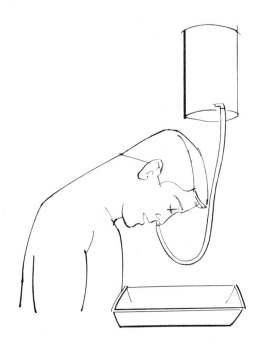

The irrigating can is hung about one foot above the patient's head, and the solution is allowed to flow first into one nostril and out the other, then into the opposite nostril. Each nostril is irrigated in this manner with about 1000 cc. of warm solution. The patient must be instructed to breathe through his mouth during the entire procedure and must be taught how to temporarily clamp off the tube during a cough. He must also be instructed not to talk during the procedure. After all the irrigating solution has been allowed to flow through the nostrils, the head is kept in the same position until all the solution is drained from the nose, and the patient is instructed not to blow his nose. This final step is necessary to prevent the infection from spreading to the eustachian tubes.

Throat Irrigations and Gargles

Irrigations of the throat are seldom used, since the advent of antibiotics. Gargles are prescribed frequently, although their effectiveness for areas beyond the tonsillar region is questioned. The solutions prescribed for gargles are numerous. Two commonly used gargles are normal saline solution and 10 grains of aspirin dissolved in 30 cc. of hot water. The solution used in gargles should be as hot as is tolerated by the patient. The nurse should instruct the patient to exhale during the gargle so as not to swallow or inhale the solution.

Mouth Irrigations and Sprays

When the patient has had extensive surgery of the mouth and neck in the treatment of carcinoma, the approach to special mouth care is somewhat different than that ordinarily associated with the phrase "special mouth care." In a radical neck dissection, the primary objective in oral hygiene is to keep the bacterial flora of the mouth at a minimum so that an infection does not develop. The pre- and postoperative routine used for these patients varies with the surgeon. Mouth care usually includes the application of solutions such as Dobell's, Dakin's and peroxide. These solutions are applied to the mouth in sprays or irrigations or both, every few hours both before and after surgery. Postoperatively a glass eye irrigation syringe (see p. 336) makes a handy irrigation device. In some institutions these irrigations and sprays constitute the mouth care. In other hospitals gauze packings may be used in addition (see p. 361).

INSTILLATIONS

Ear Drops

Years ago the standard treatment for an earache was warm oil drops and a cotton ear plug. Since the use of antibiotics, ear drops are seldom used. Oil drops are still useful in softening plugs of cerumen. Drops of hydrogen peroxide are instilled in the ear to remove excessive wax and to keep the canal clean

when the ear is draining. Cotton plugs are never used in a draining ear, since this prevents free drainage. Ear drops should always be warmed before instillation.

Nose Drops

The usual procedure of applying nose drops with the head tilted back is a waste of effort, since in this method the medication merely runs down into the throat and is swallowed. The only two effective positions for administering nose drops are the Proetz position,

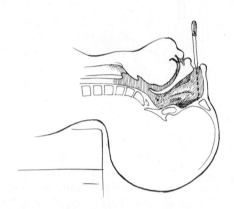

and the Parkinson position.

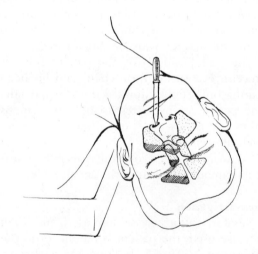

The Proetz position is best when treating the ethmoid and sphenoid sinuses; the Parkinson position when treating the frontal and maxillary sinuses and the nasal passages.

The position for holding the medicine dropper is another important aspect overlooked by many. The dropper should be slanted like this so that the solution bypasses the inferior turbinate.

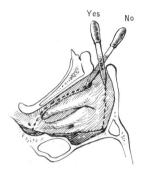

The amount of solution used for each instillation varies with the purpose. For treating congested nasal passages, about ⅓ dropperful is enough. This amount will be just enough to cover the nasal chambers and prevent the solution from going into the sinuses. When the sinuses are being treated, larger amounts are used.

TRACHEOTOMY

Since the tracheotomy is sometimes an emergency procedure performed at the patient's bedside, several details about the surgical technique will be discussed here.

When there is any suspicion that laryngeal obstruction may occur in the course of respiratory disease and after surgery, trauma or prolonged unconsciousness, a tracheotomy tray is kept at the patient's bedside for immediate use. The instruments included on the tray vary with each institution from the barest necessities to almost a complete surgical set-up. Actually, in an emergency a tracheotomy can be performed with only a scalpel. The minimal number of instruments on a tray should include a scalpel, curved blunt bistoury,

dissecting scissors, hemostat, fixation tenaculum, retractor, Trousseau tracheal dilator, and tracheotomy tube.

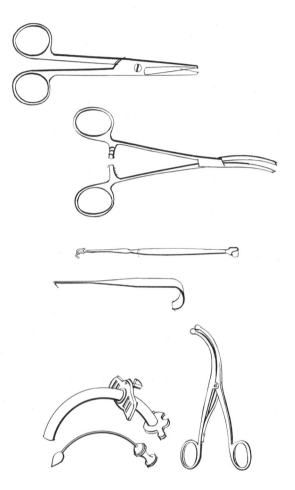

When an emergency situation calls for a tracheotomy, the best procedure is to first insert a bronchoscope or endotracheal catheter, then perform the tracheotomy in an orderly manner. A Mosher's lifesaver shown here may be used instead of the bronchoscope.

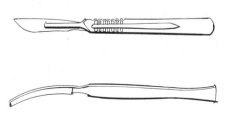

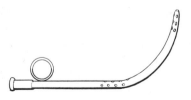

When the Mosher's lifesaver is inserted, the nurse holds and supports the head like this:

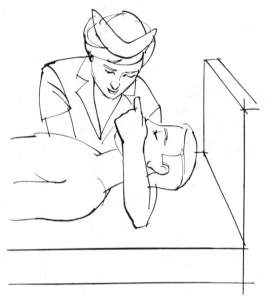

The nurse's left hand also holds the bite block which props the mouth open.

When the tracheotomy is to be performed, the patient's head should be in this position.

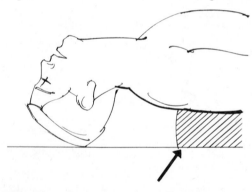

Notice the placement of a roll of fabric (any kind) under the patient's shoulder and not under the neck. This position gives the greatest prominence to the trachea. The patient is not placed in this position until the knife is about to make the incision. No anesthesia is used in an emergency procedure. When a temporary tracheotomy is performed, the tracheotomy tube is the only means of holding the air passageway open. When a permanent tracheotomy is performed, the trachea is sutured to an opening in the skin. Therefore if the tube were removed, prompt closure of this wound would not result.

During the first few days after the insertion of the tracheotomy tube, the patient is extremely restless for a number of causes. First of all, he has a large amount of bronchial secretion that makes him cough frequently. At the same time respirations sound loud, wheezy, wet and gurgling in comparison to respirations made through the nose under the same bronchial condition. These sounds tend to make the patient think that his tube is about to become clogged. When one adds these fears to the fact that the patient cannot talk or call for help, one can estimate the amount of apprehension present. For this reason and other reasons, the patient should have a nurse in constant attendance for the first 24 to 48 hours. If this is impossible, he is placed near the nurses' station where he can be seen or close enough to hear his breathing at all times. Bronchial secretions are profuse for the first few days and are slightly blood-tinged at first. The amount of blood gradually diminishes.

The nurse's prime concern for the tracheotomy tube is to keep it open. In order to do this, she must incorporate several nursing measures among a well-organized nursing plan.

To keep the tracheotomy tube open:
1. Secretions are gently and quickly wiped from the tracheotomy tube opening when the patient coughs. Whenever the patient coughs or expires forcefully, a plug of mucus may be totally or partially blown from the tube opening. If the mucous plug is only partially expelled, it will be drawn back into the tube on the next inspiration. The nurse should remove it before it is inspired. Sterile cellulose tissues (Chix) are good for wiping. Unlike facial tissue (which should never be used), they have no lint, which is dangerous if inspired. Sterile gauze squares (4 × 4) may be used, but the threads of gauze have a tendency to catch on the protruding pieces on the tracheotomy tube.* (A face-towel bib should be placed around the patient to protect the bedding.)
2. The inner cannula is suctioned frequently to keep it open and to prevent crusts from forming on the interior wall. Absolute aseptic technique is extremely important in the suctioning procedure. A suction

---

*There is a newer model tracheotomy tube which does not have any protrusions on which gauze threads can catch.

apparatus is kept next to the patient's bed with the suction catheter connected for immediate use. Here is one safe method of storing the catheter in bactericidal solution between aspirations.

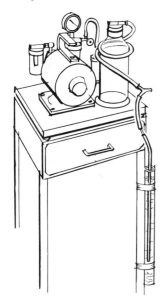

The tube, made of unbreakable plastic, is fastened to the suction machine with tape or metal clamps. A tube containing an extra catheter may be fastened to another leg of the stand. A 14 to 16 whistle-tip catheter should be cut with extra holes like this.

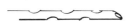

The connection to the suction should have a Y tube insert like this.

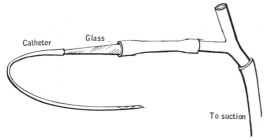

Catheter   Glass

To suction

With the Y tube insert the suctioning can be precisely regulated simply by placing the thumb over the open end of the tube. To suction the tracheotomy tube, gently insert the catheter about 5 or 6 inches, then occlude the Y tube and carefully withdraw the catheter, at the same time rotating it.

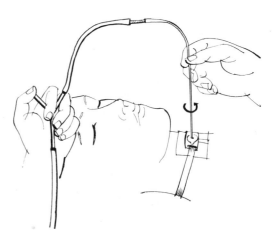

If the catheter attaches while it is being withdrawn during suctioning, release the suction by taking the thumb off the Y tube. This prevents damage to the bronchial tree. Suctioning should be continued for only brief periods of a few seconds. If one suctioning does not free the airway, use repeated short suctioning and allow a brief interval of rest between. If the mucus is extremely thick, several (3 to 5) drops of sterile water are instilled into the trachea with a medicine dropper before suctioning. During the first 24 to 48 hours postoperatively, the tracheotomy must usually be suctioned every 15 to 30 minutes. *Note:* If the pharynx also needs suctioning through the mouth, a separate catheter must be used for this in order to prevent infection in the tracheobronchial tree.

3. The inner cannula is removed and thoroughly cleansed and sterilized at frequent intervals to prevent encrusting and clogging. While one inner cannula is removed for cleansing, a second sterile inner cannula is put in place. To remove the inner cannula, turn the key or catch on the top of the tube.

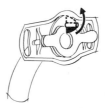

In our experience, the easiest way to get the inside of the inner cannula clean is this: Tie a doubled length of 2-inch bandage on the faucet and place a loop of thin pliable wire through the end like this:

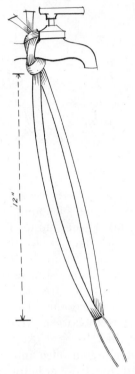

Slip the inner cannula over the gauze and wash the tube like this:

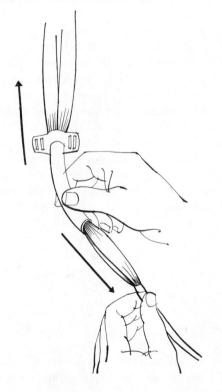

Cold running water is used for washing and rinsing. The opening is inspected to make certain it is clean; then the tube is dried and reinserted. The inner cannula is removed and cleaned at least every few hours, oftener if necessary.

Other Aspects of Tracheotomy Care

Replacement of Tube. The resident places a fresh sterile tracheotomy tube in the opening whenever necessary. This is never a nursing procedure. In some institutions, however, if the patient has a permanent tracheotomy, this may become a nursing responsibility after about 10 days. The tracheotomy tube is put in place with the inner cannula removed and the obturator in place like this:

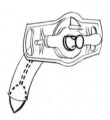

After the tube is in place, the obturator is immediately removed, the tube is tied in place, and the inner cannula is put in place.

The tube that is removed is cleansed and sterilized by boiling or autoclaving. Tracheotomy sets are made of silver, nylon and hard rubber. The silver tubes are polished before sterilization. Care must be taken in handling the silver sets because they dent easily. Each set, consisting of three pieces, must be kept together at all times. The replacement set should always be the same size as the one being worn by the patient. The size (0 to 10) is engraved on each piece.

Dressings. For the first day or so after surgery, the dressings must be changed frequently, usually every few hours. This is a nursing procedure. Two 3 × 3 sterile gauze dressings are slit and placed between the tube collar and the skin like this:

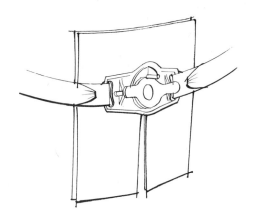

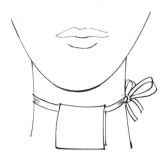

These dressings are carefully removed and replaced without untying the tapes holding the tube in place. The nurse should not loosen these tapes at any time because of the danger of the tracheotomy tube being forced out unexpectedly when the patient coughs. After a few days the dressings will become soiled less frequently. One 3 × 3 gauze dressing will then be sufficient. This is changed once daily.

The Tracheotomy Tube Tapes. The tapes are fixed on the tracheotomy tube by the nurse before the tube is inserted. Two ties of ¾ inch twill tape, each about 16 inches long, are used. A small slit is made about 1 inch from one end of each tie. The ties are slipped through the tube collar and fastened like this:

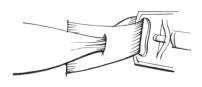

This method is used rather than knots because knots are irritating to the patient's neck.

Humidifying the Air. Warm dry air is irritating to the tracheal mucosa. For this reason it is often necessary to moisten the air. This is especially true during the winter months. A steam inhalator or mechanical humidifier (see p. 49) may be prescribed for this purpose.

Some surgeons prescribe the placement of moist gauze over the tracheotomy for the purpose of moistening and filtering the air. In this event the nurse places a moistened gauze bib over the tracheotomy opening like this:

A 4 × 8 gauze dressing is used. The twill tape is tied in a large bow at the side so that this tape does not become confused with the knotted tape that secures the tube in place. The gauze is moistened with warm sterile normal saline by means of a medicine dropper.

When the tracheotomized patient is on oxygen therapy, the air is humidified with a nebulizer attached to the oxygen setup (see Chap. 4).

Oxygen Therapy. Oxygen is administered into the tracheotomy tube by catheter or mask. The nasal catheter (see p. 36) is secured in place by ties knotted around it, then tied around the neck. A tracheotomy mask is made of clear plastic and is fastened over the tracheotomy tube like this:

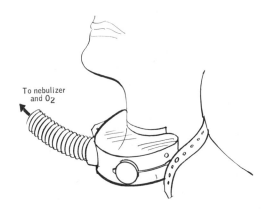

Notice that a large bore tubing is used to connect this type of mask to the oxygen supply. Also notice the additional hole in the mask, which is unstoppered in order to suction the patient.

Supplies to Be Kept at Bedside. Articles such as a duplicate tracheotomy tube, gauze dressings and wipes, dressing forceps, a sterile bowl of saline to flush the suction catheter, and any other supplies needed in the continuing care of the patient are kept at the bed-side. One other item that is most important to have on hand is the Trousseau dilator (see p. 353). This instrument is used to separate the tracheal incision. If the tracheotomy tube were to come out accidentally, the nurse would use the Trousseau dilator to hold open the tracheal incision so that the patient could get air.

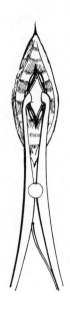

If it is impossible to keep a Trousseau dilator at the bedside, a curved hemostat can be substituted.

Decannulation. When the tracheotomy is a temporary one, the patient must learn to revert to breathing through the nose. Sometimes simply taking out the cannula and closing the tracheotomy incision creates panic because breathing through a cannula is unobstructed compared to the route through the nose. For this reason and also to make certain that the airway by the nasal route is open, the diameter of the cannula is gradually decreased. The first step is usually to put a smaller tube in place. The next step is partial occlusion of the cannula with a half cork. If this is tolerated, a three-quarter cork, then a whole cork are substituted. The decannulation corks are made from pure rubber cord. They are tied in place with braided silk, attached as shown.

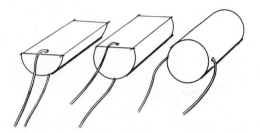

If dyspnea and restlessness develop from a larger cork it must be replaced with the previously used size. Commercial corks should never be used for this purpose because they break too easily.

SPECIAL DRESSINGS

Mastoid Dressings. A mastoid dressing consists of four or five gauze fluffs and a mastoid ring. A mastoid ring is made by folding an 18-inch square of gauze in a triangle, turning the rough edges in, then winding it loosely around the hand.

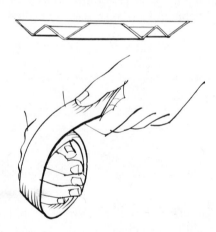

The ring dressing is placed around the patient's ear. These dressings are done up in dressing packs and sterilized for use.

After mastoid surgery the physician changes the outside dressings daily and the deep dressing about the fifth day.

Ear Dressings. When ear dressings are indicated, gauze fluffs are usually the dressings of choice. If the patient's ear protrudes a great deal, a small wad of gauze should be placed behind the ear like this:

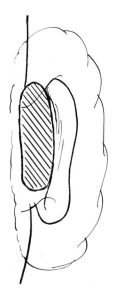

After middle and inner ear surgery it is extremely important to keep the ear dressings in place and to keep the wound surgically aseptic. After ear surgery the physician changes the dressings himself. Special instruments the physician may request for changing dressings include the bayonet forceps shown on page 349 and a Hartman forceps shown here.

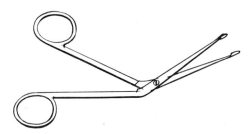

He may also need wire applicators and a brain suction tip:

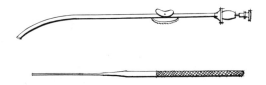

In hospitals where an extensive amount of ear surgery is done, all of the equipment needed for changing the ear dressings is done up on a tray and sterilized for use.

Ear dressings—and of course mastoid dress-

ings—are held in place like this: First, place a strip of gauze bandage around the head like this:

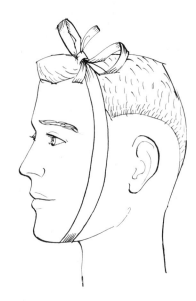

Next apply the dressings over the ear. In order for the dressings to stay in place, the patient's head must be lying on the side. If the patient is allowed to sit up, have him sit on a straight-back chair and lean his head on the overbed table:

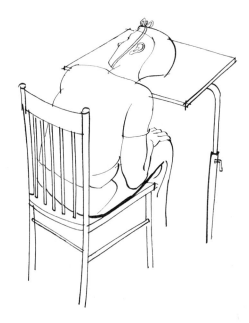

After the dressings are placed on the ear, take a roll of 2- to 3-inch bandage and unroll it like this:

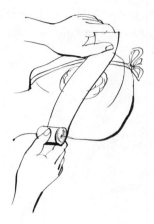

Use this strip of roller bandage to hold the dressing against the patient's ear, then ask the patient to sit up and finish wrapping the head with the patient in the sitting position. After sufficiently wrapping the head, cut the original gauze strip and tie like this:

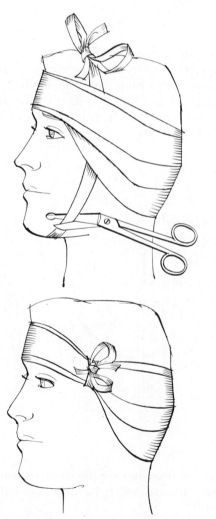

Either Kurlex or Ace bandage (see p. 125) is good for holding ear dressings in place.

Nasal Dressings and Packings. Exterior nasal dressings are seldom called for. When corrective plastic surgery is done, a splint made of aluminum with a flannel or sponge rubber backing is used. One type of splint and method of taping it in place is shown here:

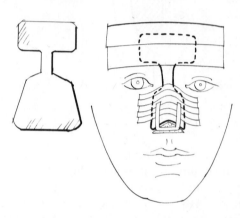

Nasal packings are used after some types of nasal surgery and in the event of uncontrollable epistaxis. Methods to control epistaxis before resorting to the use of packing include having the patient sit in an erect sitting position with the head tilted forward. This facilitates clot formation by back pressure against the bleeding vessel. Articles that the nurse should assemble for the doctor in dealing with a persistent nosebleed include:

1. Epinephrine (Adrenalin) 1:1000
2. 10% cocaine solution
3. Silver nitrate sticks
4. Instruments such as a head mirror, nasal speculum, bayonet forceps and suction tip
5. Local hemostatic agents such as Oxycel, Gelfoam and thromboplastin
6. Materials for anterior and posterior nasal packing.

Anterior nasal packing is made of gauze bandage with the edges folded in to make a strip about ¼ inch wide. This packing may be plain, with iodoform, or with petroleum jelly. These various types of packing are stored in test tubes, jars or narrow metal cans. The physician uses a bayonet forceps to put the packing in place.

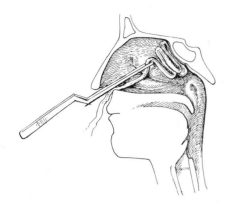

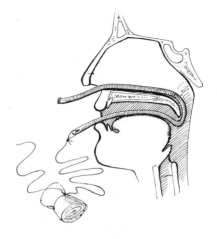

If the end of the packing tends to slip out, the nurse can tape it to the nose with a strip of ¼-inch adhesive like this:

and held in place by knotting the threads like this:

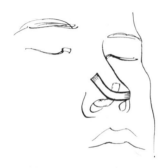

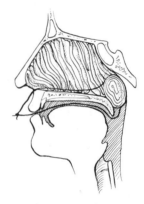

In severe nasal hemorrhage, both anterior and posterior nasal packs are used. Here are two types of posterior packs commonly used, one of cotton and one of gauze:

Depending upon the severity of the epistaxis, the packings are left in place from 1 to 3 days. After the pack is removed, the patient is observed for anterior hemorrhage from the nostrils and posterior hemorrhage in the throat.

Occasionally the surgeon may wish to pack the nose with cocaine and epinephrine before the patient goes to the operating room. In this event plain packing is used and dipped into the anesthetic solution. Whenever cocaine is used, the nurse should be on the alert for symptoms such as weakness, faintings or convulsions, the signs of cocaine poisoning.

Oral Packings.   After oral surgery packings are frequently required for several reasons. In gum surgery there is usually bleeding in the immediate postoperative period. In surgery of the gums, if the patient is conscious, sterile gauze dressings (4 × 4) are folded and placed on the gums, and the patient is in-

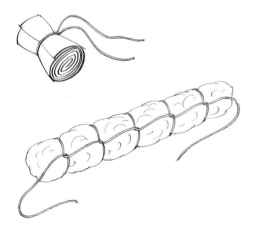

Heavy silk or cotton thread is used to secure the packing in place. The packing is put in place with a catheter

structed to bite on the dressings. The nurse changes these dressings every 1 to 3 hours as necessary.

In extensive surgery of the mouth, tongue and pharynx for carcinoma, packings may be placed along the intraoral suture line to prevent infection. This type of packing (also called a wick) is done by the nurse like this: Heavy silk thread is tied to a strip of gauze. The gauze is dipped in a mixture of activated zinc peroxide and water, just enough to make a thin paste. The excess paste is squeezed from the gauze with a tongue blade. The packing is placed along the intraoral suture line, and the silk tie is attached to the outer cheek with scotch tape, thus guarding against the loss of the packing and facilitating its removal. These packings are changed every two hours, and the mouth is sprayed before a new packing is inserted.

After extensive mouth or throat surgery, the patient may not be able to swallow for a considerable length of time. In this event a wick of gauze is placed in the patient's mouth to drain off the saliva. This prevents frequent expectoration on the part of the patient and frequent suctioning on the part of the nurse. The wick is made by folding a 4 × 8 gauze dressing lengthwise. One end is placed in the patient's mouth. The other end rests in an emesis basin.

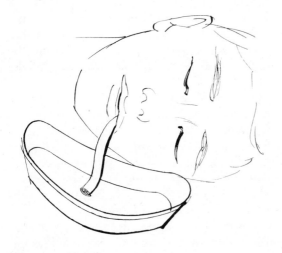

PROCEDURES TO REVIEW

Application of ice bag to reduce hemorrhage, swelling and pain in facial injuries and following plastic surgery of the nose, oral surgery, tonsillectomy and adenoidectomy. Substitution of small plastic bag or rubber gloves for ice bag in application to ear.

Use of hot water bottle in inflammatory conditions of *external* auditory canal.

Observation and care of patient with facial paralysis, a complication of mastoid and facial surgery (see p. 314).

Gastric feedings through nasal tube after laryngectomy and tongue surgery (see p. 161). The patient is also taught to do these in many instances.

Oxygen therapy (Chap. 4).

Pre- and postoperative nursing care (Chaps. 9 and 10).

Radiotherapy (Chap. 3).

Use of magic slate or pencil and paper for patients who are unable to talk as after oral surgery and tracheotomy.

General hygiene of mouth.

Isolation techniques in Vincent's angina.

Use of IPPB apparatus (see p. 55).

Care of cuffed tracheotomy tube (see p. 66).

DIETS TO REVIEW

Formulas for tube feedings.

Liquid to soft consistencies for patients with conditions of ear and throat that make it painful to chew and swallow.

MEDICATIONS TO REVIEW

Refer to medications listed at the end of Chapter 13.

BIBLIOGRAPHY

Boies, L. R., Hilger, J. A., and Priest, R. E.: Fundamentals of Otolaryngology. 4th ed. Philadelphia, W. B. Saunders Co., 1964.

Brown, A.: Medical and Surgical Nursing II. Philadelphia, W. B. Saunders Co., 1959.

Brunner, L. S., et al.: Textbook of Medical-Surgical Nursing. Philadelphia, J. B. Lippincott Co., 1964.

Falconer, M., Patterson, H., and Gustafson, E.: Current

Drug Handbook. 1968-1970. Philadelphia, W. B. Saunders Co., 1968.

Harmer, B., and Henderson, V.: Textbook of Principles and Practices of Nursing. 5th ed. New York, The Macmillan Co., 1958.

Jackson, C., and Jackson, C. L.: Diseases of the Nose, Throat and Ear. 2nd ed. Philadelphia, W. B. Saunders Co., 1959.

Krause, M.: Food, Nutrition, and Diet Therapy. 4th ed. Philadelphia, W. B. Saunders Co., 1966.

Pitorak, E. F.: Laryngectomy. Am. J. Nurs., *68*:785, 1968.

Price, A.: The Art, Science and Spirit of Nursing. 3rd ed. Philadelphia, W. B. Saunders Co., 1965.

Roe, B. B. P.: Bedside Tracheostomy. Surg. Gynec. & Obst., *115 (2)*:239, 1962.

Tabee, R. E.: A Tracheotomy Program. J. Mich. State Med. Soc., *61 (3)*:327, 1962.

Williamson, P.: Office Procedures. 2nd ed. Philadelphia, W. B. Saunders Co., 1962.

nursing techniques in the care of
Diseases of the Endocrine System

DIAGNOSTIC PROCEDURES

The diagnostic studies of importance to the nurse in endocrine disorders include laboratory studies of blood and urine, x-ray examinations, basal metabolism rate and a number of additional specific tests.

BLOOD STUDIES

The commonly used blood studies and the abnormal implications are listed on page 366.

URINE STUDIES

Urine studies include a number of tests to determine the hormonal content of urine. For hormonal excretion studies, a 24-hour specimen (see p. 257) is needed. The tests for hormones along with other studies frequently done are listed on page 365.

Urinary Collection and Testing Methods

In caring for the patient with diabetes mellitus, the nurse frequently tests the urine for sugar and albumin. The methods for doing this are discussed in Chapter 15, page 257.

Since these tests are used in regulating the patient's diet and insulin dosage, the time of the day the test is conducted is of importance. The physician prescribes whether the urine tested should be a qualitative specimen or a single specimen.

Fractional Tests. Qualitative collections are called fractionals. For fractional tests all the urine is collected between these hours:

    7 A.M. to 11 A.M.; 11 A.M. to 4 P.M.; 4 P.M. to 9 P.M.; 9 P.M. to 7 A.M.

Single Specimens. Single specimens are collected as prescribed by the physician. At first, specimens voided immediately before each meal and at bedtime may be tested. As

URINE STUDIES USED IN ENDOCRINE DISORDERS

TEST	NORMAL	DISEASE IMPLICATIONS
Albumin	None	Present in acromegaly, Addison's disease and severe diabetes mellitus.
Aldosterone*	2-23 μg. in 24 hours	Increased in some adrenal tumors. Decreased in Addison's disease.
Calcium*	200 mg. in 24 hours	Increased in acromegaly, Cushing's syndrome, hyperparathyroidism. Decreased in tetany due to hypoparathyroidism.
Catechol amines*	Less than 200 μg. in 24 hours	Elevated in pheochromocytoma.
Casts	None	Present in acromegaly and Addison's disease.
Chloride*	10-16 gm. in 24 hours	Increased in Addison's disease and dwarfism. Decreased in diabetes insipidus.
Estrogens*	4-30 gammas of estrone equivalent in 24 hours	Increased in hyperfunction of ovaries and tumors of androgenic zone of adrenals.
Gonadotropins* FSH	10-50 mouse uterine units in 24 hours	Decreased in hypopituitarism. Changes also occur in a number of testicular and ovarian diseases.
17-hydroxycorticosteroids*†	Male 3-10 mg. Female 2-8 mg. in 24 hours	Decreased in Addison's disease. Increased in adrenal cortical hyperfunction also determined in ACTH test (see p. 346).
17-ketosteroids*†	Male 8-20 mg. Female 5-15 mg. in 24 hours	Increased in tumors of androgenic zone of adrenal and some ovarian tumors. Decreased in Addison's disease and pituitary cachexia.
Pregnanediol*	Male 0-1 mg. Female 1-8 mg. in 24 hours	Increased in tumors of adrenals. Decreased in hypofunction of ovaries.
Pregnanetriol*	Male 1-2 mg. Female 0.5-2.0 mg. in 24 hours	Increased in hyperfunction of adrenals. Decreased in hypofunction of ovaries.
Sugar	None	Present in acromegaly, Cushing's syndrome, hyperthyroidism, diabetes mellitus and in some cases of pheochromocytoma.
Volume	1000-1500 cc. daily	Increased in acromegaly and diabetes insipidus.

*24-hour specimen needed.
†Tranquilizers interfere with test.

the regulation progresses, the number of specimens tested daily may be reduced to two, then one.

SPECIAL TESTS

Special tests used in diagnosing diseases of the endocrine system may include a number of the following:

Glucose Tolerance Test

This test is used mainly in diagnosing diabetes mellitus but is also of significance in the diagnosis of several other endocrine disorders. These will be discussed later.

The glucose tolerance test is of importance in detecting mild diabetes when the fasting blood sugar is normal. The test is also of value in surveying a diabetic family for the detection of diabetes. It is not used in cases of known diabetes because it is not wise to give glucose to a diabetic patient who has a blood sugar level of 200 mg. or more. The test is of most value in borderline cases where the fasting blood sugar is 140 to 160 mg. per 100 cc.

Oral Glucose Tolerance Test. (Blood and Urine Specimen Needed.) Determine the patient's weight. Nothing by mouth from 7 P.M. to after test.

Specimen 1. Obtain blood specimen and urine specimen at same time. Give glucose dissolved in lemon juice.

Blood Studies Used in Endocrine Disorders

TEST AND NORMAL RANGE	INCREASED IN	DECREASED IN
Alkaline phosphatase 1.5-4 units	Hyperparathyroidism, hyperthyroidism	
Calcium 9-11 mg.	Cushing's syndrome, hyperparathyroidism	Acromegaly, gigantism hypoparathyroidism
Catechol amines (norepinephrine 1.1-5.5 μg. liter; epinephrine 0.0-1.5 μg. liter)	Pheochromocytoma	
Chloride 350-375 mg.		Dwarfism, Addison's disease, diabetes mellitus, tumors of androgenic zone of adrenal
Cholesterol 150-280 mg.	Cushing's syndrome, hypothyroidism, severe diabetes and diabetic coma, tumors of androgenic zone of adrenal	Acromegaly, gigantism, hyperthyroidism
Eosinophil 1-3% 50-250/cu. mm.	Pituitary cachexia	
Glucose* 80-110 mg.	Acromegaly, gigantism, Cushing's syndrome, hyperthyroidism, diabetes mellitus	Dwarfism, Addison's disease, hypothyroidism
Lipids 0.4-0.6 gm.	Severe diabetes and diabetic coma	Acromegaly, gigantism, hyperthyroidism
Magnesium 1.5-2.5 mEq. per liter		Hypoparathyroidism
Nonprotein nitrogen* 25-35 mg.	Acromegaly, gigantism, Cushing's syndrome, Addison's disease, diabetes mellitus	
Phosphorus 3-4.5 mg.	Acromegaly, gigantism	
Sodium 136 to 145 mEq. per liter	Tumors of androgenic zone of adrenal	Pituitary cachexia, Addison's disease
Potassium 3.5-5 mEq. per liter	Pituitary cachexia, Addison's disease	Diabetic coma, tumors of androgenic zone of adrenal
Protein bound iodine 4-8 μg. %	Hyperthyroidism	Hypothyroidism

*Oxylated or heparinized test tube needed.

Specimen 2. Blood and urine specimens are
Specimen 3. taken again at the end of ½,
Specimen 4. 1, 2, and 3 hours
Specimen 5.
The highest blood sugar level should not be more than 30 to 60 mg. above fasting level. There should be no glycosuria. The level of blood sugar should return to the fasting level in 2 hours.

In diabetes mellitus the glucose level is high at the end of 1 hour and does not return to normal in the 2- and 3-hour specimens. The urine is usually positive for sugar in the second, third, and fourth specimens.

Intravenous Glucose Tolerance Test. (Blood and Urine Specimen Needed.) Weigh patient. Nothing by mouth after supper.
Specimen 1. Blood and urine specimen obtained. 50 ml. of 50% glucose in distilled water injected over 2-minute period.
Specimen 2. Blood and urine specimens are
Specimen 3. obtained at ½-hour intervals
Specimen 4. for 2 hours. In diabetes the

Specimen 5. blood sugar level does not return to normal in 2 hours.

Exton-Rose Glucose Tolerance Test. (Blood and Urine Specimens Needed.) Normal diet with at least 100 gm. of carbohydrates given daily for 3 days prior to test. Nothing by mouth after supper.

Specimen 1. Dissolve 100 gm. of glucose in 650 cc. of water flavored with lemon juice. Collect blood and urine specimen.

Specimen 2. Request patient to drink one half of glucose solution within 1 minute. Thirty minutes later collect blood and urine.

Specimen 3. Give remaining glucose solution. Thirty minutes later collect blood and urine specimen.

Normally the blood sugar level in the third specimen is less than that of the second specimen. No sugar should be present in the urine.

Increased sugar tolerance also occurs in hypophyseal dysfunction, Addison's disease and hypothyroidism. In these diseases the rise of sugar is only slight (up to 30 mg.), whereas in diabetes the rise is more pronounced.

Insulin Tolerance Test (Blood Specimens Only)

Determine patient's weight. Nothing by mouth after supper.

Specimen 1. Collect sample of blood. Give intravenously 0.1 unit of regular insulin per kilogram of body weight.

Specimens 2 to 7. 20 minutes later, then 30, 45, 60, 90 and 120 minutes later, collect blood specimen.

The maximum fall in blood sugar occurs within 20 to 30 minutes and in normal patients returns to the normal level within two hours. In hypopituitarism, Addison's disease and myxedema, there is an abnormal delay in the return of the blood sugar to the normal level.

Hunger, dizziness, tachycardia and sweating accompany the fall in blood sugar. If confusion and cloudiness of consciousness occur, stop the test immediately and give the patient glucose orally or intravenously. This test is not applicable in patients whose blood sugar is above or below normal.

Calcium Balance Test (Urine Test)

Patient is placed on diet containing 100 mg. of calcium per day for 6 days.

Specimens 1, 2 and 3. Collect 24-hour specimens of urine the last 3 days of the diet period.

An excretion of 300 mg. or less of calcium for the 3-day period is considered normal. In hyperparathyroidism considerably more than 300 mg. is excreted.

Sulkowitch Test (Urine Test)

Do not give the patient large amounts of fluid.

Milk should not be taken prior to the test. (In some institutions the patient is placed on a low calcium diet.)

Collect a 24-hour urine specimen and send to lab.

This is a rapid urine test for calcium that gives an indication of the blood calcium level and is of particular value in tetany and myxedema. In these two diseases the daily calcium content of the urine is markedly below that of the normal 200 mg. (or 1 to 3+).

Calcium Load Test (Urine Test)

Patient given a fixed diet for 2 days.

Two 24-hour urine specimens are collected, one on each of the 2 days.

On the second day, 1 hour after breakfast, an intravenous infusion of 1000 cc. normal saline containing 15 mg. of calcium per kilogram of body weight is administered at a steady rate over a 4-hour period.

Patient is allowed to eat lunch during the infusion.

Water by mouth ad lib.

Normally there is a considerable reduction of urinary phosphorus on the second test day. In patients with hypoparathyroidism, there is a marked increase in urinary phosphorus.

Intravenous ACTH Test (Blood* and Urine Test)

Collect a 24-hour specimen of urine (this is examined for 17-ketosteroids—see p. 385) to be used as a control specimen before test

---

*Special oxylated tube used.

is begun. The first day of the test after the 24-hour specimen is collected, a blood specimen is collected for eosinophil counts.

Immediately after this 25 USP units of ACTH dissolved in 500 ml. of normal saline is administered intravenously over an 8-hour period. A blood sample is collected when the infusion is finished.

On the second day of the test, start collecting the second 24-hour urine specimen. Give second ACTH infusion.

The purpose of this test is to determine the effect ACTH has on the eosinophil count on the first day and the effect ACTH has on the urinary steroids on the second day.

After an ACTH infusion the eosinophil count should fall 80 or more per cent. Urinary excretion of 17-ketosteroids should normally increase in excess of 4 mg. In Addison's disease the eosinophil count falls 30 per cent or less, and urinary steroids increase only slightly.

Intramuscular ACTH Test (Thorn Test) (Blood* and Urine Test)

This test is a more practical method of determining the same information as that obtained in the intravenous ACTH test.

Nothing by mouth after bedtime.

6 and 8 A.M. — Give 200 cc. water by mouth.

Specimen 1. 8 A.M. — Collect specimen of blood and urine. Urine specimen includes all urine voided between 6 and 8 A.M. Give 25 mg. ACTH intramuscularly.

10 A.M. — Give 200 cc. water by mouth.

Specimen 2. 12 noon — Blood specimen and urine specimen collected. This urine collection should contain all the urine voided between 9 and 12 A.M.

The results of this test are interpreted as is the intravenous ACTH test. A uric acid-creatinine ratio may also be done on the urine. The uric acid-creatinine ratio should normally increase above 50 per cent of the control within 4 hours. In Addison's disease there is very little increase.

Pituitary-Eosinophil Adrenal Test (Pituitary Epinephrine-Eosinophil Test) (Blood Test)

This test is still another test based on the fact that normally when ACTH is liberated,

---

*Special oxylated tube needed.

the eosinophil count drops 50 per cent or more. In this test, rather than administer ACTH to the patient, epinephrine is given to stimulate the pituitary to release ACTH.

Nothing by mouth after 8 P.M.

8 A.M. — Draw blood for eosinophil count, then give 0.3 cc. of 1:1000 epinephrine solution subcutaneously. Serve breakfast.

12 noon or 4 hours after injection — draw blood for eosinophil count. Serve lunch.

Water Tolerance Test (Water Excretion Test or Robinson, Power, Kepler Test) (Blood and Urine Test)

Day before test: Regular diet omitting extra table salt. Nothing by mouth after supper.

Specimen 1 (night urine): 10:30 P.M. — Patient voids. Discard. All urine voided after this point including a specimen obtained at 7:30 A.M. is collected as one specimen to determine the total night volume and for chemical analysis.

Day of test: Keep patient in bed except to void.

Specimens 1 to 4 (day urine): 8:30 A.M. — Patient voids. Discard. Give 20 cc. of water per kilogram of body weight and ask the patient to drink it within 45 minutes. Collect urine specimens at 9:30, 10:30, 11:30 and 12:30. Each specimen is analyzed separately. Blood is collected at 11:30 A.M. Patient resumes diet after 12:30 specimen is obtained.

Some patients with Addison's disease are unable to void more than once or twice during the entire morning.

This test is interpreted in the form of an equation based on the differences in volume and chemical analysis of the night and day urine. Normally the volume of one of the singly voided day specimens should be larger than the total night specimen. The equation is calculated in the lab and reported like this:

A = 30 or more — normal

A = 25 or less — usually indicates Addison's disease.

Water-Loading Test (Soffer-Gabrilove Test) (Urine Test)

Nothing by mouth after supper.

8 A.M. — Patient voids. Discard. Give 1500 cc. of tap water to drink over 15- to 30-minute period. Collect all urine for the next 5 hours (one specimen).

Normally the volume of the urine specimen should exceed 1000 cc. Patients with hypopituitarism, adrenal insufficiency and Addison's disease excrete less than 800 cc.

Salt Deprivation Tests (Blood and Urine Tests)

There are two salt deprivation tests: the Harrop-Weinstein-Soffer-Trescher Test and the Cutler-Power-Wilder Test. The latter is used more frequently; therefore, only this one will be described here.

Cutler-Power-Wilder Test. This test is carried out for 3 days, during which the patient is on a diet containing 1.5 gm. sodium and 4 gm. potassium per day.

Before the test is started, a 24-hour urine specimen is obtained and a blood sample withdrawn for control specimens.

First and second day of test: One cubic centimeter of 10 per cent potassium citrate per kilogram of body weight is administered, and 40 cc. of water per kilogram of body weight is given.

Third day of test: Twenty cubic centimeters of water per kilogram of body weight given prior to 11 A.M. Urine collected in one specimen between 7 and 11 A.M. Blood sample taken also during this period.

On such a diet the patient with Addison's disease has an increase in urinary sodium and chloride in excess of the intake, and there is a progressive fall in serum sodium and chlorides, whereas the blood urea nitrogen, serum potassium and hematocrit increase.

This test is hazardous, since the diet may cause a state of crisis. Observe patient for drop in blood pressure and dehydration.

Hypertonic Saline Test for Diabetes Insipidus (Carter-Robbins Urinary Excretion Test)

Stop all antidiuretic therapy.

Withhold fluid for 8 hours prior to test.

Food is not withheld.

Give orally 20 cc. water per kilogram of body weight within 1 hour.

Thirty minutes later insert catheter in bladder.

Specimens 1 and 2. Obtain two urine specimens, each 15 minutes apart (control specimens). Give 2.5 per cent sodium chloride intravenously at rate of 0.25 ml. per kilogram of body weight per minute for 45 minutes.

Specimens 3 to 7. Obtain three urine specimens every 15 minutes during infusion and two more 15 minutes apart at end of infusion (5 specimens in 1 hour and 15 minutes).

In normal individuals a decrease in urinary output occurs during and after the administration of the hypertonic saline.

If no such decrease occurs, the patient is given 0.1 unit of Pitressin intravenously. In patients with diabetes insipidus, there is no urinary decrease during the saline infusion, but when the Pitressin is administered, inhibition of urine takes place.

Radioactive Iodine Tests (See also p. 26)

Tests employing radioactive iodine are used mostly in detecting thyroid disorders; however, they do have some usefulness in other endocrine disorders. There is no preparation of the patient for these tests. The patient carries on a normal regimen during the test.

The tests employing radioiodine are not accurate up to 5 weeks after the use of thyroid drugs or the use of iodide contrast media in x-ray studies.

Radioiodine Uptake. The patient is given a tracer dose of 3 to 5 μc. of radioiodine orally in distilled water. This is a colorless, tasteless drink. The fraction of this amount that accumulates in the thyroid is measured with an automatic scaler 5, 12 or 24 hours later. There should be an uptake in the thyroid of 5 to 30 per cent in 5 hours and 20 to 40 per cent in 24 hours. In hyperthyroidism the curve rises to over 30 per cent in 5 hours and to 50 per cent or higher in 24 hours. In hypothyroidism the uptake is below normal.

TSH Test (Thyrotropin Test). Radioiodine uptake is determined for a base study, then TSH (thyrotropin) is administered intramuscularly in a dose of 20 to 30 mg. for three consecutive days. This normally causes an increase in radioiodine uptake of 20 per cent. This test is of importance in differentiating hypothyroidism from pituitary myxedema. In hypothyroidism the increase is about 7 per cent; in piutitary myxedema about 32 per cent. Also in lymphadenoid goiter TSH does not increase iodine uptake but does in nodular goiter.

Thyroid Suppression Test (Werner Test). In normal persons the administration of 1 grain of thyroid three times daily or triiodothyronine 75 to 150 µg. daily for one week causes a 30 per cent drop in the 24-hour radioiodine uptake. There is little or no decrease in patients with hyperthyroid.

Red Blood Cell Radioiodine Uptake (Hamolsky Test). Red blood cell uptake normally averages 15 per cent per 100 hematocrit; in hyperthyroidism it is considerably higher. This test is done on the blood; the patient does not take any radioactive material.

Radioiodine Excretion. This is another method used in measuring radioiodine uptake. The radioactive substance is administered, then the total urinary output is collected for 24 or 48 hours thereafter. The amount of radioiodine excreted in the urine is measured. The amount that has not been excreted is considered the uptake amount.

Conversion Ratio. The rate of protein-bound radioactive iodine (see below) appearance in the serum after administration of a tracer dose is determined. This is done by comparing the protein-bound fraction with the amount in total plasma 24 hours after the administration of the tracer dose. Over 50 per cent conversion is strong evidence of hyperthyroidism.

Thyrobinding Index Test (TBI Test). In this test the amount of radioiodine which the patient's blood takes up in an anion exchange is measured. No radioactive substance is given to the patient. This test is done in the laboratory. Normal is 0.86 to 1.20. Hyperthyroid is above normal, and hypothyroid is below normal.

Scintillation or Thyroid Scanning. This is done to determine the size and location of a thyroid tumor (see p. 26).

P.B.I.: Protein-Bound Iodine (Blood Test)

The total blood iodine is broken down into several types of iodine. One is called protein-bound iodine. The normal amount is 3.5 to 8 µg. per 100 cc. Increased amounts are found in hyperthyroidism, decreased amounts in myxedema and hypothyroidism. Withhold breakfast.

B.E.I.: Butanol Extractable Iodine (Blood Test)

This test is supposed to be more specific than the P.B.I. The normal is 3.5 to 6.5 µg. per 100 cc. Increases and decreases are the same as for the P.B.I. Withhold breakfast.

T.R.P. Test (Tubular Resorption of Phosphate)

The patient is placed on a low phosphorus diet for several days, and the urine is examined for phosphorus content to test kidney function.

Pregnancy Tests

These are all done with samples of urine. The urine must be the first specimen voided in the morning, and the container must be absolutely clean. The urine is kept refrigerated until used. If the patient has vaginal bleeding, she must be catheterized because human blood in the urine will kill the animal.

Aschheim-Zondek Test. The urine is injected in mice. The test takes 96 hours.

Friedman Test. The urine is injected in a rabbit. The test takes 24 to 48 hours.

Male Frog Test. The urine is injected in the frog. This test takes 3 to 12 hours depending on the species of frog used.

The pregnancy tests are also used for the male patient on occasion. In malignant tumors of the testes, the urinary excretion of chorionic gonadotropins becomes so elevated that the pregnancy test is positive. After removal of a testicular neoplasm, the prognosis of the patient is considered to be good if pregnancy tests remain negative.

Basal Metabolism Rate or B.M.R.

The basal metabolism rate is not in itself an important diagnostic tool because there are too many factors that may cause error in the calculations. The test is useful in connection with other testing methods.

Preparation of Patient

1. Weigh patient and measure height.
2. Nothing by mouth for 15 hours prior to test.
3. Patient remains on complete bed rest during this period. Do not disturb patient for any nursing activities except to give him the bedpan when needed. If the patient is in a private room, keep the door closed during the night and in the morning before the test so that he is not awakened. In the ward keep the curtains pulled around the bed. Place a Do Not Disturb sign on the door or curtains.
4. The B.M.R. apparatus is brought to the patient's room for the test.
5. Make certain the patient understands what he may and may not do.

The normal ranges from +10 to −10.

Interpretation of Test

The B.M.R. is increased in
   Hyperthyroidism
   Exophthalmic goiter
   Thyroiditis
   Early acromegaly
   Diabetes insipidus
   Pituitary basophilism (sometimes)
   Hyperadrenalism
   Leukemia
   Hodgkin's disease
   Fever
   Pernicious anemia
The B.M.R. is decreased in
   Hypothyroidism
   Myxedema
   Cretinism
   Thyrogenous obesity
   Hypoadrenalism including Addison's disease
   Hypopituitarism

X-ray Examinations

X-ray procedures used in diagnosing diseases of the endocrine glands include plain films of bones to determine the stage of maturation and growth.

X-ray examinations in addition to plain films done to detect tumors of the adrenals include retrograde pyelogram (see p. 261), intravenous urogram (see p. 261), translumbar aortogram (see p. 261) and extraperitoneal pneumography.

In extraperitoneal pneumography, air is introduced into the extraperitoneal space through a needle inserted along the anterior coccyx, between the anus and the coccyx. The preparation of the patient for this procedure includes withholding food and cleansing the colon.

Vaginal Smears

Vaginal secretions are examined in order to evaluate ovarian function. A pipette is used to aspirate the secretion. Several designs of pipettes are shown here:

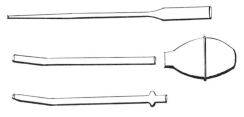

A rubber bulb tip is attached to one end of the pipette, and the vaginal secretion is aspirated and placed on a clean dry slide. The slide is then dropped immediately in a jar of fixative that consists of equal parts of ether and 95 per cent alcohol. When several smears are taken, the smears can be prevented from touching each other by placing a paper clip on the end of each slide like this:

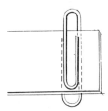

The jar containing the fixative and smears must be kept closed to prevent evaporation.

Estrogen deficiency is recognized by the total or relative absence of cornified cells. There should normally be 60 per cent cornification in the adult female.

Semen Analysis

Semen obtained by coitus interruptus or masturbation may be examined to determine abnormalities in the testes. For more details concerning this method, see page 264.

THERAPEUTIC AND REHABILITATIVE PROCEDURES

FACTS USEFUL IN CARING FOR THE DIABETIC

INSULIN SYRINGES

Two types of insulin syringes are recommended: the Official Insulin Syringe and the 1.0 cc. syringe.

The Official Insulin Syringe is available in the long and short types. The long type is recommended because the patient can see the spaces better with this than with the short type.

The USE U-40 ONLY syringes are printed in red; the USE U-80 ONLY syringes are printed in green to match the color of the label on these same strength vials of insulin. If used for U-40 insulin, each space on the 1.0 cc. syringe holds four units. If used for U-80 insulin, each space holds 8 units. This type is easy to read but may be complicated for some patients.

Others types of insulin syringes should not be recommended to the patient because their use is too complicated. The recommended insulin syringes are noted here:

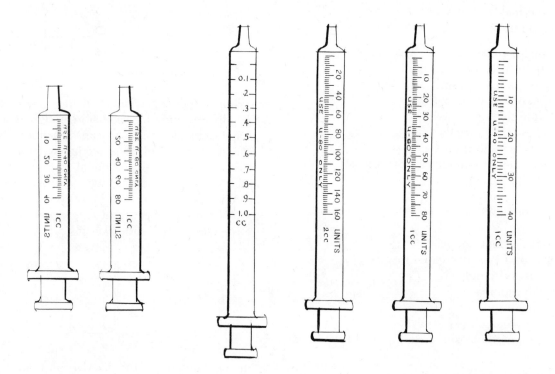

INSULIN NEEDLES

Hypodermic needles either 25 or 26 gauge are used in three lengths:

½ inch

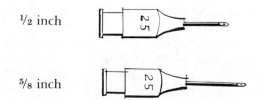

⅜ inch

5/8 inch

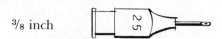

Needles must be sharpened frequently. To sharpen the needle, place it in a cork like this:

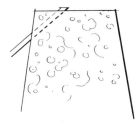

Then pass the point gently over an oilstone.

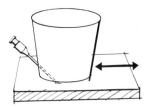

AUTOMATIC INJECTORS

There are available automatic injectors. One type, Busher, injects the needle, and the patient pushes the plunger in. In the Kayden-Vim injector the needle and the plunger are both automatically pushed forward. These apparatuses are seldom used.

INJECTION KITS

There are kits available that contain all the equipment necessary to give an insulin injection. These are handy when one is traveling.

INSULINS

Regular Insulin

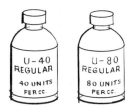

This is a rapid-acting insulin in a round bottle. It is a clear colorless solution. The peak of effect is 2 to 3 hours. The duration of effect is 6 to 8 hours. It is used for emergency situations and in combination with slow or intermediate acting insulins. The diet usually consists of three meals 5 or 6 hours apart.

Globin Insulin

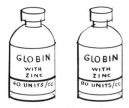

An intermediate-acting insulin in a round bottle. A clean, amber-colored solution. Peak of effect: 8 to 16 hours. Duration of effect: 12 to 24 hours. Used for patients who are sensitive to protamine. Diet: three meals 5 to 6 hours apart with midafternoon snack.

NPH Insulin

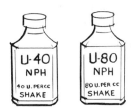

This is an intermediate-acting insulin in a square bottle. It has a milky appearance and contains a suspension of crystals of insulin together with protamine and zinc. Mix thoroughly before using. The peak of effect is 8 to 12 hours. Duration of effect is 28 to 30 hours. This type of insulin is used most frequently. The diet usually consists of three meals 5 or 6 hours apart with midafternoon snack.

Lente Insulin

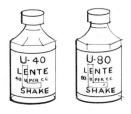

An intermediate-acting insulin in a round bottle with a six-sided shoulder. This insulin has a cloudy-milky appearance and contains only insulin and zinc. There are three kinds of lente available—semilente, lente and ultralente. Semilente has a big S on the label, and ultralente has a big U on the label. Notice that plain lente shown here has a big L on the label. The action of semilente is shorter and more rapid than lente. The action of ultralente is slower and longer than lente. These two additional types are used in mixtures with lente for better control. The action of lente is the same as NPH. Shake before using. The label on lente insulin has an expiration date. The diet usually consists of three meals 5 or 6 hours apart, with midafternoon snack.

PZI Insulin

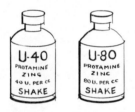

This is a long-lasting insulin in a round bottle. It has a cloudy milky appearance and contains insulin, zinc and protein (protamine). Mix thoroughly before using. The peak of effect is 12 to 24 hours. The duration of effect is up to 48 hours. The diet usually consists of three meals spaced 5 to 6 hours apart with a bedtime snack.

Insulin being used daily need not be stored in the refrigerator. Extra vials not being used should be kept in the refrigerator until use. The proper method of shaking insulin so that bubbles do not appear in the vial is demonstrated on page 383.

INSULIN MIXTURES

Various combinations of insulin may be recommended. A frequently used mixture is regular with protamine zinc, NPH or lente. Two kinds may be mixed in one syringe. Regular insulin should always be drawn into the syringe first because if a portion of the other insulins becomes mixed with regular insulin, the action of regular insulin may be altered.

When mixing the various types of lente insulin, there is no need for a special sequence.

See also page 383 for the procedure of mixing insulins.

INSULIN INJECTIONS

Insulin is given subcutaneously. These two methods of holding the skin are acceptable:

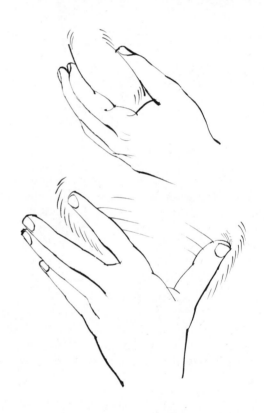

Both of these methods of holding the syringe are acceptable because a short needle is used.

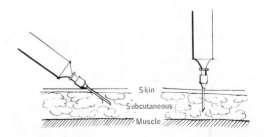

ROTATING INJECTIONS

Injections should never be given within an inch of the same spot a second time in one month. A recommended method of rotating the areas is like this:

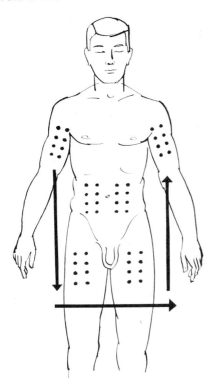

Each area has eight different spots for injection. Start with the top outer spot of each area, then do the other spots in a systematic manner like this:

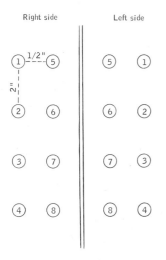

TEACHING THE DIABETIC PATIENT

The most important aspect in the long-term approach to diabetic care is that of educating the patient and his family so that they will understand the disease and its treatment. A great portion of responsibility for teaching the patient rests upon the nurse.

The instruction involved in the care of the diabetic approaches the level of classroom instruction. In other words, in order to teach the diabetic all he needs to know about diabetes, the teacher must know how to teach. An experienced instructor once made the statement that knowing how to perform a procedure and teaching others how to perform a procedure are two entirely different matters, each requiring an amount of skill. How true this is! For this reason, in this discussion we are emphasizing how to teach rather than what to teach.

Here are a few practical pointers on how to get the point across.
1. The nurse must be well versed in the subject she is teaching. If she doesn't know all the answers, she should know where to find them.
2. The nurse must explain things in a language that the patient understands. Words such as cubic centimeters, hypodermic, urinalysis, glucose, calories, metabolism, etc., which are part of the daily conversation of nurses, mean nothing to the patient.
3. Never assume that the patient already knows something about the subject. This is a common error in dealing with adults. Regardless of the patient's educational background, the nurse must approach the instruction with the attitude that the patient knows absolutely nothing about the subject.
4. Never assume that because facts are being explained and demonstrated to the patient, he is learning them. Sooner or later every professional teacher discovers to his horror that it is possible to have spent hours of instruction on a particular subject only to find out later that not a bit of it got through to the pupil. The only way to find out how much the patient is learning is to test him. Ask questions and ask him to

demonstrate what he learned. Never ask a question such as "Do you understand?" which requires only a "Yes" or "No" for an answer.

5. Don't give the patient too much information at one time. It is impossible to retain large amounts of new information.
6. Use visual aids in teaching. The patient understands and can remember more by seeing sketches, diagrams and pictures.
7. The instruction must be well planned and organized in advance. Impromptu lectures and demonstrations are never organized and invariably important points are omitted.
8. The environment must be quiet and free from interruption. Close the door to a private room, pull the curtains around the bed in a semi-private room, or take the patient to a clinical classroom.

What to Teach the Patient

Every hospital should have an organized plan of instruction for teaching the diabetic patient and his family. Unfortunately, few do. For this reason we are including a simple guide of instruction that can be used by the nurse who must rely on her own resources.

In teaching patients, we have discovered that it is better to start with a few basic, simple facts and stick to these until the patient masters them, then branch out into more detail later. The amount of detail given to each patient of course varies. The patient who is mentally alert can absorb more than one who is less alert. The subjects to be covered also vary. The patient who is in the hospital only 3 to 5 days simply cannot learn everything he should know in this length of time. In some communities the follow-up program of instruction for diabetics after discharge is quite thorough and efficient. In other communities there may be no resource for further instruction in the home. In this event the responsibility of the nurse is the greatest. The nurse should familiarize herself with the community public health program and the hospital clinic program so that she knows what, if anything, the patient will be taught after discharge.

Subjects that may be covered are:

1. A simple explanation of diabetes and its treatment.

2. How to collect and test urine for sugar and acetone.
3. How to give insulin injections and care for equipment.
4. How to prepare the diet.
5. The importance of exercise and special care of the feet.
6. The symptoms of diabetic acidosis and insulin reactions. Use of diabetes identification card.
7. Personal and social factors such as nationality, recreation, cost of medical care, marriage, pregnancy and heredity.

Aids to Instruction

The patient should be given reading material as an adjunct to oral explanation and demonstration. A number of pamphlets are available free from the American Diabetes Association, 1 East 45th Street, New York, N.Y. 10017. The nurse should have this literature on hand to give to the patient. In addition, the A.D.A. also has available a number of teaching charts useful in instruction. The nurse, however, can make her own teaching aids. (These will be illustrated later.) The patient should receive written instructions on all subjects of importance. A number of hospitals have mimeographed instructions that are given to each diabetic patient. If these are not available, the nurse must write the instructions for the patient.

The patient should also have a notebook in which to write notes during the instruction sessions. If he cannot obtain one of his own, the nurse can make him one.

Diabetic handbooks, written especially for the patient, are extremely helpful. I am familiar with several of these books and would like to recommend that one especially be on the "must" list for every diabetic. *Diabetic Care in Pictures,* by H. Rosenthal and J. Rosenthal, 3rd ed., J. B. Lippincott Co., 1960; price $5.00. Two other such books are *Diabetic Manual,* by E. P. Joslin, 10th ed., Lea & Febiger, 1959; price, $3.75, and *A Modern Pilgrim's Progress with Further Revelations for Diabetics,* by G. G. Duncan, 2nd ed., W. B. Saunders Co., 1967; price, $3.75.

A Guide for Instruction

Instruction of the patient should start as soon as possible. Here is a guide that, it is hoped, will help the nurse in knowing how to teach the patient. Each lesson should be presented on a different day. The lesson should be presented at a time when one or several members of the patient's family can attend. During afternoon visiting hours is an excellent time, usually convenient to both the nurse and the patient.

First Lesson: Orientation

Purpose: To acquaint the patient with the instruction program.

It can start like this:

"So you are a diabetic! I have taken care of a lot of persons who are diabetic. In fact, you might be surprised at the number of patients who are diabetic. One thing to be thankful about is that your disease is not hopeless. It is a disease that can be controlled. I know that you have a lot of questions about your condition, and because of this I'm going to spend some time with you every day so that you will have an opportunity to ask questions and so I can answer these questions and teach you just how this disease can be controlled."

Of course the patient will have comments to make during the first session. His reaction to an opening statement such as "So you are a diabetic" will give a clue to several important things. He may not know what "diabetic" means. He may only be familiar with terms such as "sugar" or "sugar diabetes." His attitude, whether it be acceptance, rejection or plain ignorance of the condition, will be shown in this session. All of his reactions and comments at this point will give clues as to how the nurse can approach the future teaching of the patient. The patient will also have a number of questions during this session. It is better not to answer any question about the technicalities of the disease or its treatment at this stage. Tell him that these will all be covered later.

During this session:

1. Give pamphlets pertaining to next lesson and ask him to read them. Reading material is a must.
2. Ask him to obtain a looseleaf notebook before the next session.
3. Give him pencil and paper and tell him to list questions pertaining to reading assignment.

Second Lesson: Definition and Treatment of Diabetes

Purpose: To give the patient an idea of just what diabetes is and how it can be controlled. Misconceptions about the disease should be cleared up at this session.

Barest essentials are presented like this:

"The body normally needs sugar for energy. Insulin is needed in the body so that sugar can be used up for energy. The body normally manufactures its own insulin.

"In diabetes the body does not make enough insulin, so the sugar cannot be used to give energy. The result is that the body gets weaker and weaker. It needs more energy and sends a message to the stomach for more food." Sketch this on a blackboard or paper:

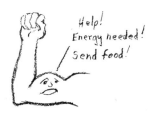

"You eat more and more food, but this does not help. The body still does not get enough energy because there is no insulin to help." Sketch this:

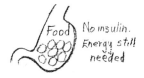

"The more food you eat, the more sugar accumulates in the blood and urine." Sketch this:

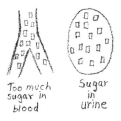

"Soon the blood has so much sugar that it must call for help. It wants water to dissolve the sugar. So you drink lots of water." Write this next to the previous sketch:

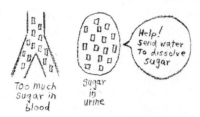

"This is what happened to you, isn't it? Your body felt weak and tired; you became terribly hungry and ate more and more. You were very thirsty and drank a lot of water, then naturally had to go to the bathroom a lot. In addition, the doctor discovered that you had too much sugar in your blood and some sugar in your urine.

"Now we will figure out how you can straighten this whole mess out. You yourself can do it, you know. That is the wonderful part about this disease. You can be healthy again and keep yourself healthy."

Now ask the patient these questions. They will (1) tell you what he has learned; (2) enable him to understand the aim of treatment:

Point to the entire sketch which should look like this:

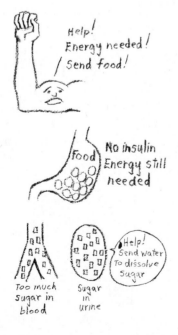

then ask these questions:

Q: Here is the muscle; why is it crying for help?

A: Weak, no energy, no insulin.

Q: How can we help this weak muscle?

A: Find some way to give it a supply of insulin.

Point to sketch:

Q: Here is the blood. What happened to it?

A: Too much sugar, needed water.

Q: How did too much sugar get into the blood?

A: Ate a lot of food.

Q: How can we help the blood?

A: Eat less food.

Q: How do you suppose you will know whether or not your blood and urine are OK?

A: Special tests on both.

Now proceed to summarize. Write these in patient's notebook:

"1. Today we learned what happens to the body when it has diabetes." (List symptoms.)

"2. We learned what you can do to help the body:

"A. Give it insulin.

"B. Eat less food.

"C. Check on blood and sugar often to make sure they are all right.

"3. There's one other thing that will be important that was not mentioned. That is exercise. Exercise is just as important as food and insulin. You will learn more about that another time."

Answer patient's questions pertaining to this lesson.

Give literature to read pertaining to next session.

Lesson Three: Checking the Blood and Urine

Purpose: To teach the patient how to test urine and the importance of scheduled blood tests and daily urine tests.

Approach:

Q: Yesterday we learned how you can help your body. Can you remember how?

A: Insulin, less food, exercise and check blood and urine.

"Today we are going to learn how to keep

a check on the blood and urine. This is important because it is the only way you have of knowing whether or not you are healthy (or keeping your condition in control)."

Proceed with subject.

1. Blood: "You will visit your doctor from time to time, and he will tell you when to have a blood test. You will go to the laboratory for these tests. They will take a sample of blood and test it for sugar. The blood should have some sugar in it, 80 to 120 (milligrams is omitted on purpose). If the blood has more than 120 of sugar, this is too much."

2. Urine: "This test you will be doing all by yourself. The urine test is by far the most important test. I am going to tell you three ways that you can test your urine for sugar, then you can select the one you like best."

Show this chart made in advance or draw on patient's notebook.

SOLUTION

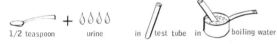

1/2 teaspoon   urine   in test tube   in boiling water

TABLET

+ urine + water   in test tube

TAPE

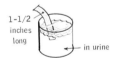

1-1/2 inches long   in urine

Briefly explain the chart. This gives the patient a general ideal of the methods. Do not mention the trade names of testing substances as yet. Then give the advantages and disadvantages of each.

Solution: Buy by the pint
By far the cheapest
Doesn't spoil

Tablet: Tablets sold in bottles
Easier to do but is more expensive
Tablets spoil easily

Tape: Comes in a container like a tape measure that pulls out
Easiest to do
Expensive

Get the prices of these materials (Benedict's solution, Clinitest and Tes-tape) from a local drugstore. Tell the patient what the price of each is and let him estimate the weekly cost of each on a basis of four daily tests (one pint of Benedict's solution contains about 125 teaspoonsful). Benedict's solution is actually the one most preferred. The patient will usually express his preference at this point. Next demonstrate the method the patient prefers.

For example, if the patient prefers the use of the solution, tell him that the name of the solution is Benedict's Sol. Then show him how to do the test. Keep the steps in the demonstration simple, and stress throughout the importance of doing the test exactly as instructed. The materials for the demonstration are assembled before the session begins.

"We will need boiling water to do the test. Put a metal cup of water on a hot plate and start heating. To test the urine for sugar, we need ½ teaspoon Benedict's solution. Put this in a test tube.

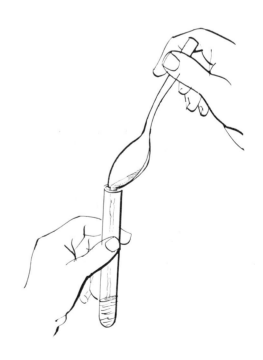

"Next add four drops of urine. There must be exactly four drops, and the dropper must be held straight up and down."

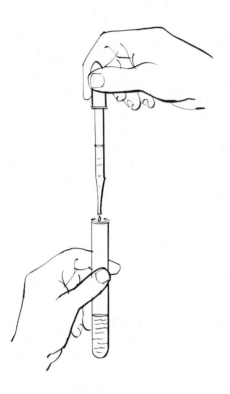

"Then shake the tube. If it is not shaken, the test will not come out right."

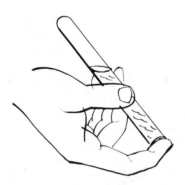

"Place the tube in boiling water, and keep it there for 5 minutes." During this 5 minutes tell the patient that after the solution boils, it will change color. The color will tell how much sugar is in the urine. Show the color chart, and describe the colors and their implications in terms of no sugar, a little sugar, a medium amount of sugar and a lot of sugar.

Ask the patient: "Do you know how much

sugar a healthy person should have in the urine?" Answer: None.

"I wonder if our mixture has been in the boiling water long enough. Do you remember how long it is to be kept there?"

Remove the test tube from the boiling water with a test tube forceps, shake again and ask the patient:

"What color would you say that is?

"Now look at the color chart. How much sugar would you say there is in this urine?" Now allow the patient to do the entire test himself. Allow him time to figure out which step comes next, but if he has too much difficulty, simply tell him what to do next. For this test substitute orange juice for urine. Refer to the orange juice as "This is the urine we are going to use for this test." If he remarks that it does not look like urine, simply say, "No, it really isn't, but we are going to pretend it is."

The orange juice will show a 4+ reaction and will further test the patient's ability to read the test. After completing the test, have the patient write the steps of the test in his notebook under the heading "Benedict's test." If the patient does not appear fatigued, proceed with a demonstration of acetest. It is better, however, if time of hospitalization permits, to do this at a separate session (see p. 376).

Then tell the patient that from now on he is going to test his own urine in the hospital. A nurse will help him at first. He is also to keep a record of the test.

Place a heading on a page in his notebook like this:

Date   Time   Benedict's Test
At this time he can be told that instead of writing out the colors of the reaction, + marks are used. Refer to the color chart.

It is important that the patient start testing his own urine with supervision following this session. Otherwise he will forget the procedure.

Lesson Four: Giving an Injection

This is by far the most difficult subject to teach because everyone is terrified at the thoughts of giving an injection and much more so of giving the injection to oneself. The minute the nurse announces the subject of this lesson, the patient will become tense, knowing that the end result of this session is that he will be expected to give himself a needle. He will most likely be in such a state of anxiety that he cannot concentrate on the instructions. The nurse also becomes tense because she anticipates the worst and fears that she will not be able to persuade the patient to give himself the injection. All this anxiety on the part of the nurse and the patient can easily be prevented this way. On the morning of the day that this session is to take place, prepare the patient's injection, walk into his room, and announce: "You are going to help give your own insulin this morning." Hand him the alcohol sponge, and tell him to cleanse the skin. Then hand him the syringe and tell him that you want him to hold the syringe while you give the injection. Hold both his hands like this:

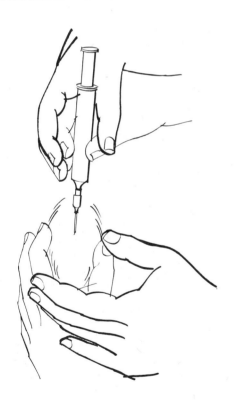

Holding his hand, push the needle in, then use your left hand to pull back on the plunger to check for blood. Then tell the patient to push the plunger in, at the same time guiding his fingers through the proper motions. Then depress the skin over the needle, and ask the patient to pull out the needle by himself. This

surprise attack works wonders. Do not tell the patient about it in advance. Also make a notation on the patient's medicine card that this is to be done so that the medicine nurse (if there is one) does not give the insulin. At a suitable time later in the day, the patient can be taught how to prepare and give the injection.

In preparation for this lesson, fill an empty vial (of the type insulin the patient is receiving) with water. If a cloudy insulin (PZI, NPH or lente) is being used, add a little milk to the water. An empty insulin vial is best because of the label and the color, etc., which the patient must learn to compare. Be sure to label this bottle so that someone else does not mistake it for insulin in the meantime.

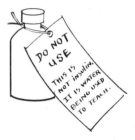

If an empty insulin vial is not available, use a vial of sterile water for practice and take the patient's vial of insulin along to show him how it looks.

Start the lesson like this: "Today I am going to show you how to put insulin in a syringe. First, I would like to show you how a syringe looks. Here is a drawing of the syringe you will be using."

Show a large drawing on 8 × 11 paper like this. If possible, have lettering done in red.

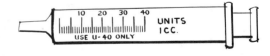

"You see, there are quite a few things written on a syringe. All of these numbers and words are important. The first thing we want to read is this—Use U-40 only. All kinds of insulin come in different numbers like U-40 and U-80. You are using number 40 insulin, so you must be sure that the syringe you use is also a number 40."

Show the patient the number on the insulin vial. Show him also that both are printed in red.

"If you were using number 80 insulin, the color on the bottle would be green, and the color of the letters on a number 80 syringe would be green.

"Always use a syringe that says 'U-40 ONLY' when you use number 40 insulin.

"Next notice there are lines on the syringe. Some lines are long, and some are short. Some of the long lines point to the numbers 10, 20, 30 and 40. These lines and numbers tell how much insulin to put in the syringe. For instance, if the doctor told you to take 20 units of insulin, you would fill the syringe up to this line." (Point to 20 line.)

"If the doctor told you to take 30 units of insulin, you would fill the syringe to here.

"If the doctor told you to take 25 units, to which line would you fill the syringe? Yes, you will notice that each long line between the 10, 20, 30 and 40 line stands for five. What number does each of the small lines stand for?

"If the doctor told you to take 18 units of insulin, how far would you fill the syringe?"

Give several more hypothetical questions using numbers other than 10, 20, 30 and 40. Next show the patient two syringes, a U-40 and a U-80, and say: "Pick out the syringe that you will use."

Allow the patient to compare his syringe with the drawing. Show him all the numbers on his syringe and show how the plunger pulls out. Give several more hypothetical doses, and have him indicate the answers by pulling the plunger to the correct number.

"We are ready to prepare the syringe for use. Before you use the syringe, it must be boiled to kill all the germs. Germs are very sturdy creatures and must be boiled for a full 5 minutes in order to kill them."

Be sure to mention this because many individuals think that merely rinsing in steaming water kills germs. Depending upon the patient, this should be elaborated.

Prepare the equipment as shown and start the sterilization. Point out that water must cover the syringe.

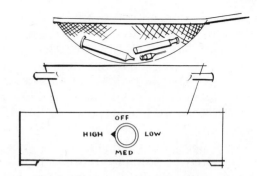

While waiting for this, write the list of the equipment the patient will need in his notebook:

2 insulin syringes, long—USE U-40 ONLY (two are needed in the event one breaks). (The long syringe is easier to read than the short one.)

3 No. 25 ⅝-inch needles

Isopropyl alcohol

Absorbent cotton

Arkansas oilstone for sharpening needles

(All are available in a kit manufactured by Becton-Dickinson Co.)—Buy at drugstore.

Show the patient a No. 25 needle; show where the number is written and explain that this means size in diameter. Explain the necessity of other articles. If the sterilized equipment has not cooled enough to handle at this point, the nurse may continue with another syringe to illustrate which parts of equipment should not be touched when assembling syringe and needle. Mention that the inside of the insulin vial must remain sterile.

"If germs are on the needle and the needle is pushed into the bottle of insulin, germs will stay on the inside of the bottle." Nurse and patient wash hands.

Demonstrate assembly of syringe.

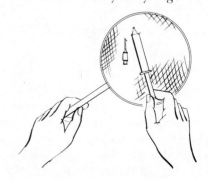

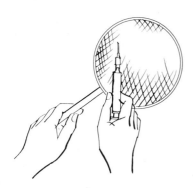

Again stress areas to be touched and those not to be touched. Show how to place syringe down with needle on alcohol sponge, then show how to shake insulin (NPH, PZI and lente).

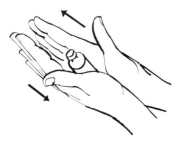

Cleanse top of vial and demonstrate withdrawal of insulin. Do not go into reasons why air must be put in syringe before inserting needle into vial. Withdraw the amount of insulin the patient is getting. Allow patient to practice withdrawing insulin, starting with the shaking of insulin. Next demonstrate the injection, using an orange. Allow the patient to practice this, then ask patient to demonstrate the entire procedure from start to finish.

Some physicians permit the use of alcohol for sterilizing. In this event teach the patient this procedure for sterilizing the equipment.
1. Equipment used:

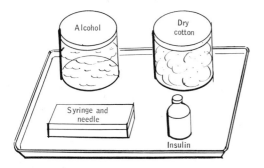

2. Put the needle in the alcohol and keep it there one minute.
3. Sterilize the inside of the syringe by drawing alcohol into the syringe and emptying it four times.

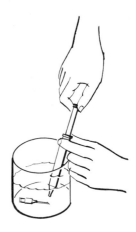

4. Take the needle out of the alcohol with fingers.

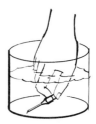

5. Boil syringe and needle once weekly.
   If the patient receives two types of insulin (regular plus PZI or NPH), the nurse demonstrates the method of placing two insulins in one syringe like this:
1. Wipe top of both vials.

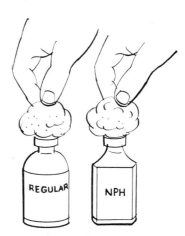

2. Put air in cloudy insulin vial first.

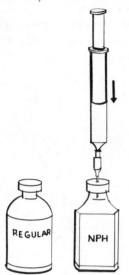

3. Withdraw regular insulin into syringe, then cloudy insulin.

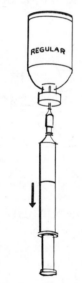

4. Put air bubble in syringe and mix.

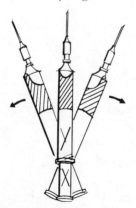

After this session the patient should be allowed to give his own insulin.

The diabetic who does not take insulin should also be instructed how to give injections because in the event of any minor illness at home, he may need insulin. The nurse may allow this patient to give her an injection of sterile water.

Lesson Five: The Diabetic Diet

This is taught by the hospital dietitian.

Additional lessons should cover the remaining subjects mentioned on page 376. If there is not time during the hospitalization to have separate daily lessons on the remaining subjects, make certain that the patient and his family are given ample time to read over instructions concerning those subjects so that questions may be answered and discussed by the nurse before the patient's discharge.

PROCEDURES TO REVIEW

Maintenance of cool, quiet atmosphere for hyperthyroid patient

Assistance in eating if incoordination is present in hyperthyroidism

Pre- and postoperative procedures with attention toward observation for hemorrhage and maintenance of adequate airway for thyroid surgery (see p. 65)

Tracheotomy when necessary after thyroid surgery (see p. 353)

Recording salt intake and urinary output in Addison's disease

Observation for signs of circulatory disturbances important in adrenal disease

Radiotherapy (see p. 18)

Buerger's exercises (see p. 243) used for diabetic

DIETS TO REVIEW

High calorie, high protein, high vitamin; high vitamin and high mineral with no coffee or tea used in hyperthyroidism

Calculation of diabetic diet and importance of reporting vomiting or refusal of any part of diet

High sodium, low potassium in Addison's disease

MEDICATIONS TO REVIEW

Pituitary Hormones. Gonadotropic hormones (APL, Antuitrin-S, Follutein); corticotropin (ACTH); thyrotropin (T.S.H., Thytropar); growth hormone (GH, STH); posterior pituitary extract; fractionated posterior pituitary extracts: Vasopressin (Pitressin), oxytocin (Pitocin, Syntocinon); melanophore stimulating hormone (MSH).

Thyroid. Thyroid USP: Proloid, thyroxin, sodium levothyroxin (Synthroid), sodium liothyronine (Cytomel), iodine, radioactive iodine (I^{131}), propylthiouracil, methimazole (Tapazole), iodothiouracil (Itrumil).

Parathyroid. Parathyroid extract (Parathor-mone).

Adrenal. Cortisone, hydrocortisone, prednisone, prednisolone, triamcinolone (Aristocort, Kenacort), methylprednisolone (Medrol), dexamethasone (Decadron, Deronil, Gammacorten).

Pancreatic Islets. Glucagon: for hypoglycemia; insulins: Regular, NPH, protamine zinc, and lente; oral preparations: tolbutamide (Orinase), chlorpropamide (Diabinese), phenformin (DBI).

Testes. Testosterone propionate in oil, testosterone cyclopentylpropionate (Depo-Testosterone), testosterone phenylacetate (Perandren phenylacetate), testosterone enanthate (Delatestryl), fluoxymesterone (Halotestin, Ultandren, Ora-Testryl).

Ovaries. Estrogens: estrone (Theelin), estradiol (Progynon), estradiol valerate (Delestrogen), diethylstilbestrol, dienestrol, ethynyl estradiol (Estinyl, Eticylol), conjugated estrogens (Premarin), crystalline equine estrogenic factors (Menagen); Progestins: progesterone in oil, hydroxyprogesterone caproate (Delalutin), ethisterone (Lutocylol, Pranone), norethindrone (Norlutin), medroxyprogesterone acetate (Provera), Enovid.

BIBLIOGRAPHY

Beeson, P. B., and McDermott, W.: Cecil-Loeb Textbook of Medicine. 12th ed. Philadelphia, W. B. Saunders Co., 1967

Brown, A.: Medical and Surgical Nursing II. Philadelphia, W. B. Saunders Co., 1959.

Davidsohn, I., and Henry, J. B.: Todd-Sanford Clinical Diagnosis by Laboratory Methods. 14th ed. Philadelphia, W. B. Saunders Co., 1969.

Davis, L.: Christopher's Textbook of Surgery. 9th ed. Philadelphia, W. B. Saunders Co., 1968.

Duncan, G. G.: Diseases of Metabolism. 5th ed. Philadelphia, W. B. Saunders Co., 1964.

Falconer, M., Patterson, H., and Gustafson, E.: Current Drug Handbook. 1968-1970. Philadelphia, W. B. Saunders Co., 1968.

Goodale, R.: Clinical Interpretation of Laboratory Tests. 5th ed. Philadelphia, F. A. Davis Co., 1964.

Harmer, B., and Henderson, V.: Textbook of Principles and Practices of Nursing. 5th ed. New York, The Macmillan Co., 1958.

Krause, M.: Food, Nutrition, and Diet Therapy. 4th ed. Philadelphia, W. B. Saunders Co., 1966.

Lisser, H., and Escamilla, R. F.: Atlas of Clinical Endocrinology. 2nd ed. St. Louis, C. V. Mosby Co., 1962.

Price, A.: The Art, Science and Spirit of Nursing. 3rd ed. Philadelphia, W. B. Saunders Co., 1965.

Welbourn, E. R.: Surgery and the Endocrine System. Nurs. Mir., *122*:1, 1966.

Williams, R. H.: Textbook of Endocrinology. 4th ed. Philadelphia, W. B. Saunders Co., 1968.

Index